BRAIN AND SPACE

BRAIN AND SPACE

Edited by

JACQUES PAILLARD

Emeritus Professor,
University of Aix-Marseille II,
France

OXFORD   NEW YORK   TOKYO
OXFORD UNIVERSITY PRESS
1991

Oxford University Press, Walton Street, Oxford OX2 6DP
Oxford New York Toronto
Delhi Bombay Calcutta Madras Karachi
Petaling Jaya Singapore Hong Kong Tokyo
Nairobi Dar es Salaam Cape Town
Melbourne Auckland
and associated companies in
Berlin Ibadan

Oxford is a trademark of Oxford University Press

Published in the United States
by Oxford University Press, New York

British Library Cataloguing in Publication Data
Brain and space.
1. Man. Brain. Neurophysiological aspects
I. Paillard, Jacques
612.82
ISBN 0–19–854284–4

Library of Congress Cataloging in Publication Data
Brain and space / edited by Jacques Paillard.
1. Space perception.   2. Cognition.   3. Brain.   I. Paillard,
Jacques, 1920–
QP491.B77   1991   612.8'2—dc20   90–19179
ISBN 0–19–854284–4

Set by
Footnote Graphics, Warminster, Wiltshire
Printed in Great Britain by
Bookcraft (Bath) Ltd
Midsomer Norton, Avon

Preface

In December 1989, an international scientific meeting was held in Marseilles on the topic 'Brain and Space', which was judged to be ripe for heuristic interdisciplinary discussion. It brought together many of the leading scientists in the field. The quality of their contributions prompted the publication of this book which reflects the state of the art in a domain long neglected in neurobiological approaches to brain function.

The nature of space and of spatial relationships has been a matter of endless philosophical controversy, an intriguing question for clinical neurologists, and a major field of experimental investigation in neuropsychology. Until comparatively recently, however, the topic has not been subjected to a thoroughgoing analysis of neural mechanisms and their behavioural counterparts by a collaborative effort from the relevant disciplines in neuroscience. Accordingly, the aim of this book is to bring together contemporary and interdisciplinary contributions to the study of spatial processing and its neural support.

The text is divided into five main sections which address five leading themes of contemporary integrative neuroscience. Part 1 is devoted to the important field of oculomotor control, which links the problem of gaze control to that of sensorimotor mapping of visual space. Part 2 deals with the neural control of skeletal movements in relation to the various reference-frames that are used to organize and guide our spatially oriented motor activities. The specific role of proprioception as a link between body space and extra-personal space is emphasized here, together with a revival of the classical neurological concept of the body schema. Part 3 gives prominence to recent developments of our knowledge of the cortical parietal association areas and their contribution to the mapping of spatial information of multimodal origin, with special emphasis on the neuropsychology of spatial disorders. Part 4 highlights evidence from the rapidly growing field of research on the hippocampal structures and their role in the cognitive mapping of space and in spatial memory. Part 5 reflects the impetus given by recent developments in artificial intelligence (neuromimetics) and neoconnectionism to the modelling of brain function. It examines how neural networks can map spatial relationships, combine different space co-ordinate systems, and generate an internal representation of the physical world.

All but one of the chapters are original contributions. The exception is a chapter by David Sparks on the neural coding of the location of targets for saccadic eye movements. It incorporates extracts from a recently published and seminal article in *The Journal of Experimental Biology* and thus represents a substantial and comprehensive introduction to the first section of the book.

Interdisciplinary convergence on a clearly defined topic is an increasingly important strategy for theoretical progress in the neurosciences. This book has been designed in that spirit and should urge neuroscientists, neurologists, and psychologists to consider new theoretical approaches, and to design new experimental paradigms to explore the variety and the diversity of the spatial constraints that shape our brain activity. It also provides fresh material for practitioners in various applied fields, including physical education, physiotherapy, and sport physiology. In addition, it could provide new insights for philosophers in one of their favourite domains of controversy.

I am much indebted to many colleagues and friends—especially François Clarac, Jean Massion, Jean Requin, and Bernard Soumireu-Mourat—for their help in the conception and organization of both the scientific meeting and this book. They initiated the project, and found the support necessary (from the Centre National de la Recherche Scientifique in France and from Universities and regional institutions in Marseilles) to bring it to fruition.

I am also grateful to all the contributors, who were extraordinarily prompt in providing their finished manuscripts so that there has been a minimal delay between the original conception of the project and its completion. Thanks are due to the staff of the Oxford University Press for their continual support and expert assistance at all stages of the editorial process, and also to Freda Newcombe for her invaluable help.

Marseilles   J.P.
July 1990

Contents

Contents

Contributors

Michael A. Arbib *Center for Neural Engineering, University of Southern California, Los Angeles, CA 90089–2520, USA.*

Alain Berthoz *Laboratoire de Physiologie Neurosensorielle, CNRS, 15 Rue de l'École de Médecine, 75270 Paris Cedex 06, France.*

Edoardo Bisiach *Istituto di Clinica Neurologica, Università di Milano, Via Francesco Sforza 35, 20122 Milano, Italy*

E. M. Bostock *Department of Psychology, Queens College, CUNY, Queens, USA.*

T. Brandt *Neurologische Klinik der Universität München, Postfach 70 12 60, 8000 München 70, Germany.*

Marie-Christine Buhot *Laboratoire de Neurosciences Fonctionnelles, U1bis, CNRS, 31 Chemin Joseph-Aiguier, 13402 Marseille Cedex 9, France.*

Yves Burnod *Département des Neurosciences de la Vision, Institut des Neurosciences, Université de Paris VI, Paris, France.*

Yves Coiton *Laboratoire de Neurobiologie Humaine, Départment de Psychophysiologie, Faculté Saint Jérôme, URA CNRS 372, av. Escadrille Normandie Niemen, 13396 Marseille Cedex 13, France.*

Carol L. Colby *Laboratory of Sensorimotor Research, National Eye Institute, Building 10, Room 10C101, Bethesda, MD 20892, USA.*

Paul Dassonville *Brain Research Institute, UCLA Medical Center, Los Angeles, CA 90024, USA.*

Vincent Delreux *Laboratoire de Neurophysiologie, Faculté de Médecine, NEFY, UCL 5449, Université de Louvain, B-1200 Brussels, Belgium.*

Marianne Dieterich *Neurologische Klinik der Universität München, Postfach 70 12 60, 8000 München 70, Germany.*

Michel Dufossé *Laboratoire de Neurosciences Fonctionnelles, CNRS and Institut Méditerranéen de Technologie, 13402 Marseille, France.*

Jean-René Duhamel *Laboratory of Sensorimotor Research, National Eye Institute, Building 10, Room 10C101, Bethesda, MD 20892, USA.*

Jean-Claude Gilhodes *Laboratoire de Neurobiologie Humaine, Département de Psychophysiologie, Faculté Saint Jérôme, URA CNRS 372, av. Escadrille Normandie Niemen, 13396 Marseille, France.*

Michael E. Goldberg *Laboratory of Sensorimotor Research, National Eye Institute, Building 10, Room 10C101, Bethesda, MD 20892, USA.*

Daniel Guitton   *Montreal Neurological Institute, McGill University, 3801 University Street, Montreal, Quebec, H3A 2B4, Canada.*

V. S. Gurfinkel   *Institute of Information-Transmission Problems, Academy of Sciences, Ermolovoy Street, Moscow 101 474, USSR.*

Marc Jeannerod   *Vision et Motricité, INSERM U94, 16 Av. du Doyen Lépine. 69500 Bron, France.*

John F. Kalaska   *Centre de Recherche en Sciences Neurologiques, Département de Physiologie, Université de Montreal, CP 6128, Succursale A, Montreal, Québec H3C 3J7, Canada.*

John L. Kubie   *Department of Anatomy and Cell Biology, Box 31, SUNY at Brooklyn, 450 Clarkson Ave., Brooklyn NY 11203, USA.*

Philippe Lefèvre   *Laboratoire de Neurophysiologie, Faculté de Médecine, NEFY, UCL 5449, Université de Louvain, B-1200 Brussels, Belgium.*

Yu. S. Levick   *Institute of Information-Transmission Problems, Academy of Sciences, Ermolovoy Street, Moscow 101 474, USSR.*

Pietro Morasso   *Department di Informatica Sistemistica e Telematica, Universita di Genova, 16 145 Genova, Italy.*

Robert Muller   *Department of Physiology, Box 31, SUNY at Brooklyn, 450 Clarkson Ave., Brooklyn, NY 11203, USA.*

D. P. Munoz   *National Institute of Health, National Eye Institute, Laboratory of Sensorimotor Research, Bldg. 10, Room 10C101, Bethesda, MD 20892, USA.*

John O'Keefe   *Department of Anatomy and Developmental Biology, University College London, Gower Street, London WC1E 6BT, UK.*

Jacques Paillard   *Laboratoire de Neurosciences Fonctionnelles, U2bis, CNRS, 31 Chemin Joseph-Aiguier, 13402 Marseille Cedex 9, France.*

Daniel Pélisson   *Vision et Motricité, INSERM U-94, 16 av. du Doyen Lépine, 69500 Bron, France.*

Bruno Poucet   *Laboratoire de Neurosciences Fonctionnelles, U1bis, CNRS, 31 Chemin Joseph-Aiguier, 13402 Marseille Cedex 9, France.*

T. Probst   *Neurologische Klinik der Universität München, Postfach 70 12 60, 8000 München 70, Germany.*

G. J. Quirk   *Department of Physiology, Box 31, SUNY at Brooklyn, 450 Clarkson Ave., Brooklyn, NY 11203, USA.*

Graham Ratcliff   *Harmaville Rehabilitation Center, PO Box 11460 Guys Run Road, Pittsburgh, PA 15238, USA.*

Jean-Pierre Roll   *Laboratoire de Neurobiologie Humaine, Département de Psychophysiologie, Faculté Saint Jérôme, URA CNRS 372, av. Escadrille Normandie Niemen, 13396 Marseille, France.*

Régine Roll   *Laboratoire de Neurobiologie Humaine, Département de Psychophysiologie, Faculté Saint Jérôme, URA CNRS 372, av. Escadrille Normandie Niemen, 13396 Marseille, France.*

Edmund T. Rolls *Department of Experimental Psychology, Oxford University, South Parks Road, Oxford OX1 3UD, UK.*

André Roucoux *Laboratoire de Neurophysiologie, Faculté Médecine, NEFY, UCL 5449, B-1200, Université de Louvain, Brussels, Belgium.*

Vittorio Sanguineti *Department di Informatica Sistemistica e Telematica, Universita di Genova, 16 145 Genova, Italy.*

E. Save *Laboratoire de Neurosciences Fonctionnelles, U1bis, CNRS, 31 Chemin Joseph-Aiguier, 13402 Marseille Cedex 9, France.*

John Schlag *Department of Anatomy and Cell Biology, Brain Research Institute, UCLA Medical Center, Los Angeles, CA 90024, USA.*

Madeleine Schlag-Rey *Department of Anatomy and Cell Biology, Brain Research Institute, UCLA Medical Center, Los Angeles, CA 90024, USA.*

David L. Sparks *Department of Psychology, University of Pennsylvania. Philadelphia PA 19104 6196, USA.*

John F. Stein *University Laboratory of Physiology, University of Oxford, Parks Road, Oxford OX1 3PT, UK.*

J. S. Taube *Department of Psychology, Dartmouth College, Hanover, New Hampshire 03755 USA.*

Catherine Thinus-Blanc *Laboratoire de Neurosciences Fonctionnelles, U1bis, CNRS, 31 Chemin Joseph-Aiguier, 13402 Marseille Cedex 9, France.*

Sylvie Vanden Abeele *Laboratoire de Neurophysiologie, Faculté de Médecine, NEFY, UCL 5449, Université de Louvain, B-1200 Brussels, Belgium.*

Jean-Luc Velay *Laboratoire de Neurobiologie Humaine, Département de Psychophysiologie, Faculté Saint Jérôme, URA CNRS 372, av. Escadrille Normandie Niemen, 13396 Marseille, France.*

PART 1

Gaze control and the mapping of space

1

The neural encoding of the location of targets for saccadic eye movements

DAVID L. SPARKS

Introduction

As an introduction to the session on the superior colliculus (SC), David Sparks described three classes of models of the saccadic system that have evolved over the past 20 to 25 years and discussed the possible role of the SC in these models. A major goal of the talk was to provide background information for the other speakers by describing the functional organization of the SC and outlining the neural representations of saccade targets that are thought to exist. As much of this material was reviewed in a recent paper (Sparks, 1989), most of that paper is reproduced in this chapter. The last section updates this information and provides a set of additional references.

Retinocentric models

Spatial perception and sensory-guided movements are thought to depend upon several different neural representations of the environment (see Howard 1982; Jeannerod 1982; Paillard 1987, for references). These include representations of the positions of the various body components, representations of the spatial location of objects in the external environment, and representations of the location of objects with respect to the body. Information about the organization of these neural representations and where they might reside in the central nervous system (CNS) comes from a variety of sources. Sensory and cognitive psychologists have a long-standing interest in the question of how changing patterns of sensory stimulation produced by object movement or by movements of the observer are integrated into a coherent, stable, perceptual representation (see, for example, Neisser 1967; Treisman 1977: Hochberg 1978; Treisman and Gelade 1980). Other researchers focusing on motor behaviour hypothesize that the neural control of limb movements is based upon an abstract code of the location of objects in space (see MacNeilage 1970; Larish and Stelmach 1982). Accumulating clinical data concerning disorders of spatial perception and spatially guided movements have led to refinements in the classification of neurological disturbances of spatial cognition (De Renzi

D. L. Sparks

1982). Computational models of how the brain might represent spatial relationships have now begun to appear (see, for example, Feldman 1985; Grossberg and Kuperstein 1986; Kuperstein 1988).

Despite the increasing interest in spatially guided behaviour and the neural representation of the spatial location of objects, relatively few neurophysiological experiments have investigated these phenomena directly. Much of what is known about the neural mechanisms for encoding the location of an object in space comes from studies of the neural control of eye movements. In this chapter, I describe models of the saccadic eye movement system, making assumptions about the co-ordinate frames in which saccade targets are localized, present evidence that supports or fails to support these models, and summarize the available neurophysiological data concerning neural representations of target location.

Models of the saccadic system

Retinocentric models

Early models of the saccadic system (Young and Stark 1963; Robinson 1973) assumed that the visual system computed a signal of *retinal error* (RE, the distance and direction of the target image from the fovea) and that this signal was relayed directly to the oculomotor system, which generated a command to correct for RE (see Fig. 1.1A). In these models, saccades were assumed to be pre-programmed or ballistic because the trajectory of the saccade was determined at its onset.

Early studies of the functional organization of the SC were interpreted as supporting retinocentric models. Schiller and Koerner (1971) hypothesized that the location of a visual target relative to the fovea was coded by the site of neural activity in the retinotopic map of the superficial layers of the SC. The discharge of visual neurons in the superficial layers was assumed to activate underlying regions of the SC containing neurons that discharge before saccades. As the motor map of saccadic eye movements found in the deeper layers is aligned with the retinotopic map of the overlying superficial neurons, the ensuing saccade would direct the foveal projection towards the region of the visual field containing the target. However, subsequent experiments have revealed a number of problems with this hypothesis (Sparks and Mays 1981; Sparks 1986) and there is evidence that an alternative, spatial model of the saccadic system is correct.

Spatial models

More recent models of the saccadic system assume that visual targets for saccadic eye movements are localized with respect to the head or body and

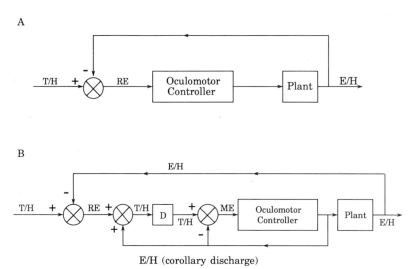

Fig. 1.1. Simplified versions of retinocentric (A) and spatial (B) models of the saccadic system. T/H, target position with respect to the head; E/H, position of the eye in the orbit; RE, retinal error; D, delay; ME, motor error. See text for further details. (Adapted from Sparks and Mays 1983a.)

not with respect to the retina. A simplification of one such model (Zee *et al.* 1976) is shown in Fig. 1.1B. With the head stationary, the appearance of a visual target creates an RE signal that depends upon the position of the eye in the orbit (E/H). The RE signal and a copy of the command signal to move the eye are combined to form a representation of *target position with respect to the head* (T/H). After a delay (D), a signal of the current position of the eye in the orbit is substracted from T/H, resulting in a signal of *motor error* (ME). Motor error is the direction and amplitude of the saccade required to bring the image of the target onto the fovea. If eye position changes in the interval between the computation of RE and the command to move the eye, ME will be different from RE; otherwise, RE and ME are the same.

Spatial models differ from retinocentric models in three important ways (Sparks and Mays 1983a). First, in spatial models, the direction and amplitude of a saccade are not determined by retinal information alone, but retinal signals are continuously combined with information about eye position to localize the target in a head or body frame of reference. Second, in spatial models, the motor command moves the eye to a certain position in the orbit; in retinocentric models, the command produces a movement of a certain distance and direction. Third, in some spatial models, the saccade is not preprogrammed or ballistic but guided to its destination by a neural circuit that continuously compares actual and desired eye position.

Evidence for spatial models

The assertion that saccade targets are localized in spatial (head or body) rather than retinal co-ordinates is supported by psychophysical and neurophysiological evidence. Saccades can be made on the basis of cues other than RE. Auditory cues that are localized in a head frame of reference (Zahn *et al.* 1978) and somatosensory cues can be used to initiate saccades. Hallet and Lightstone (1976) found that subjects could make a saccade to the location of a visual stimulus that was flashed, briefly, during a saccade. As the position of the eye changed after the flash, RE information alone could be used to compute the direction and amplitude of the subsequent saccade to the position of the flashed target. The computation of the distance and direction of the second saccade must take into account information about the direction and amplitude of the first saccade.

Mays and Sparks (1980a, 1981; Sparks and Mays 1983b) conducted experiments that also strongly support the view that saccade targets are localized in a non-retinocentric frame of reference. On a typical trial, the fixation target was extinguished and an eccentric target was illuminated for 50 to 100 ms. Randomly, in 30 per cent of the trials, after the target was extinguished but before the animal could begin a saccade, the eye was driven to another position in the orbit by electrical stimulation of the SC. Under these circumstances, if the monkey attempts to look to the position where the target appeared, where will it look? Retinocentric models assume that the direction and amplitude of a saccade are based entirely upon an RE signal, and predict that the animal should produce a saccade with a predetermined distance and direction. Thus, the animal should produce a saccade that would direct gaze to a point in space that differs from the target location by an amount equal to the direction and amplitude of the stimulation-induced saccade. Spatial models assume that RE signals will be combined with information about the change in eye position produced by collicular stimulation and predict that the animal will look to the actual position of the target in space. Note that, except for the fixation target and the briefly flashed target, the task was performed in total darkness. Thus, the targets could not be localized using visual background cues as an external frame of reference. Also, the target was extinguished before the stimulation-induced saccade. If the animal made a saccade to the position of the target, it could not be based upon a visual update of target position.

Mays and Sparks (1980a, 1981) found that regardless of the position of the target and regardless of the direction and amplitude of the saccade required to compensate for the stimulation-induced movement, the monkey made a saccade to the approximate position of the target in space. This finding supports spatial rather than retinocentric models because, on stimulation trials, saccades to the actual target locations could not be directed by RE alone. Furthermore, as the occurrence of the stimulation trials was completely unpredictable, compensation for the stimulation-induced perturbation could not have been predetermined; rather, the target must have been localized using both retinal information and information about the stimulation-induced change in eye position.

The original findings of Mays and Sparks using the stimulate/compensate method have been extended in a number of ways. Sparks and Porter (1983) found that neurons in the SC discharging before saccades to visual targets also discharge before saccades compensating for stimulation-induced perturbations in eye position. This indicates that the computation of the trajectory of the compensatory saccade occurs at a relatively high level in the oculomotor circuitry. Schiller and Sandell (1983) found that animals compensate for displacements of the eye produced by electrical stimulation of the frontal cortex (frontal eye fields) as well as stimulation of the SC, and that neither the frontal eye fields nor the SC are necessary for compensation. Guthrie *et al.* (1983) found that animals compensate for stimulation-induced changes in eye position after extra-ocular muscle proprioceptive signals have been eliminated surgically. This finding gives indirect support to the hypothesis that a central copy of the saccadic command provides precise information about the position of the eye in the orbit.

Neural representations of saccade targets

Identification of neurons encoding saccade targets in different co-ordinate systems

Spatial models of the saccadic system imply that there are at least three neural representations of a visual target to which a saccade is made (Fig. 1.2A): the first is a representation of the target as an RE signal; the second represents the target location in a head or body frame of reference and is based upon a combination of retinal and eye positional information; and the third is a representation of ME, the difference between current and desired eye position. Sparks and Mays (1983a) described the response properties required of neurons encoding the position of a target in these three different ways, and the conditions necessary to identify these neurons.

Activation of neurons signally RE is dependent upon excitation of receptors in a particular region of the retina. Accordingly, the receptive field moves with each change in gaze (Fig. 1.2B). Note, however, that neurons appearing to be responsive to activation of a particular region of the retina may actually be signalling ME. The distinction between neurons encoding RE and ME depends upon a critical test, described below.

D. L. Sparks

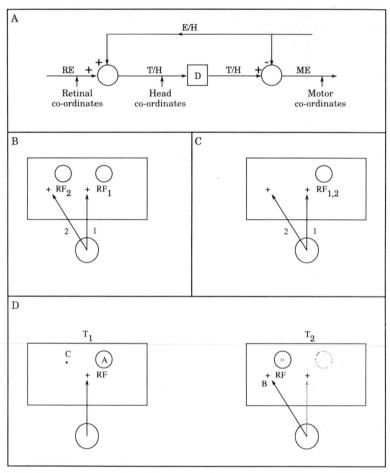

Fig. 1.2. Response properties of three types of hypothetical neurons. (A) Spatial models imply that there will be at least three neural representations of a saccade target: representations in retinal, head and motor co-ordinates. RE, retinal error; T/H, target position with respect to the head; E/H, position of the eye in the orbit; ME, motor error; D, delay. (B) Neurons signalling the position of the target in retinal coordinates have a retinal receptive field. With fixation of point 1, the neuronal discharge changes when stimuli activate a specific region of the retina (receptive field 1, RF_1). If the position of gaze changes (fixation of point 2), the receptive field moves (RF_2) since a specific region of the retina must still be activated to produce a neuronal response. (C) Neurons encoding the position of a target in head coordinates discharge whenever a stimulus appears in a specific region of the visual environment ($RF_{1,2}$), regardless of gaze direction (fixation 1 or fixation 2). The response of these neurons depends upon both retinal and eye-position information. (D) Response properties of neurons encoding motor error. Neurons conveying a motor error signal alter their discharge rate when there is a specific difference between current and desired eye position. This difference may occur because of the appearance of a visual target that produces a motor error (left) or because of a change in eye position after the brief appearance of a visual target (right). RF, response field of motor error neuron; A, B, C, target positions. T_1, Time period 1, central-fixation; T_2, Time period 2, after a leftward saccade. (Adapted from Sparks and Mays 1983a.)

Neurons representing a saccade target in a head or body frame of reference respond to targets in a specific region of the visual environment, regardless of the position of the eye in the orbit. Thus, as shown in Fig. 1.2C, the plot of the receptive field of such a neuron while the animal is fixating point 1 will be the same as the plot of the receptive field while the animal is fixating point 2. These neurons are responsive to stimuli occupying a particular region of visual space, regardless of the retinal locus of the target image and regardless of the position of the eye in the orbit. The spatial properties of these neurons would not be detected in an acute recording study nor in a chronic recording experiment in which the receptive field was plotted with a single fixation point.

Neurons coding an ME signal alter their discharge rate when there is a certain difference between current and desired eye position. Motor error can be produced in two ways; by the appearance of a visual target located a certain distance and direction from the fixation point; or by a change in eye position after the appearance of a visual target. These situations are shown in Fig.1. 2D. On the left, the response field of a hypothetical ME neuron is represented as a circle (RF). With fixation straight ahead, the neuron discharges in response to a saccade target (A) presented in the circular response field. The neuron discharges not because a particular region of the retina was activated but because, after the appearance of target A, the difference between current and desired eye position requires a saccade with a particular direction and amplitude. Note that if this is the only test applied, the discharge of the cell appears simply to reflect RE. A saccade target presented at position C outside the response field will not activate the neuron as long as fixation of the centre point is maintained. Suppose, however, after target C has disappeared, gaze is shifted to a new fixation point (B) but a saccade to the remembered location of target C is still required (Fig. 1.2D). After the first saccade, the difference between current and desired eye position is in the response field of the neuron, and the neuron generates an increase in firing rate to signal this new ME. In this case, the ME signal is created not by the appearance of a new target but by the change in eye position after the original target has disappeared.

Experimental data

Representations of retinal error and motor error

Mays and Sparks (1980b) reported that the SC contains an RE signal and a representation of ME. Monkeys were trained to perform a task like the one illustrated in Fig.1.2D. After fixation of an initial centre target for a variable period, the offset of the centre fixation target was followed by successive presentations of two targets, B and C. Although the total duration of both targets B and C was less than the reaction time of the monkey, reward was contingent on the animal making a saccade to position B within 300 ms and a second saccade from B to C before an additional 500 ms elapsed. Thus, two saccades were made in succession; the first to B and the second from B to C.

Visually responsive neurons isolated in the superficial layers of the SC were activated by stimulation of a particular region of the retina. They responded only to the appearance of a visual stimulus in their receptive field, and the location of the receptive field shifted with each change in gaze. Thus, the site of neuronal activity in the retinotopic map of the superficial layers represents a map of RE.

One type of neuron that signals ME (the quasi-visual or QV cell) was identified in the intermediate layers of the SC. If these cells are tested while the animal maintains a single fixation position, they appear to be visually responsive, to have visual receptive fields, and to respond to targets in their receptive field whether or not a saccade is made towards the target. But on trials requiring a change in fixation (Fig. 1.2D, right), QV cells begin to fire after the eye has reached position B and continue to fire until after the saccade from B to C. The cells firing in this case are not those whose receptive field contained the original target C, but cells whose receptive field would contain target C if the target were flashed again in the same spatial location after the eyes reached position B. In other words, the activity of QV cells reflects motor error. Quasi-visual cells discharge whenever a saccade with a particular direction and amplitude is appropriate, regardless of whether the movement becomes appropriate because of the onset of a visual stimulus or because of an eye movement occurring after the disappearance of the target. Unlike neurons in the superficial layers that are activated if, and only if, a particular region of the retina is stimulated, QV cells can be activated by stimulation of any region of the retina if, after a subsequent movement of the eye, a saccade with a particular trajectory is required to look to the target. As there are many combinations of sites of retinal stimulation and subsequent eye movements requiring a movement in the response field of a single QV cell, all regions of the retina must be mapped, at least indirectly, to each QV cell.

The hypothesis that the activity of QV cells encodes ME was tested in a separate experiment (Sparks and Porter 1983) by recording their activity during trials in which the monkey compensated for stimulation-induced perturbations in eye position. Quasi-visual cells increased their discharge rate whenever there was a certain difference between current and desired eye position, regardless of whether this ME was produced by the sudden appearance of a visual target or by a stimulation-induced change in eye position after target offset. Based upon these and other findings, I have

concluded that the discharge of QV cells signals ME and holds this information in spatial register until a saccade occurs or is cancelled. Moreover,
the mapping of target location in motor coordinates is a dynamic one: if the
eyes move after a brief target disappears, the site of QV cell activity shifts
to a location representing the new ME.

Cells with properties almost identical to the QV cells of the SC have now
been discovered in the lateral bank of the intra-parietal cortex (Gnadt and
Andersen 1988). By using the double saccade task of Mays and Sparks
(1980b), they found that the response of some cells in the parietal cortex is
encoded in motor rather than sensory co-ordinates. Moreover, on using a
delayed saccade task, they discovered that these cells remain active
throughout the memory interval, confirming the suggestion of Mays and
Sparks (1980b) that cells of this type hold in spatial register the metrics of
planned eye movements throughout the stimulus/response interval.

Experiments with auditory targets also support the view that the responses of sensory cells in the deeper layers of the SC are encoded in motor
rather than sensory co-ordinates (Jay and Sparks 1984, 1987). Monkeys
trained to look to either visual or auditory targets in a completely darkened
room were placed with their heads fixed in the centre of a semicircular
track. Movement of a speaker (with a light-emitting diode attached) along
the track and rotation of the track allowed targets to be presented at most
locations on an imaginary sphere surrounding the animal. Three fixation
lights separated by 24° were placed along the horizontal meridian. At the
beginning of each trial, one of the three fixation lights was randomly
activated. After a variable interval, an auditory (broad-band noise burst)
or visual target was presented and the animal was required to look to the
target location in order to receive a liquid reward. A delayed saccade task
was used to separate, temporally, sensory and motor activity.

The major objective of the experiment was to plot the receptive fields of
sound-sensitive cells in the SC of alert monkeys while varying the direction
of visual fixation. If the receptive fields of auditory neurons in the SC are
based upon inter-aural cues and are organized in head-centred co-
ordinates, the direction of fixation would have no effect. But, if the response of auditory neurons is organized in ME co-ordinates, then the
response should depend upon both speaker position and fixation direction.
We found that the position of the eye in the orbit had a distinct effect upon
the response of sound-sensitive cells in the SC. When the magnitude of the
neural response was plotted as a function of the stimulus location in space,
the receptive fields of the neurons shifted with the position of the eye in the
orbit. But when the magnitude of the neural response was plotted as a
function of the direction and amplitude of the movement required to look
to the auditory target, the plots obtained with the different fixation positions were closely aligned. Thus, the discharge of sound-sensitive neurons

in the SC is not determined solely by the position of the auditory stimulus in space but depends upon ME, the trajectory of the saccade required to look to the target.

The mapping of the location of auditory targets in the SC is also dynamic. With each movement of the eye in the orbit, the population of neurons responsive to a stationary auditory stimulus in a particular location of the external environment changes to a new site within the SC, a site representing the new movement required for target acquisition.

Representations of target position in space

Neurons coding the position of a target in head or body coordinates were not found in the monkey SC. Nor have cells with properties identical to the hypothetical neuron illustrated in Fig.1.2C been observed in other brain areas. This is not surprising, because few experiments have been conducted that would allow the detection of neurons encoding the location of a visual target in other than retinal co-ordinates. Nevertheless, spatial models of the saccadic system require a neural representation of the target in a head frame of reference and, presumably, the properties of QV cells in the SC and of QV-like cells in the parietal cortex are based upon a subtraction of an eye position signal from a stored representation of the position of the target in space. Neurons that could be used to construct a map of visual space in head or body co-ordinates have been found in the internal medullary lamina (IML) of the thalamus and in the parietal cortex.

Schlag *et al.* (1980) and Schlag and Schlag-Rey (1983) found cells in the IML of the cat that responded only when the animal looked directly at a visual target or within a few degrees of it. These cells had central receptive fields but the visual response was more vigorous if the target appeared in a particular region of the visual field. These cells are described as discharging with a frequency related to eye position when a target appears in the receptive field of the cell (Schlag and Schlag-Rey 1983). Most of these cells display a discharge frequency related to eye position even in the dark, although the vigour of the response is reduced in the dark. A second type of cell in the IML with responses dependent upon gaze angle has large receptive fields that include the central retina. Consequently, gaze can be directed as much as 10° away from the target without a significant reduction in the visual response of the cell. As visual responses are similar whether or not the animal fixates the target, firing rate is more related to the absolute position of the stimulus in space than to either eye position or retinal error.

The signals observed in the IML may be relayed to the parietal cortex, another brain region implicated in spatial perception and spatially guided behaviour. The discharge of many light-sensitive cells of the inferior parietal lobule is influenced by the direction of gaze (Hyvarinen and Poranen 1974; Lynch *et al.* 1977; Andersen and Mountcastle 1983). For many of these cells, visual stimuli delivered to the same region of the retina produce more or less vigorous responses, depending upon the location of the fixation target in the visual field. These neurons are said to have gaze fields, i.e. the increase in spike frequency during stimulus presentation is only observed if gaze is directed to a restricted region of the visual field. Control experiments by Andersen and Mountcastle (1983) indicate that these effects are not produced by changes in visual background associated with changes in the angle of gaze, by changes in fixation distance, or by variations in the intensity of stimuli viewed from different angles. It should be noted, however, that some of these cells show increased firing rates during particular directions of gaze, even in total darkness (Sakata *et al.* 1980).

The properties of cells in area 7a of the parietal cortex have now been described in more detail (Andersen *et al.* 1987; Andersen and Zipser 1988). First, they mapped the receptive fields of light-sensitive neurons. Next, they presented a stimulus in the centre of the cell's retinotopic receptive field while the animal fixated targets at nine different locations in the visual field. Changes in the position of fixation produced systematic variations in the magnitude of the visual response. Moreover, the responses of the cell to stimuli presented at different points in the receptive field were all altered by an amount proportional to gaze angle, indicating a multiplicative interaction of the visual and eye position signals. The receptive fields of these cells remain retinotopic as the peaks and symmetry of the receptive fields do not change; but the overall responsiveness of the cells is modulated by eye position.

These studies indicate that the visual response of many cells in the parietal cortex is jointly dependent on eye position and the location of the visual receptive field. But these cells do not encode absolutely the spatial location of visual stimuli; the spatial location of the visual stimulus cannot be determined from the cell's discharge unless the position of the eye in the orbit is known. Computer simulations developed by Zipser and Andersen (1988) show that a code of the position of a visual target in head co-ordinates can be achieved by considering the simultaneous activity of several neurons having the same retinotopic receptive fields but different sensitivity to the angle of gaze. Thus, the convergence of the outputs of groups of cells in the parietal cortex onto cells in other regions of the parietal lobe or in still other brain structures could be used to generate a topographically coded representation of the location of a visual target in head or body coordinates. Zipser and Andersen suggest that this additional step of convergence is unnecessary for a signal of target position in head co-ordinates because this information can be extracted from the response of sub-populations of neurons in area 7a.

Some neurons in the frontal cortex display sensory activity seemingly related to the position of a stimulus with respect to a specific body region. Rizzolatti *et al.* (1981) isolated visually responsive neurons in the rostral part of area 6 just posterior to the arcuate sulcus. They described these neurons as 'peripersonal' cells because they were excited by visual stimuli within the animal's reach and also had tactile receptive fields on the hands or around the mouth and face. Visual receptive fields in front of or below the mouth were accompanied by tactile responsiveness to mouth and face or forearm stimulation. More recently, Gentilucci *et al.* (1983) described visually responsive neurons in the post-arcuate region that are said to have visual receptive fields independent of eye position. The location of the visual receptive field appears to remain in register with the tactile receptive field even when the eyes move. This implies that the neurons are activated by visual stimuli in a particular region of 'egocentric' space, regardless of the site of retinal activation.

In summary, converging lines of clinical and experimental data implicate the posterior parietal cortex, the frontal and peri-arcuate cortex, the thalamic IML, and the SC in the spatial localization of visual targets. The evidence that a topographically organized map of the visual environment organized in head or body co-ordinates resides in one or more of these brain regions is not yet compelling. Many of the early electrophysiological studies used informal and uncontrolled test procedures or failed to use methods capable of detecting neurons encoding the location of visual targets in other than retinal co-ordinates. Additional experiments continuing to explore, systematically, the implicated brain areas using electrophysiological methods capable of detecting neural representations of the visual environment organized in non-retinal coordinates are needed.

Additions to the original paper by Sparks (1989)

The models of the saccadic system described above assume that the head is fixed. But how are the movements of the eyes and head co-ordinated? Bizzi and colleagues studied this question in a series of influential experiments conducted in the 1970s (see Bizzi *et al.* 1972). During large gaze shifts made when the head is not restrained, a stereotyped sequence of eye and head movements occurs. Saccadic eye movements begin first and then, after 20 to 30 ms, the head begins to move in the same direction. After the combined eye and head movements direct the line of sight to the target, gaze position remains relatively constant even though the head continues to move. This occurs because the vestibulo-ocular reflex (VOR) is still active, producing a counter-rotation of the eyes with a velocity that exactly opposes head velocity.

Based upon these and other findings, eye and head movements were thought to be programmed independently (Morasso *et al.* 1973). During gaze shifts involving both eye and head movements, displacements of the retinal image due to head movements are automatically nullified by the VOR. According to this view, the commands required to generate saccadic eye movements could be identical whether or not the head moved. If the head moves, vestibularly induced compensatory eye movements are added linearly to the saccade signal.

Despite the simplicity of the linear summation hypothesis, there are a number of reasons for thinking that a single strategy for co-ordination of eye and head movements cannot be responsible for all types of gaze shifts. Self-paced eye and head movements between visual targets at fixed locations differ from gaze shifts made to targets appearing at unpredictable times and locations (Bizzi *et al.* 1972). During the predictive movements, the head begins to move well before the eyes. The head movement is achieved by a gradual increase in the activity of the agonist muscles, not the sudden burst of agonist neck muscle activity recorded when unexpected stimuli are presented. That the interval between the onset of eye and head movements depends upon target eccentricity, predictability, and visibility (see Guitton 1988 for references) suggests that, temporally, command signals driving the eye are only loosely coupled with those driving the head.

How are the gaze shifts programmed when the target lies beyond the oculomotor range of the observer. The oculomotor range of cats ($\pm 25°$) is smaller than that of monkeys ($\pm 45°$) and, in cats with their heads free, almost all saccades larger than 4° are accompanied by head movements (see Guitton 1988 for references). Moreover, highly motivated subjects (cats and humans) usually generate single-step, saccade-like gaze shifts when looking to targets beyond their oculomotor range. During the initial phase of these large gaze shifts, the eyes and head move in the same direction and may continue to do so until the eyes reach their oculomotor limit or until the line of sight is directed at the target. Usually the head continues to move and, at this point, the eyes move in the opposite direction, compensating for the still ongoing head movement. This pattern of eye and head movement suggests that initially the VOR is inactive but is activated later, after the target is acquired.

Dual modes for gaze control have now been observed in monkeys. Tomlinson and Bahra (1986a,b) report that for movements of less than 20° in amplitude, gaze shifts are accomplished almost exclusively by eye movements, but for larger saccades, approximately 80 per cent of the total change in gaze is due to movement of the head. The hypothesis that the VOR is inactivated during large gaze shifts has been tested in experiments in which the head is braked suddenly and unexpectedly during a saccade. Based upon the experiments of Tomlinson and Bahra (1986b), the VOR appears to be inactive for most of the duration of large-amplitude (>40°) gaze shifts. During quite small gaze shifts (<10°), the VOR is clearly functioning; however, as the size of the gaze shift is increased, there appears to be a region where the VOR operates with reduced gain before it enters the large gaze shift region where the VOR is turned off entirely. In related experiments, Laurutis and Robinson (1986) reported that there was no compensation for mechanical perturbations in head position during gaze shifts larger than 40°. Guitton and Volle (1987) performed similar experiments and obtained results similar to those of Tomlinson and Bahra, and of Laurutis and Robinson, from two subjects but found considerable variability in the interaction between the VOR and saccade signals in the remaining two subjects.

The different patterns of eye and head movements produced by electrical stimulation of rostral and caudal regions of the SC also illustrate different modes of eye–head co-ordination. Electrical stimulation of neurons at a single site in rostral regions of the deep layers of the cat's SC produces saccades of approximately the same direction and amplitude, regardless of the initial starting position of the eye (Roucoux and Crommelinck 1976). In contrast, stimulation of neurons located in caudal regions of the SC evokes movements that bring the eye to a given position in the orbit even when the stimulation-induced movement begins at different initial positions. When these experiments were repeated in animals free to move their heads (Harris 1980; Roucoux *et al.* 1980), application of brief stimulation trains through electrodes in the rostral SC evoked gaze shifts consisting of eye movements only; evoked head movements were not observed. Brief trains of electrical stimulation applied caudally evoked contralateral eye and head movements that produced gaze shifts of particular directions and amplitudes. The stimulation-induced head movements had short and constant latencies (25–30 ms) and were high-velocity movements. Unlike those produced by stimulation at rostral sites, the saccades associated with these head movements were not modified by the VOR. Thus, there are at least two modes for controlling gaze: one produced by eye movements alone, and a second involving combined eye and head movements. In the first mode, movements of the head are compensated for by an active VOR. In the second mode, vestibular compensatory movements are absent.

Findings such as these have led to models of the saccadic system which assume that gaze not eye position is being controlled. In these models, a signal of gaze error is used to drive an eye movement generator and a head movement generator. Mechanisms are need for apportioning the gaze error signal to the separate generators and papers in this volume by Guitton and Roucoux address some of the issues involved in designing models for the co-ordinated control of eye and head movements.

References for additional material

Bizzi, E., Kalil, R., and Morasso, P. (1972). Two modes of active eye-head coordination in monkeys. *Brain Research* **40**: 45–8.

Guitton, D. (1988). Eye–head coordination in gaze control. In *Control of head movement* (ed. B. W. Peterson and F. J. Richmond), pp. 196–207. Oxford University Press.

Guitton, D. and Volle, M. (1987). Gaze control in humans: eye–head coordination during orienting movements to targets within and beyond the oculomotor range. *Journal of Neurophysiology*, **58**, 427–59.

Harris, L. R. (1980). The superior colliculus and movements of the head and eyes in cat. *Journal of Physiology*, **300**, 367–91.

Laurutis, V. P. and Robinson, D. A. (1986). The vestibulo-ocular reflex during human saccadic eye movements. *Journal of Physiology*, **373**, 209–34.

Morasso, P., Bizzi, E., and Dichgans, J. (1973). Adjustment of saccade characteristics during head movements. *Experimental Brain Research*, **16**, 492–500.

Roucoux, A. and Crommelinck, M. (1976) Eye movements evoked by superior colliculus stimulation in the alert cat. *Brain Research*, **106**, 349–63.

Roucoux, A., Crommelinck, M., and Guitton, D. (1980). Stimulation of the superior colliculus in the alert cat. II. Eye and head movements evoked when the head is unrestrained. *Experimental Brain Research*, **39**, 75–85.

Sparks, D. L. (1989). The neural encoding of the location of targets for saccadic eye movements. *Journal of Experimental Biology*, **146**, 195–207.

Tomlinson, R. D., and Bahra, P. S. (1986a). Combined eye–head gaze shifts in the primate. I. Metrics. *Journal of Neurophysiology*, **56**, 1542–57.

Tomlinson, R. D. and Bahra, P. S. (1986b). Combined eye–head gaze shift in the primate. II. Interactions between saccades and the vestibuloocular reflex. *Journal of Neurophysiology*, **56**, 1558–70.

References

Andersen, R. A. and Mountcastle, V. B. (1983). The influence of the angle of gaze upon the excitability of the light-sensitive neurons of the posterior parietal cortex. *Journal of Neuroscience*, **3**, 532–48.

Andersen, R. A. and Zipser, D. (1988). The role of the posterior parietal cortex in coordinate transformations for visual-motor integration. *Canadian Journal of Physiology and Pharmacology*, **66**, 488–501.

Andersen, R. A., Essick, G. K., and Seigel, R. M. (1987). Neurons of area 7 activated by both visual stimuli and oculomotor behavior. *Experimental Brain Research*, **67**, 316–22.

De Renzi, E. (1982). *Disorders of space exploration and cognition*. Wiley, Chichester.

Feldman, J. A. (1985). Four frames suffice: A provisionary model of vision and space. *Behavioral and Brain Sciences*, **3**, 265–89.

Gentilucci, M., Scandolara, C., Pigarev, I. N., and Rizzolatti, G. (1983). Visual responses in the postarcuate cortex (area 6) of the monkey that are independent of eye position. *Experimental Brain Research*, **50**, 464–8.

Gnadt, J. W. and Andersen, R. A. (1988). Memory related motor planning activity in posterior parietal cortex of macaque. *Experimental Brain Research*, **70**, 216–20.

Grossberg, S. and Kuperstein, M. (1986). *Neural dynamics of adaptive sensory-motor control: ballistic eye movements*. Elsevier, Amsterdam.

Guthrie, B. L., Porter, J. D., and Sparks, D. L. (1983). Corollary discharge provides accurate eye position information to the oculomotor system. *Science*, **221**, 1193–5.

Hallet, P. E. and Lightstone, A. D. (1976). Saccadic eye movements towards stimuli triggered by prior saccades. *Vision Research*, **16**, 99–106.

Hochberg, J. E. (1978). *Perception*. Prentice-Hall, Englewood Cliffs, NJ.

Howard, I. P. (1982). *Human visual orientation*. Wiley, Chichester.

Hyvarinen, J. and Poranen, A. (1974). Function of the parietal associative area 7 as revealed from cellular discharges in alert monkeys. *Brain*, **97**, 673–92.

Jay, M. F. and Sparks, D. L. (1984). Auditory receptive fields in the primate superior colliculus that shift with changes in eye position. *Nature*, **309**, 345–7.

Jay, M. F. and Sparks, D. L. (1987). Sensorimotor integration in the primate superior colliculus: II. Coordinates of auditory signals. *Journal of Neurophysiology*, **57**, 35–55.

Jeannerod, M. (1982). How do we direct our actions in space? In *Spatially oriented behavior* (ed. A. Hein and M. Jeannerod), pp. 1–13. Springer-Verlag, New York.

Kuperstein, M. (1988). An adaptive neural model for mapping invariant target position. *Behavioral Neuroscience*, **102**, 148–62.

Larish, D. D. and Stelmach, G. E. (1982). Spatial orientation of a limb using egocentric reference points. *Perception and Psychophysics*, **32**, 19–26.

Lynch, J. C., Mountcastle, V. B., Talbot, W. H., and Yin, T. C. T. (1977). Parietal lobe mechanisms for directed visual attention. *Journal of Neurophysiology*, **40**, 362–89.

MacNeilage, P. F. (1970). Motor control and serial ordering of speech. *Psychological Review*, **77**, 183–96.

Mays, L. E. and Sparks, D. L. (1980a). Saccades are spatially, not retinocentrically, coded. *Science*, **208**, 1163–5.

Mays, L. E. and Sparks, D. L. (1980b). Dissociation of visual and saccade-related responses in superior colliculus. *Journal of Neurophysiology*, **43**, 207–32.

Mays, L. E. and Sparks, D. L. (1981). The localization of saccade targets using a combination of retinal and eye position information. In *Progress in oculomotor research* (ed. A. Fuchs and W. Becker), pp. 39–47. Elsevier, New York.

Neisser, U. (1967). *Cognitive psychology*. Appleton-Century-Crofts, New York.

Paillard, J. (1987). Cognitive versus sensorimotor encoding of spatial information. In *Cognitive processes and spatial orientation in animal and man* (ed. P. Ellen and C. Thinus-Blanc), pp. 43–77. Martinus Nijhoff, Dordrecht.

Rizzolatti, G., Scandolara, C., Matelli, M., and Gentilucci, M. (1981). Afferent properties of periarcuate neurons in macaque monkeys. II. Visual responses. *Behavioural Brain Research*, **2**, 147–63.

Robinson, D. A. (1973). Models of the saccadic eye movement control system. *Kybernetik*, **14**, 71–83.

Sakata, H., Shibutani, H., and Kawano, K. (1980). Spatial properties of visual fixation neurons in posterior parietal association cortex of the monkey. *Journal of Neurophysiology*, **43**, 1654–72.

Schiller, P. H. and Koerner, F. (1971). Discharge characteristics of single units in superior colliculus of the alert rhesus monkey. *Journal of Neurophysiology*, **34**, 920–36.

Schiller, P. H. and Sandell, J. H. (1983). Interactions between visually and electrically elicited saccades before and after superior colliculus and frontal eye field ablations in the rhesus monkey. *Experimental Brain Research*, **49**, 381–92.

Schlag, J. and Schlag-Rey, M. (1983). Interface of visual input and oculomotor command for directing the gaze on target. In *Spatially oriented behavior* (ed. A. Hein and M. Jeannerod), pp. 87–103. Springer-Verlag, New York.

Schlag, J., Schlag-Rey, M., Peck, C. K., and Joseph, J.-P. (1980). Visual responses of thalamic neurons depending on the direction of gaze and the position of targets in space. *Experimental Brain Research*, **40**, 170–84.

Sparks, D. L. (1986). The neural translation of sensory signals into commands for the control of saccadic eye movements: The role of the primate superior colliculus. *Physiological Reviews*, **66**, 118–71.

Sparks, D. L. and Mays, L. E. (1981). The role of the monkey superior colliculus in the control of saccadic eye movements: A current perspective. In *Progress in oculomotor research* (ed. A. Fuchs and W. Becker), pp. 137–44. Elsevier, New York.

Sparks, D. L. and Mays, L. E. (1983a). The role of the monkey superior colliculus in the spatial localization of saccade targets. In *Spatially oriented behavior* (ed. A. Hein and M. Jeannerod), pp. 63–86. Springer-Verlag, New York.

Sparks, D. L. and Mays, L. E. (1983b). The spatial localization of saccade targets. I: Compensation for stimulation-induced perturbations in eye position. *Journal of Neurophysiology*, **49**, 45–63.

Sparks, D. L. and Porter, J. D. (1983). The spatial localization of saccade targets. II: Activity of superior colliculus neurons preceding compensatory saccades. *Journal of Neurophysiology*, **49**, 64–74.

Treisman, A. (1977). Focused attention in the perception and retrieval of multidimensional stimuli. *Perception and Psychophysics*, **22**, 1–11.

Treisman, A. M. and Gelade, G. (1980). A feature-integration theory of attention. *Cognitive Psychology*, **12**, 97–136.

Young, L. R. and Stark, L. (1963). Variable feedback experiments testing a sampled data model for eye tracking movements. *IEEE Transactions, Human Factors*, **4**, 38–51.

Zahn, J. R., Abel, L. A., and Dell'Osso, L. F. (1978). Audio-ocular response characteristics. *Sensory Processes*, **2**, 32–7.

Zee, D. S., Optican, L. M., Cook, J. D., Robinson, D. A., and Engel, W. K. (1976). Slow saccades in spinocerebellar degeneration. *Archives of Neurology*, **33**, 243–51.

Zipser, D. and Andersen, R. A. (1988). A back-propagation programmed network that simulates response properties of a subset of posterior parietal neurons. *Nature*, **331**, 679–84.

2

Spatio-temporal patterns of activity on the motor map of cat superior colliculus

D. GUITTON, D. P. MUNOZ, and D. PÉLISSON

Introduction

Reticular circuits responsible for generating saccadic eye movements are thought to be commanded directly by only two supra-reticular structures acting in parallel: the superior colliculus (SC) and the frontal eye field (FEF). The prime evidence supporting this hypothesis is that simultaneous bilateral destruction of the SC and FEF severely impairs monkeys' ability to generate saccades (Schiller *et al.* 1980). Each structure appears to dominate the control of saccades generated in a specific behavioural context.

Both FEF and SC neurons discharge before visually guided saccades (FEF: Bruce and Goldberg, 1985; SC; see below). This suggests redundancy in the control of such movements. Indeed, bilateral removal of the FEF alone does not generate long-term deficits in the ability of monkeys to generate saccades to visual targets. By comparison, bilateral SC lesions alone also do not generate strong long-term deficits in accuracy, but nevertheless cause increases in the latency of such saccades and the elimination of very short-latency (100 ms) 'express' saccades (Schiller *et al.* 1987). It appears, therefore, that there is some redundancy in the control of visually guided saccades and that the SC provides the shortest latency route for their generation. By comparison, there seems to be no redundancy in the control of 'cognitively driven' saccades: frontal lobe patients with presumed FEF damage cannot perform an 'anti-saccade' task which requires a reflex-like saccade to a target to be suppressed in favour of an instructed saccade (Guitton *et al.* 1985). In this context, frontal lobe structures are thought to impose inhibition on collicular mechanisms which, if not checked, would generate short-latency saccades to the visual target, thereby confining subjects to the 'fatality of a [collicular driven] reflex' (Holmes 1938).

The SC has attracted considerable attention because of this pivotal role in the control of saccades to sensory targets. Additional interest stems from an interesting neuronal computation performed by the SC and its reticular target structures: the so-called spatio-temporal transform. This computation is inherent to the theme of this book. It addresses the problem of how the nervous system transforms spatially coded discharges in the SC's motor map (see below) to temporally coded discharges used by motoneurons that drive the extra-ocular muscles.

Sensorimotor aspects of the superior colliculus

The mammalian SC is a laminated structure consisting of seven alternating fibre and cell body layers which are oriented parallel to the surface. Anatomical, physiological, and behavioural considerations suggest that these layers can be separated into two major subdivisions: the so-called superficial and deep layers.

Neurons in the superficial layers of the SC have sensory responses that are exclusively visual in origin (see reviews by Chalupa 1984 and R. Grantyn 1988). Each cell responds to a small region of the visual field, the cell's receptive field. Such visually responsive neurons are disposed across the SC's surface in a map which has an orderly topographical organization. The location of a neuron can be identified according to the position, in the visual field, of the centre of its receptive field. This retinotopic representation of the contralateral visual field subtends, on the SC's surface, from $0°$ up to about $80°$ in peripheral vision (Feldon *et al.* 1970).

The deeper layers of the SC are also organized into a map. Many neurons show sensory responses to visual targets, and the resulting retinotopic map is in spatial register with the overlying one in the superficial layer (Schiller and Koerner 1971; Schiller and Stryker 1972; Mays and Sparks 1980; see Sparks and Mays 1990 for review). Some of the visually responsive neurons, and also other neurons, discharge high-frequency bursts of action potentials immediately before the initiation of saccadic eye movements in the head-fixed animal (Schiller and Koerner 1971; Schiller and Stryker 1972; Wurtz and Goldberg 1972; Sparks 1978; Sparks *et al.* 1976; Sparks and Mays 1980; Peck 1987; reviews by Wurtz and Albano 1980; Sparks 1986; Sparks and Mays 1990). These saccade-related burst neurons are 'vector-tuned': each cell discharges maximally for a given amplitude and direction of movement. The more the saccade vector differs from the optimal, the weaker is the saccade-related discharge. The range of possible movement vectors defines the movement field of the cell. Usually, one neuron is active for a specific but large range of movements. It follows that any one movement is preceded by activity in a large ensemble of neurons. (A circular zone, about 3 mm in diameter, is usually active.) This zone of collicular activity is centred at a location on the retinotopically coded motor map that is appropriate to drive a saccade of the appropriate vector (i.e. amplitude and direction). This brings the eye from its current fixation point onto the target that activates the cell's receptive field (if it has one).

The movement vectors defining the motor map are in spatial register with the vectors specifying the position of the centre of the cell's receptive field with respect to the fixation position, i.e., the motor and visual maps are coextensive.

On the basis of these well-known observations it has been proposed that the SC provides the brain-stem premotor circuitry with a *topographically coded command specifying initial eye motor error* (Sparks *et al.* 1976; Sparks and Mays 1980 (reviewed in Fuchs *et al.* 1985); Sparks 1986; Sparks and Mays 1990). Whether this proposal is sound is the principal subject of this chapter.

The organization of the motor map in the deeper layers of the SC presents a special problem. The oculomotor range (the angular limits of ocular motility) of most animals is less than ±80°, so that eye movements alone will be insufficient to reach a target at, say, 80° in peripheral vision. This problem is extremely well illustrated in the cat, whose visuo-oculomotor system has been well studied and whose gaze control systems appears to be similar to that of humans (Guitton 1988). The cat has restricted ocular motility, yielding an oculomotor range (OMR) of only ±25°. Consequently, combined co-ordinated eye–head movements must be used to attain targets situated in a large portion of visual space. The same is true of the squirrel monkey—another frequently used species in oculomotor research—whose OMR is similar to that of the cat.

The first question that arises from these considerations is whether the topographically coded command issued by the motor map of the cat's SC specifies initial *gaze* motor error rather than initial eye motor error as hypothesized for the monkey. We have investigated this problem by recording from the main output cells of the deep layers involved in controlling orienting movements: the tecto-reticular (TRN) and tecto-reticulo-spinal neurons (TRSN), together called TR(S)Ns. TR(S)Ns are located in the deeper collicular layers and project via the crossed predorsal bundle to many mesencephalic, pontine, and medullary centres implicated in the control of eye and head movements (Grantyn and Grantyn 1982; Grantyn and Berthoz 1985). Electrophysiological experiments in the anaesthetized cat have demonstrated di- or polysynaptic activation of abducens motoneurons (Precht *et al.* 1974; Grantyn and Grantyn 1976) and neck muscle motoneurons (Anderson *et al.* 1971) following electrical stimulation of the contralateral SC. Microstimulation of the deeper collicular laminae in the alert cat elicits co-ordinated eye–head orienting movements (Hess *et al.* 1946; Syka and Radil–Weiss 1972; Guitton *et al.* 1980; Roucoux *et al.* 1980; Crommelinck *et al.* 1990). These effects are mediated by the crossed TR(S) pathway, which therefore forms a potentially powerful neural substrate for providing a common, gaze-related drive to eye and head premotor centres.

In a series of experiments (Munoz 1988; Munoz and Guitton 1985, 1986,

1988, 1989), we have investigated the role of TR(S)Ns in the control of orienting behaviour in the alert cat whose head is unrestrained.

TR(S)N discharge characteristics

TR(S)Ns were studied using procedures which have already been described (Guitton *et al.* 1984; Munoz 1988; Munoz and Guitton 1985, 1986, 1989). The animals were trained to perform several visuomotor tasks while their heads were restrained ('head-fixed') or unrestrained ('head-free'). Cells were identified antidromically by their response following stimulation of the predorsal bundle, rostromedial to the abducens nucleus. The name TR(S)N signifies that an unknown fraction of the cells we studied projected as far as the upper cervical spinal cord.

Almost all TR(S)Ns responded to some form of visual stimulation. TR(S)Ns had visual receptive fields that conformed to the retinotopic map of visual space present in the superficial collicular laminae (Feldon *et al.* 1970). TR(S)Ns located in the rostral SC had centrally placed visual receptive fields that included a representation of the area centralis, while TR(S)Ns situated in the caudal SC had receptive fields in the contralateral hemifield, away from centre. We will refer to these cells as *fixation* TR(S)Ns and *orientation* TR(S)Ns, respectively, based on the location of their visual receptive fields.

Fixation TR(S)Ns

The salient features of fixation TR(S)N discharges can be explained from the data presented in Fig. 2.1. The behavioural paradigm used is schematically represented in Fig. 2.1C–F. This fixation TR(S)N, located in the rostral right SC, had a visual receptive field (dashed circle) that was centred about the point of fixation (marked by 'X'). A food target (represented by the small, filled circle) was presented from either the left (Fig. 2.1C,D) or the right (Fig. 2.1E,F) side of an opaque rectangular barrier in front of the cat. The animal, whose head was restrained in these trials, fixated upon the food target (Fig. 2.1C,F) or looked away to the opposite side of the barrier (Fig. 2.1D,E). Fig. 2.1A (target left) and B (target right) show, from top to bottom, the vertical (E_v) and horizontal (E_h) eye position traces, the electromyographic (EMG) activity recorded from the left splenius neck muscle, and the instantaneous firing frequency of the cell (F4). The letters under the unit traces correspond to the appropriate behavioural situations illustrated in Fig. 2.1C–F.

When the food target was on the left of the barrier (Fig. 2.1A), the cell was activated in a sustained manner whenever the animal looked left to

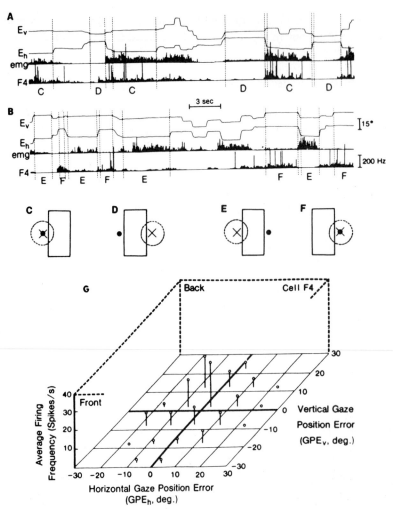

Fig. 2.1. Activity of a fixation Tr(S)N recorded in a head-fixed cat when the target was located on the left (A) or right (B) side of a barrier. From top to bottom in (A) and (B) are shown: vertical (E_v) and horizontal (E_h) eye positions, electromyographic (emg) activity of the left splenius muscle, and instantaneous, firing frequency histogram of a TR(S)N located in the rostral right SC (F4). Letters under the unit traces correspond to the appropriate schematics (C–F) describing the different behavioural situations. A barrier (represented by a filled rectangle) was placed in front of the animal and a food target (filled circle) protruded from the left (C, D) or the right (E, F) side of the barrier. The cat looked (fixation point denoted by X) at either the target (C, F) or the other edge of the barrier (D, E). The visual receptive field of the neuron is represented by a dashed circle. (G) Gaze-position error field of cell F4 obtained when the target was visible in the head-fixed condition. Intersection of the thick lines marks 0° gaze-position error (i.e., fixation of the target). Note that cell F4 was maximally active when the visual axis was directed at the target.

fixate the target, thereby placing it in the cell's visual receptive field. The cell's activity in Fig. 2.1A was considerably reduced or absent for right-ward eye positions when the cat looked away from the target. When the target was positioned on the right side of the barrier (Fig. 2.1B), the cell was activated for rightward eye deviations when, once again, the target was in the cell's visual receptive field. When the eye moved to the left, how-ever, the level of cell discharge was reduced.

Note that this sustained discharge pattern was not correlated to the tonic EMG ativity recorded from the contralateral splenius neck muscle. The left splenius muscle was tonically active with ipsilateral (leftward) eye positions, as has been demonstrated by Vidal *et al.* (1982). However, the sustained discharges of fixation TR(S)Ns and contralateral dorsal neck muscles were congruent only when the target was on the left (Fig. 2.1A); these activities were inversely related when the target was on the right (Fig. 2.1B). Thus the sustained discharges of fixation TR(S)Ns occur in-dependently of tonic EMG activity recorded from contralateral neck muscles even though studies of TR(S)N axonal and collateral trajectories show that there may be only two synapses between the SC and contra-lateral neck muscle motoneurons (Anderson *et al.* 1971). However, fixa-tion and orientation TR(S)Ns may project to different target structures (Munoz 1988; Munoz and Guitton 1989).

The sustained discharges illustrated in Fig.2.1A and B were also present in the head-free condition (not shown). This pattern of activity was there-fore not related to any particular position of the eyes or head, nor pattern of contralateral neck muscle activity. Rather, it was related to the angular separation between the target and the visual axis, which we have called 'gaze position error' (Munoz and Guitton 1985).

The average firing frequency of the cell is plotted against gaze position error in Fig.2.1G. Different target positions were used. The gaze position error and average firing frequency were calculated for each period of fixation, and the data were grouped into 10° horizontal by 10° vertical bins. The cell illustrated in Fig. 2.1 clearly had a preferential gaze position error at or near 0°. That is, it fired maximally when the cat looked straight at the target, and the discharge decreased for larger values of gaze position error, when the visual axis was directed away from the target. The ensemble of gaze position error vectors for which this TR(S)N was activated is called the neuron's 'gaze position error field'. Gaze position error fields coincided with visual receptive fields for all the cells studied.

Note that all the TR(S)Ns we studied had large gaze position error fields. The smallest fields, which were displayed by fixation TR(S)Ns, were none the less about 20° in diameter. The broad tuning of TR(S)N gaze position error fields implies that a large number of TR(S)Ns are active for a given gaze position error (McIlwain 1986).

Orientation TR(S)Ns

Orientation TR(S)Ns, defined as those cells whose visual receptive fields lacked a representation of the area centralis, were recorded in the caudal part of the SC. They also exhibited a sustained discharge pattern which was related to the position of the visual axis relative to a target of interest. Figure 2.2, whose format is identical to Fig. 2.1, illustrates the results obtained from a typical orientation TR(S)N. The method is schematically represented in Fig. 2.B and C. The food target (filled circle) was on the left of the barrier. The cell was located in the caudal right SC and had its visual receptive field (dashed circle) situated near the horizontal meridian, to the left of the point of fixation (marked by 'X'). This orientation TR(S)N was activated with a sustained discharge when the visual axis was directed to the right thereby placing the target in the cell's receptive field. When the cat looked to the left, the neuron was silenced. This same pattern of activity was recorded in both head-fixed and head-free conditions (Munoz and Guitton 1985). Note from the traces in Fig. 2.2A that there was an independence between the sustained discharge of this orientation TR(S)N and the contralateral (left) splenius neck muscle. Thus, like the fixation TR(S)Ns, the sustained discharges of orientation TR(S)Ns were not related to any pattern of muscle activation. This pattern of TR(S)N activity was instead related to the position of the visual axis relative to the target (i.e. gaze position error). The gaze position error field of this cell, which was measured in a head-free condition, is plotted in Fig. 2D. This cell was maximally activated when the visual axis was directed approximately 30° right and 10° above the target of interest.

TR(S)N sustained discharges are not visual or movement-related

In the preceding sections, we have described the characteristics of fixation and orientation TR(S)N susained discharges which were related to the coding of gaze position error. It might be argued that these discharge patterns were visually evoked, being caused by the presence of the target in a cell's visual receptive field. To rule out this hypothesis, we recorded from TR(S)Ns while cats oriented to a predicted target (Fig. 2.3). The food target was initially visible to the right side of the barrier and the head-free cat fixated on it (Fig. 2.3A). Then the target was hidden behind the barrier (Fig. 2.3B) and the trained animal oriented to the left side of the barrier (Fig. 2.3C), where it anticipated target reappearance.

Figure 2.3D illustrates the associated response of an orientation TR(S)N recorded in the caudal right SC. This cell had its visual receptive field situated on the horizontal meridian, to the left of the fixation point, so that when the cat fixated upon the right edge of the barrier, the left edge was in the cell's visual receptive field. This TR(S)N was silent at the start of the

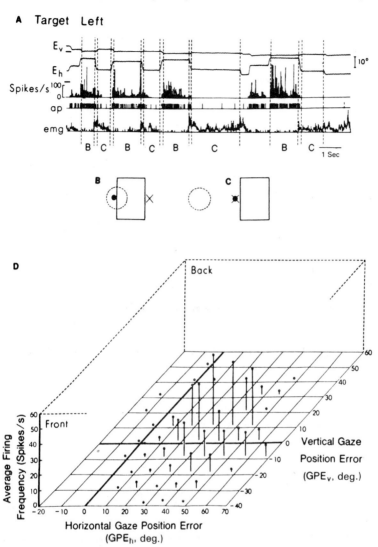

A Target Left

E_v

E_h

Spikes/s

ap

emg

B C   B   C   B   C   B   C

B

C

D

Back

Front

Average Firing Frequency (Spikes/s)

Vertical Gaze Position Error (GPE$_v$, deg.)

Horizontal Gaze Position Error (GPE$_h$, deg.)

Fig. 2.2. (A): Activity of an orientation TR(S)N recorded in a head-fixed cat when the target was located on the left. From top to bottom are shown: vertical (E_v) and horizontal (E_h) eye positions, instantaneous firing frequency histogram (spikes/s) and unit histogram (ap) of a TR(S)N located in the caudal right SC, and electromyographic (EMG) activity of the left splenius muscle. (B, C): Schematics of behavioural situations (same format as Fig. 2.1). The target (filled circle) was located on the left side of the barrier. The cell's visual receptive field (dashed circle) was located to the left of the point of fixation (marked by X). (D): Gaze-position error field of the cell obtained when the target was visible in the head-free condition. Note that this cell was maximally active when the visual axis was directed to the right and above the target.

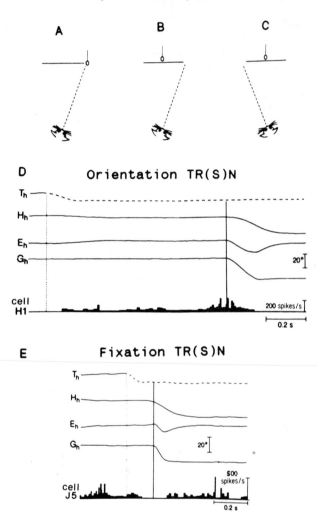

Fig. 2.3. Orientation and fixation TR(S)N activity associated with the preparation and the execution of a head-free orienting movement. (A–C): Schematics of the behavioural situation: the food target was moved from the right side of the barrier to behind it, where it stayed hidden until the end of the trial; the cat oriented its gaze to the left in anticipation of target reappearance. (D, E): Orientation and fixation TR(S)N discharge recorded from separate animals. Shown from top to bottom are the target (T_h), head (H_h), eye (E_h) and gaze (G_h) horizontal positions, and the instantaneous, firing frequency histograms. Dashed vertical lines denote target disappearance. Target trace is dashed when target is hidden. Solid vertical lines denote onset of gaze shift.

trial, when the cat fixated upon the target. Shortly after the target disappeared (where T_h becomes dashed), the cell was activated in a sustained manner. This pattern of activity continued until the head-free animal oriented to the left edge of the barrier. Note that, although the visual input to the cell was the same in (A) and (B) (namely, the left edge of the barrier passed through the cell's visual receptive field), the cell was only active in condition (B). For this reason we believe that TR(S)N sustained discharges are not simple visual responses; rather, they are related to the coding of gaze position error (or the position of the gaze when referred to target—either visible or predicted—position). We have also recorded sustained discharges from TR(S)Ns when cats were in total darkness, provided that the animals were anticipating the ultimate appearance of the food target in the cells' gaze position error field.

TR(S)N sustained discharges were independent of any orienting movement. Figure 2.3D shows that the sustained discharge began shortly after the disappearance of the target even though the cat delayed its response to the predicted target for almost one second after the food disappeared from the right side of the barrier. In such a trial, the sustained discharge could be clearly separated from the weak burst which was associated with and preceded movements towards a predicted target. In cases where there was no movement, the sustained discharge gradually disappeared (Munoz and Guitton 1985).

The sustained discharges of fixation TR(S)Ns were also dependent on the animal's locus of attention, and not only on visual input. Figure 2.3E illustrates the activity of a fixation TR(S)N, located in the area centralis representation of the rostral left SC, when a cat whose head was free generated a leftward orienting movement towards a predicted target. This cell was active at the start of the trial, when the animal attentively fixated a visible target on the right of the barrier (see Fig. 2.3A), the rate of discharge began to decrease. Firing resumed at the termination of the gaze shift (Fig. 2.3C), when the visual axis was directed to the left side of the barrier, even though the visual target was still not visible. Thus fixation TR(S)Ns were maximally active when the animal attentively fixated a visual target (left part of Fig. 2.3E; see also Fig. 2.1), but sustained discharges were also recorded for predicted targets (right part of Fig. 2.3E) in which case the animal's locus of attention was a more significant causative factor than the visual input. Note also that the decrease of fixation TR(S)N activity associated with movement execution (Fig. 2.3E) is the inverse of the movement-related pattern of increased activity of orientation TR(S)Ns (Fig. 2.3D). Neurons with properties similar to fixation TR(S)Ns have been also reported in the foveal representation of the monkey's SC (D. P. Munoz and R. H. Wurtz, personal communication).

Movement-related discharges of TR(S)Ns

We will now present evidence linking the movement-related discharge patterns of orientation TR(S)Ns to the metrics of eye, head, and gaze orienting movements. To facilitate a description of this relationship, we will consider orienting responses that are triggered by both predictive and visual cues (Munoz and Guitton 1986, 1989). An example of such an orienting movement is shown in Fig. 2.4A, along with the neuronal activity of an orientation TR(S)N whose sustained discharges were described in Fig. 2.4D. This cell had a visual receptive field located to the left of the point of fixation. Each trial began with the cat fixating a food target located on the right side of the barrier, thereby placing the left edge of the barrier in the neuron's visual receptive field. The target was then moved behind the barrier and reappeared on the left. The leftward orienting movement was triggered either before or after target reappearance. Each trial terminated with the cat fixating the target on the left. The left and right vertical dashed lines in Fig. 2.4A correspond to target disappearance and reappearance, respectively. The solid vertical line denotes onset of the leftward orienting movement which, in this example, nearly coincided with the reappearance of the target.

The TR(S)N began its sustained discharge shortly after the target disappeared from the right side and continued to fire until the end of the leftward gaze shift. This gaze shift was initiated about 15 ms after target reappearance; therefore it could not have been triggered by this event. Rather, the initial slowly rising gaze, eye, and head velocity profiles are typical of a slow movement to a *predicted* target (see below). After the initial increase in velocity there is, in each of the eye, head, and gaze traces, a deceleration phase which suggests that peak velocity is soon to be attained. However, as evidenced by the inflection point on each velocity trace (marked by arrows), the trajectory of the orienting response was modified in mid-flight with all velocity profiles showing a re-acceleration. The discharge pattern of the TR(S)N showed similar changes. At the onset of the gaze shift, the neuron was only firing at a low frequency—a pattern of activity characteristic of movements to the predicted target. Shortly after target reappearance, but within the gaze shift, the cell discharged a high-frequency burst of spikes whose onset preceded the modification of the gaze and eye trajectories by 9 ms and of the head trajectory by 29 ms. (Note that it was possible to mimic these modified trajectories with different patterns of electrical stimulation applied to the deeper laminae of the cat SC; Munoz 1988.)

Both the eye and head trajectories were affected by the TR(S)N burst. The levels of acceleration and neuronal firing frequency could be related.

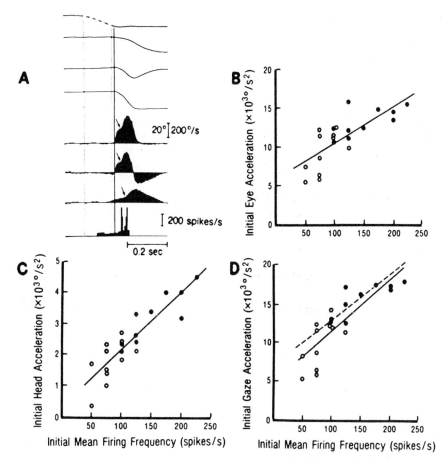

Fig. 2.4. Dependence of eye, head, and gaze velocity on TR(S)N burst frequency. (A): A food target, visible on the right side of a barrier, was moved (left vertical dashed line) quickly behind the barrier and reappeared on the left side (right vertical dashed line). The cat generated a leftward gaze shift that began (vertical solid line) about synchronously with target reappearance. This gaze shift was triggered by 'predictive' cues. Traces represent from top to bottom: horizontal target (T_h), head (H_h), eye (E_h), and gaze (G_h) position traces; horizontal gaze ($\dot{G}_h$), eye ($\dot{E}_h$), and head ($\dot{H}_h$) velocity traces; cell firing frequency. (B–D): Relation between initial eye, head, and gaze accelerations, respectively, and initial discharge frequency of cell shown in (A)—see text for details.

To do this, the average initial firing rate of the cell was determined during a 40 ms interval: from 20 ms before to 20 ms after the onset of a gaze saccade. Average acceleration of the eye and gaze were evaluated for the first 20 ms after onset of optimal amplitude and direction gaze saccades. Average head acceleration was also measured across a 20 ms interval, taken between 20 ms and 40 ms after onset of the gaze movement. This delay between the interval of eye and head accelerations was chosen since we found that head acceleration tended to lag behind eye acceleration by about 20 ms (Guitton *et al.* 1990).

Figure 2.4B–D shows the relation between discharge intensity of this orientation TR(S)N (cell H1) and the initial acceleration of about 20 leftward gaze shifts, all of about the same amplitude (24°–32°). The data were obtained for movements to both visible (filled circles) and predicted (empty circles) targets. The initial rate of discharge of this cell was well correlated with the initial average acceleration of the eye (Fig. 2.4B), head (Fig. 2.4C), and therefore gaze (Fig. 2.4D). Regression analyses generated the solid lines with correlation coefficients of 0.77, 0.89, and 0.84, respectively. The dashed line in Fig. 2.4D was obtained from a regression analysis of similar data obtained when the animal's head was fixed ($r = 0.61$, $N = 19$). The other orientation cells that we analysed showed similar correlations.

Spatio-temporal pattern of activity on TR(S)N motor map

We have illustrated above three fundamental properties of the motor map formed by TR(S)Ns:

1. The initial *location* of activity on the map codes the initial gaze vector, not eye vector.
2. The *quantity* of activity specifies the speed of the eye, head, and gaze movements.
3. The retinotopic position of the active ensemble of TR(S)Ns differs if measured, respectively, at the start (orientation TR(S)Ns) and end (fixation TR(S)Ns) of a gaze shift.

At the end of a gaze shift, activity on the motor map disappears from its initial location in the caudal SC and reappears 'instantaneously' at the fixation area of the SC's rostral pole (Figs. 2.1–4). Put another way, the retinotopic location of the active ensemble of TR(S)Ns differs if measured at the start and end of a gaze shift, respectively. In view of this it was natural to ask where the retinotopic location of the active ensemble was *during* a gaze shift.

To answer this question we studied the timing of TR(S)N discharges with respect to the onset and termination of gaze shifts which had a large range of amplitudes, but whose directions were restricted to each cell's preferred direction.

We recorded enough data from 16 TR(S)Ns in six cats to be able to develop the hypothesis described below. Figure 2.5A and B illustrates the movement-related discharges recorded from a typical TR(S)N, cell Q24

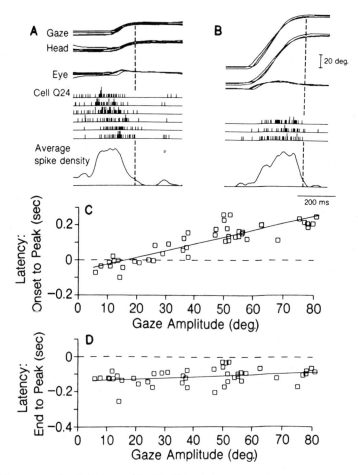

Fig. 2.5. Movement-related discharge of a TR(S)N. (A): Superimposed traces of five-co-ordinated eye–head movements producing a 15° rightward, horizontal gaze displacement preferred by this cell. The corresponding discharge patterns of a TR(S)N, cell Q24, is shown below the eye trace. The occurrence of an action potential, or spike, is represented by a small vertical line. Additional small lines superimposed on top of others indicate extra spikes within the same time-bin. Vertical dashed line indicates termination of gaze shift. Below the array of cell discharges is the average spike-density function obtained by replacing each spike with a gaussian curve 20 ms wide, and summing the transformed array. (B): 80° gaze shift; three superimposed traces. Other details explained above in (a). (C): Latency from *onset* of a gaze shift to peak discharge of cell, plotted against amplitude of gaze displacement. Each square represents data from one gaze shift. Horizontal dashed line corresponds to zero latency. Solid line obtained from a regression analysis. Note that cell Q24 burst before all gaze shifts smaller than about 15°. (D): Latency from *end* of gaze shift to peak discharge plotted against total gaze displacement. Note that the cell discharges maximally at about the same time relative to the end of all gaze shifts.

(located in the left SC), which discharged in response to rightward gaze shifts. The traces are aligned with respect to the termination of gaze shifts. This TR(S)N was active before and during gaze shifts that were about 15° in amplitude (Fig. 2.5A). Contrary to the classic notion of vector-tuned neurons in the SC, this cell also discharged in relation to gaze shifts that were much larger in amplitude (for example, 80°; Fig. 2.5B). However, for these large amplitude movements, the cell began to discharge only after movement onset. Peak discharge was attained late in the gaze shift. Similar discharge profiles were obtained from TR(S)Ns when the orienting movements were executed in complete darkness. Note that this cell's peak discharge preceded the onset of the *eye* saccade for small amplitude gaze shifts (Fig. 2.5A), but occurred during the plateau phase in the eye's trajectory that followed the eye saccade for large amplitude gaze shifts (Fig. 2.5B).

We plotted the latency to the peak of the burst discharge (from onset (Fig. 2.5C) or termination (Fig. 2.5D) of each *gaze* shift), versus the total amplitude of the gaze displacement. Only movements that consisted of a single-step gaze shift to the target along the cell's preferred direction were considered. Points lying below the horizontal dashed line in Fig. 2.5C represent trials in which peak discharge was attained before movement onset. As total gaze displacement increased, the latency from movement onset to peak discharge increased, whereas the latency from the end of each gaze shift to peak discharge remained constant (as was seen in Fig. 2.5A and B). Hence cell Q24's discharge peaked at about a *fixed value of gaze error* and the rising slope in Fig. 2.5C is due to the duration of gaze shifts increasing with amplitude (the 'main sequence' relationship).

In conclusion, the data presented in Fig. 2.5 suggest that the zone of TR(S)N activity is *moving* across the cat's SC motor map during the course of an orienting gaze shift. First a zone of TR(S)N activity is established in the caudal region of one SC, at a location on the retinotopically coded SC motor map specified by the vector error (say, 80°) that exists between the initial position of the visual axis and the target of interest. The location of this initial activity determines the vector of initial gaze motor error. As the gaze shift runs its course, this zone of TR(S)N activity migrates towards the rostral pole. Its instantaneous location on the map specifies the remaining gaze motor error. When the gaze shift terminates (i.e. when gaze motor error is zero), the active zone invades the rostral pole, where fixation-related TR(S)Ns are located.

An alternative interpretation is that a circular wave of activity propagates in a radial direction from an origin at the initial site of activation. Our data are not compatible with this mechanism. There is no burst activity in TR(S)Ns located on the side of the initially active zone furthest from the fixation zone, which would occur if this interpretation were correct.

We suggest that the topographically coded signal of instantaneous gaze motor error is due to the location of the cat's SC within a gaze feedback loop. This hypothesis is favoured by our observation (Fig. 2.4) that a sudden increase in the discharge frequency of TR(S)N phasic bursts speeds up a gaze shift without affecting its accuracy. Such a finding is difficult to incorporate in current models of the SC, but would be consistent with a feedback control system wherein the SC provides the gaze error signal and the higher velocities eliminate gaze error more quickly, such that movement duration is shorter but accuracy maintained.

Acknowledgements

This work was supported by the Medical Research Council of Canada (MRC) and le Fonds de la Recherche en Santé du Québec. D. Pélisson was supported by the Fondation Simone et Cino del Duca (Paris), the MRC, and l'Office Franco-Québecois pour la Jeunesse. D. Munoz was supported by an MRC studentship. The generous, industrious, and good-humoured assistance of Ms. Jane Thibaudeau is gratefully acknowledged.

References

Anderson, M. E., Yoshida, M., and Wilson, V. J. (1971). Influence of superior colliculus on cat neck motoneurons. *Journal of Neurophysiology*, **34**, 898–907.

Bruce, C. J. and Goldberg, M. E. (1985). Primate frontal eye fields. I. Single neurons discharging before saccades. *Journal of Neurophysiology*, **53**, 603–35.

Chalupa, L. M. (1984). Visual physiology of the mammalian superior colliculus. *Comparative neurology of the optic tectum* (ed. H. Vonegas), pp. 775–818. Plenum Press, New York.

Crommelinck, M., Paré, M., and Guitton, D. (1990). Gaze shifts evoked by superior colliculus stimulation in the alert cat. *Society for Neuroscience Abstracts*, **16**, 444.1, 1.082.

Feldon, S., Feldon, P., and Kruger, L. (1970). Topography of the retinal projection upon the superior colliculus of the cat. *Vision Research*, **10**, 135–43.

Fuchs A. F., Kaneko, C. R. S., and Scudder, C. A. (1985). Brainstem control of saccadic eye movements. *Annual Review of Neuroscience*, **8**, 307–37.

Grantyn, A. and Berthoz, A. (1985). Burst activity of identified tectoreticulo-spinal neurons in the alert cat. *Experimental Brain Research*, **57**, 417–21.

Grantyn, A. and Grantyn, R. (1976). Synaptic actions of tectofugal pathways on abducens motoneurons in the cat. *Brain Research*, **105**, 269–85.

Grantyn, A. and Grantyn R. (1982). Axonal patterns and sites of termination of cat superior colliculus neurons projecting in the tecto-bulbo-spinal tract. *Experimental Brain Research*, **46**, 243–56.

Grantyn, R. (1988). Gaze control through superior colliculus: structure and function. In *Neuroanatomy of the oculomotor system* (ed. J. Büttner-Ennever) pp. 273–333. Elsevier, New York.

Guitton, D. (1988). Eye–head coordination in gaze control. In *Control of head movement* (ed. B. W. Peterson and F. J. Richmond), pp. 196–207. Oxford University Press.

Guitton, D., Crommelinck, M., and Roucoux, A. (1980). Stimulation of the superior colliculus in the alert cat. 1. Eye movements and neck EMG activity evoked when the head is restrained. *Experimental Brain Research*, **39**, 63–73.

Guitton, D., Douglas, R. M., and Volle, M. (1984). Eye–head coordination in cat. *Journal of Neurophysiology*, **52**, 1030–50.

Guitton, D., Buchtel, H. A., and Douglas, R. M. (1985). Frontal lobe lesions in man cause difficulties in suppressing reflexive glances and in generating goal-directed saccades. *Experimental Brain Research*, **58**, 455–72.

Guitton, D., Munoz, D. P., and Galiana, H. L. (1990). Gaze control in the cat: Studies and modelling of the coupling between orienting eye and head movements in different behavioral tasks. *Journal of Neurophysiology*, **64**, 509–31.

Hess, W. R., Burgi, J., and Bucher, V. (1946). Motorishe funktion des tektal und tegmentalgebietes. *Monatschrift für Psychiatrie und Neurologie*, **112**, 1–52.

Holmes, G. (1938). The cerebral integration of ocular movements. *British Medical Journal*, **2**, 107–12.

Mays, L. E. and Sparks, D. L. (1980) Dissociation of visual and saccade-related responses in superior colliculus neurons. *Journal of Neurophysiology*, **43**, 207–32.

McIlwain, J. T. (1986). Point images in the visual system: New interest in an old idea. *Trends in Neuroscience*, **9**, 354–8.

Munoz, D. P. (1988). On the role of the tecto-reticulo-spinal system in gaze control. Unpublished Ph.D. thesis. McGill University, Montreal, Canada.

Munoz, D. P. and Guitton, D. (1985). Tectospinal neurons in the cat have discharges coding gaze position error. *Brain Research*, **341**, 184–8.

Munoz, D. P. and Guitton, D. (1986). Presaccadic burst discharges of teco-reticulo-spinal neurons in the alert head-free cat. *Brain Research*, **398**, 185–90.

Munoz, D. P. and Guitton, D. (1988). Rostral output neurons of superior colliculus are active during attentive fixation. *Society for Neurosciences Abstracts*, **14**, 956.

Munoz, D. P. and Guitton, D. (1989). Fixation and orientation control by the tecto-reticulo-spinal system in the cat whose head is unrestrained. *Revue Neurologique* (Paris), **145**, 8–9, 567–79.

Peck, C. K. (1987). Saccade-related burst neurons in cat superior colliculus. *Brain Research*, **408**, 329–33.

Precht, W., Schwindt, P. C., and Magherini, P. C. (1974). Tectal influences on cat ocular motoneurons. *Brain Research*, **82**, 27–40.

Roucoux, A., Guitton, D., and Crommelinck, M. (1980). Stimulation of the superior colliculus in the alert cat. II. Eye and head movements evoked when the head is unrestrained. *Experimental Brain Research*, **39**, 75–85.

Schiller, P. H. and Koerner, F. (1971). Discharge characteristics of single units in superior colliculus of the alert rhesus monkey. *Journal of Neurophysiology*, **34**, 920–36.

Schiller, P. H. and Stryker, M. (1972). Single-unit recording and stimulation in superior colliculus of the alert rhesus monkey. *Journal of Neurophysiology*, **35**, 915–24.

Schiller, P. H., True, S. D., and Conway, J. L. (1980). Deficits in eye movements following frontal eye field nd superior colliculus ablations. *Journal of Neurophysiology*, **44**, 1175–89.

Schiller, P. H., Sandell, J. H., and Maunsell, J. H. R. (1987). The effect of frontal eye field and superior colliculus lesions on saccadic latencies in the rhesus monkey. *Journal of Neurophysiology*, **57**, 1033–49.

Syka, J. and Radil-Weiss, T. (1972). Electrical stimulation of the tectum in freely moving cats. *Brain Research*, **28**, 567–72.

Sparks, D. L. (1978) Functional properties of neurons in the monkey superior colliculus: coupling of neuronal activity and saccade onset. *Brain Research*, **156**, 1–16.

Sparks, D. L. (1986) Translation of sensory signals into commands for control of saccadic eye movements: role of the primate superior colliculus. *Physiological Review*, **66**, 118–71.

Sparks, D. L. and Mays, L. E. (1980). Movement fields of saccade-related burst neurons in the monkey superior colliculus. *Brain Research*, **190**, 39–50.

Sparks, D. L. and Mays, L. E. (1990). Signal transformations required for the generation of saccadic eye movements. *Annual Review of Neuroscience*, **13**, 309–36.

Sparks, D. L., Holland, R., and Guthrie, B. L. (1976). Size and distribution of movement fields in the monkey superior colliculus. *Brain Research*, **13**, 21–34.

Vidal, P. P., Roucoux, A., and Berthoz, A. (1982). Horizontal eye position-related activity in neck muscles of the alert cat. *Experimental Brain Research*, **46**, 448–53.

Wurtz, R. H. and Albano, J. E. (1980). Visual–motor function of the primate superior colliculus. *Annual Review of Neuroscience*, **3**, 189–226.

Wurtz, R. H. and Goldberg, M. E. (1972). Activity of superior colliculus in behaving monkey. III. Cells discharging before eye movements. *Journal of Neurophysiology*, **35**, 575–86.

3

Eye–head co-ordination: influence of eye position on the control of head movement amplitude

VINCENT DELREUX, SYLVIE VANDEN ABEELE,
PHILIPPE LEFEVRE, and ANDRÉ ROUCOUX

Introduction

Orienting the gaze towards a visual stimulus is usually by a combined eye and head movement. How the position of the target in space is transmitted to the motor systems of the eye and head is still a matter of debate. Among the unsolved questions, the nature of the frame of reference into which motor commands sent to the neck muscles are coded is particularly intriguing. Common sense suggests that the retinal error (the position of the target on the retina, i.e. a signal coded within a retinocentric frame of reference) should not be sent as such to the motor plant of the head. This error should at least take into account eye position in the orbit (craniocentric coding) and perhaps head position with respect to the trunk (so-called body-centric coding). Experimental data also lead to consideration of such changes in co-ordinates. Roucoux *et al.* (1981) and Vidal *et al.* (1982) demonstrated, in the cat, the existence of strong electromyographic activity in many neck muscles, closely related to eye position in the orbit. One of the suggestions made was that this 'oculo-cephalic' reflex was, in fact, revealing the presence of an extraretinal signal (an efference copy?) supposed to 'add' to the motor signal for the head in order to transpose it from a retinocentric into a craniocentric frame of reference. There are now many experimental data which demonstrate that the eye saccade command is generated within a craniocentric frame of reference (Hallett and Lightstone 1976; Mays and Sparks 1980) or at least controlled through a feedback loop carrying eye position (Robinson 1975) or even eye plus head or gaze position (Munoz and Guitton 1989). By analogy, truncocentric control of head movements, taking head position into consideration, might be postulated. Neck proprioceptors and also semicircular canals are able to generate this information, meaning one does not have to postulate a role for an efference copy.

It is well known that the amplitude of head-orienting movements is almost always smaller than the eccentricity of the target and that the final position of the head is linearly related to target position (Gresty 1974; Bizzi *et al.* 1971; Biguer *et al.* 1984; Tomlinson and Bahra, 1986). These studies, however, do not give any hint about the eventual influence of extraretinal factors, as all the movements studied began with eyes and head aligned. Other studies have established that head position plays a role in the internal reconstruction of extrapersonal space. Marteniuk (1978) and Biguer *et al.* (1988) have indeed demonstrated the influence of head position signals on the final position of the arm in oculo-manual, open-loop, pointing tasks (see Jeannerod 1988 for a review).

Our aim now was to describe the role in the control of orienting head movements of extraretinal factors such as eye position in the orbit or head position on the trunk.

Methods

Eye and head movements were measured in seven adult human subjects with normal or corrected vision, and without oculomotor deficit, aged between 19 and 39 years. They sat in front of a hemispherical screen having a radius of 1 m. Targets were small light-emitting diodes (LED; 1.5 mm in diameter) affixed to the back of the screen at various eccentricities along the horizontal meridian. The subjects were in total darkness; their shoulders and trunk were immobile. Binocular horizontal eye movements were recorded with the electro-oculographic technique by means of bitemporal electrodes (Ag–AgCl Meditrace), with the reference electrode placed on the forehead. Head movements were recorded by the magnetic field technique, a small coil being attached to a light, tightly fitting helmet. Eye movements were automatically calibrated between the trials by asking the subjects to fixate successively given targets while keeping their head perfectly still (immobility of the head was checked by means of the coil signal). Head movements were calibrated before each session by asking the subjects to align their head with equally spaced LEDs. This was done with a small light attached to the helmet that projected a narrow beam onto the screen; this device was adjusted so as to project the beam onto the 0 target (straight ahead) while subjects held their heads in their natural resting or 'primary' position. The head and eye position signals were digitized (500 Hz sampling-DC to 100 Hz band-width) and stored on tape. These data were computer analysed. In the reconstruction of gaze (eye position in space) the distance between the rotation centres of the eyes and of the head was taken into account.

Two types of experiments were done:

Experiment 1. The subjects were first asked to fixate the central LED for 3 s with eyes and head aligned; for this purpose, the helmet light beam was turned on. Then the central target and the helmet light were simultaneously turned off while one of the peripheral targets was turned on. The latter target remained on for 3 s. After this, two other targets were successively presented, each for 3 s. The targets were randomly selected among three LEDs located in the left visual hemifield, at 30° and 60°, as well as in the midline (0°). Examples of successive fixations are: 0–30–60–0, 0–60–30–0, 0–60–30–60, etc. Subjects were instructed to make 'natural' eye–head movements at the targets, without any particular constraint. The helmet light remained off during the rest of the sequence. In total, subjects made at least 10 identical orienting movements (see Fig. 3.1).

Experiment 2. The subjects were first asked to fixate for 3 s, with eyes and head aligned, one of the three LEDs (0°, 30°, or 60° on the left side). The helmet light was on. Then the helmet light and the initial target were turned off while another of the three LEDs (selected at random) was turned on. The instruction given to the subjects was to orient their eyes and head 'naturally'. In total, subjects made, for each initial target, 10 movements towards each of the two other targets. The possible movements were: 30–60, 30–0, 0–30, 0–60, 60–30 and 60–0 (see Fig 3.2).

Results

Amplitude as well as the final position of the head were measured for each movement.

Experiment 1

For a given amplitude of gaze movement, the amplitude of the head movement was relatively constant. The total mean head amplitude for all subjects and for an amplitude of 30° was 18.9° for the 0–30 targets, 20.1° for the 30–60 targets, 17.3° for 60–30 targets and 20.9° for 30–0 targets. For an amplitude of 60°, the mean was 38.9° for 0-60 targets and 37.6° for 60–0 targets. As a consequence, for a given target eccentricity, the position reached by the head was very similar, whatever the direction of the movement (centrifugal or centripetal) or its amplitude. There appeared to be no relation between the initial position of the eyes in the orbit and the amplitude of the head movement. For instance, for a movement between 0–30 targets, the craniocentric error (initial error between the target and the head antero-posterior axis) was 30°, whereas the head movement had an

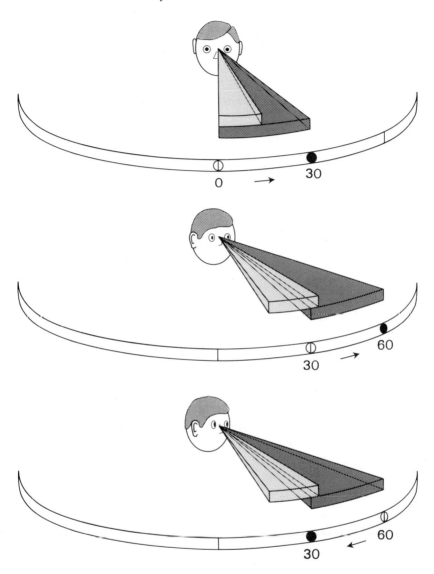

Fig. 3.1. Schematic illustration of three successive fixations made in experiment 1. The targets presented are 0–30, 30–60 and 60–30°. Notice that, in this series of fixation movements, the final position of the preceding movement is the initial position of the next. In dark grey—gaze movement; in light grey—head movement.

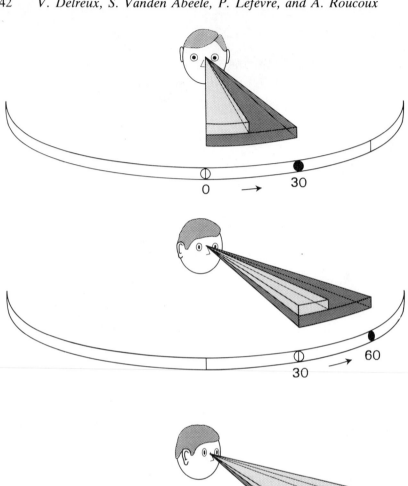

Fig. 3.2. Schematic illustration of three orienting movements made in experiment 2. In this condition, eyes and head are realigned upon each initial target. In dark grey—gaze movement; in light grey—head movement.

amplitude of 18.9°. For a movement between 30–60 targets, the craniocentric error was 41.1°, and the head movement had an amplitude of 20.1°.

The alternative conclusions that can be drawn from this set of experiments are:

(1) either the amplitude of the head movement is coded in terms of a final position with respect to a given target in external space;
(2) or the head movement is coded in amplitude; this amplitude is a fraction of the gaze error as measured by the retinal error. The mean percentage of retinal error sent to the head, for our population of subjects, was 65 per cent.

Table 3.1 illustrates some of the results of experiment 1 for each subject. The amplitude of the head movement, expressed as a fraction of retinal

Table 3.1. Mean amplitudes of head movements, for the seven studied subjects (S1 to S7), in degrees and in percentage of the initial gaze error, for the most significant centrifugal movements, in experiment 1 and 2; the mean for all subjects is indicated, as well as the standard deviation (SD)

Subjects	Experiment 1						Experiment 2	
	0–60		0–30		30–60		30–60	
	deg.	%	deg.	%	deg.	%	deg.	%
S1	50.0	83	23.5	78	27.5	92	21.1	70
S2	35.3	59	18.1	60	17.3	58	23.2	77
S3	35.0	58	17.0	57	19.2	64	6.9	23
S4	35.0	58	17.4	58	19.0	63	10.4	35
S5	39.0	65	20.0	67	20.0	67	13.8	46
S6	35.3	59	17.4	58	15.4	51	13.8	46
S7	42.5	71	19.1	64	22.5	75	18.6	62
Mean	38.9	65	18.9	63	20.1	67	15.4	51
SD	5.7	*	2.3		3.9		5.9	

error, was fairly constant for a given subject. However, variations between subjects was higher. Subject 1, for instance, had a mean retinal error/head amplitude ratio of 0.84 whereas subject 6 had a mean ratio of 0.56.

Experiment 2

The results of experiment 2 differed for centrifugal and centripetal movements, which will thus be described separately.

Centrifugal movements

The findings were broadly similar to those of experiment 1. The total mean amplitude of head movements for all subjects and targets 0–30 was 17.2°; for 0–60 targets, 37.2°; and for 30–60 targets, 15.4°. This last figure is lower than the corresponding value in experiment 1 (20.1°). The individual means are given in Table 3.1. It appears that three subjects (3, 4, 5) had a much lower mean than the others. If their data are neglected, the mean rises to 19.2°, a value very close to that in experiment 1.

Centripetal movements

Findings are shown in Table 3.2. For targets 60–30, the head movements ended around 30° (the global mean for all subjects was 30.8°). For targets 60–0, the mean end position of the head was 2.0° (to the left), and for targets 30–0, the mean final position of the head was 3.5° (to the left). In all these movements, the retinal error/head amplitude ratio was very close to 1.

Table 3.2. Comparison of centripetal final position of head movements in experiment 1 and 2; the mean and standard deviation for all subjects are indicated

	60–30	60–0	30–0
Experiment 1			
Mean	21.6	1.3	0.7
SD	3	2.7	2.1
Experiment 2			
Mean	30.8	2	3.5
SD	2.4	1.7	2.3

Discussion

Amplitude of head movement

Our data confirm the classical observation that the amplitude of the orienting head movement is related to the eccentricity of the target. The head movement represents a fraction of the initial gaze error, which is estimated at 63 per cent by Biguer *et al.* (1984) and 75 per cent by Gresty (1974), in man. In the monkey, Bizzi *et al.* (1971), and Tomlinson and Bahra (1986) describe similar patterns. However, our study underlines the intersubject variability of the retinal error/head amplitude ratio. The distinction between 'head movers' and 'non-head movers' was introduced by Afanador and Aitsebaomo (1982) and confirmed by Roll *et al.* (1986). These differences between individuals may be represented by a gain factor between the retinal input and the head motor output; this gain might be different from one subject to the other. This gain might also vary from one behavioural situation to another (Fuller 1990) or might be a function of the eccentricity of the target, as suggested by microstimulation studies of the superior colliculus in the cat (Roucoux *et al.* 1980). This should be further investigated.

Influence of eye position

The results of the two experiments together suggest that the initial eye position in the orbit does not influence the amplitude of head movement. The results of experiment 1 exclude a craniocentric coding of head movement. But they do not allow of a distinction between two other modes of head movement control: truncocentric/body-centric (final position coded with respect to target position in external space) or retinocentric (head rotation amplitude proportional to initial gaze error, which is identical to the retinal error). Figure 3.3A illustrates the gaze and head movements between targets 30–60 in experiment 1 for subject 7. Fig. 3.3B shows the same gaze movement in experiment 2. It is clear that, at the end of the movement, when target 60 was fixated, the head position was quite different in the two conditions: 41.6 in experiment 1 versus 48.6 in experiment 2. As a consequence, the only possible explanation is a retinocentric coding.

Close inspection of Table 3.1 shows that three subjects behaved differently in experiment 2 (subjects 3, 4, 5). No clear explanation can be given for these particular behaviours; further investigation is needed.

The particular case of centripetal movements

Centripetal movements recorded in experiment 1 obey the proposed mechanism of a retinocentric coding coupled with an attenuation of 65 per cent (Fig. 3.3B). They also suggest that there is no important hysteresis in final head position. In experiment 2 (Fig. 3.3D), however, all centripetal movements followed a different rule, whatever the final position, the primary position, or the intermediate target 30. The rule seems to be a realignment of eyes and head on the target. Here, the intersubject variations were small. To the best of our knowledge, this phenomenon has not been described before. Three explanations may be proposed:

1. Obeying the retinocentric mechanism would entail a rather unusual relative position of eyes and head: the head would be more eccentric than the eye, and in the case of the primary position, the eyes would be deviated

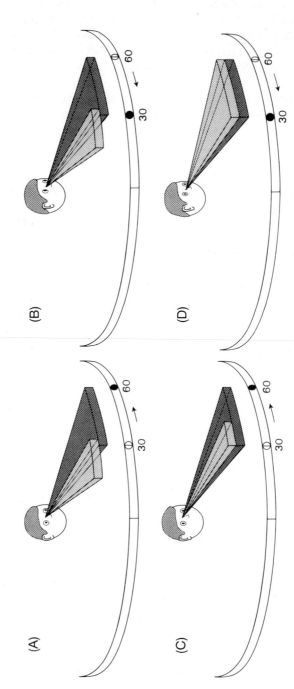

Fig. 3.3. Comparisons between different 30° gaze movements for subject 7: centrifugal (A and C) and centripetal (B and D) movements made between targets 30–60, in experiment 1 (A and B), and experiment 2 (C and D).

(possibly up to 20°) towards one side in the orbit, while the head would be deviated on the trunk, by an equal amount, towards the opposite side. This is a very unnatural situation, which would be avoided by an oculo-cephalic reflex (Vidal *et al.* 1984); this would tend to realign the eye in the orbit, thanks to an eye position-related signal sent to the neck muscles ipsilateral to the eye deviation.

2. Instructing the subjects to realign their eyes and head voluntarily and rather unnaturally on a peripheral target does require a high level of attention that could perturb the subsequent orientation behaviour. It is known that the behavioural context may modify the patterns of eye–head orientation (Fuller 1990).

3. The customary sharing of the final gaze position between the eyes and the head might facilitate the encoding of the target position in space and the reconstruction of the body-related frame of reference (Biguer *et al.* 1984). Aligning eyes and head in an eccentric fixation could distort this congruence between factors such as eye position, head position, vestibulo-ocular gain, retinal error/eye, and head amplitude ratio, etc. Recentring the eye at the end of the movement would allow the 'resetting' of these factors.

In conclusion, it appears that the coding of the head amplitude in gaze orientation might obey a relatively simple law: a retinocentric coding with a retinal error/amplitude gain varying between 0.4 and 0.8, on average, depending on the subjects, the behavioural context, and probably on the eccentricity of the target. Exceptions to this rule are perhaps apparent and should be further studied carefully.

References

Afanador, A. J. and Aitsebaomo, A. P. (1982). The range of eye movements through progressive multifocals. *Optometric Monographs*, **73**, 82–8.

Biguer, B., Prablanc, C., and Jeannerod, M. (1984). The contribution of coordinated eye and head movements in hand pointing accuracy. *Experimental Brain Research*, **55**, 462–9.

Biguer, B., Donaldson, I. M. L., Hein, A., and Jeannerod, M. (1988). Neck muscle vibration modifies the representation of visual motion and direction in man. *Brain*, **111**, 1405–24.

Bizzi, E., Kalil, R. E., and Tagliasco, V. (1971). Eye–head coordination in monkeys. Evidence for centrally patterned organization. *Science*, **173**, 452–4.

Fuller, J. H. (1990). Comparison of head movement strategies among mammals. In *Head–neck symposium*, Vol. 2, (ed. A. Berthoz, W. Graf, and P. P. Vidal). John Wiley, Chichester (in press).

Gretsy, M. A. (1974). Coordination of head and eye movements to fixate continuous and intermittent targets. *Vision Research*, **14**, 395–403.

Hallett, P. E. and Lightstone, A. D. (1976). Saccadic eye movements towards stimuli triggered by prior saccades. *Vision Research*, **16**, 99–106.

Jeannerod, M. (1988). Directional codind of reaching. In *The neural and behavioural organisation of goal-directed movements*, pp. 132–70. Clarendon, Oxford.

Marteniuk, R. G. (1978). The role of eye and head position in slow movement execution. In *Information processing in motor learning and control* (ed. G. E. Stelmach), pp. 267–88. Academic Press, New York.

Mays, L. E. and Sparks, D. L. (1980). Saccades are spatially, not retinocentrically, coded. *Science*, **208**, 1163–5.

Munoz, D. and Guitton, D. (1989). Gaze control in the head free cat. II. Spatio-temporal variations in the discharge of the S.C. output neurons. *Society for Neuroscience Abstracts*, **15**, 807.

Robinson, D. A. (1975). Oculomotor control signals. In *Basic mechanisms of ocular motility and their clinical implications* (ed. P. Bach-y-Rita and G. Lenner-strand), pp. 337–78. Pergamon, Oxford.

Roll, R., Bard, C., and Paillard, J. (1986). Head orienting contributes to the directional accuracy of aiming at distant targets. *Human Movement Science*, **5**, 359–71.

Roucoux, A., Guitton, D., and Crommelinck, M. (1980). Stimulation of the superior colliculus in the alert cat. II. Eye and Head movements evoked when the head is unrestrained. *Experimental Brain Research*, **39**, 75–85.

Roucoux, A., Crommelinck, M., Guérit, J. M., and Meulders, M. (1981). Two modes of eye-head coordination and the role of the vestibulo-ocular reflex in these two strategies. In *Progress in oculomotor research* (ed. A. Fuchs and W. Becker), pp. 309–18. Elsevier, New York.

Tomlinson, R. D. and Bahra, P. S. (1986). Combined eye–head shifts in the primate. II. Interactions between saccades and the vestibulo-ocular reflex. *Journal of Neurophysiology*, **56**, 1558–70.

Vidal, P. P., Roucoux, A., and Berthoz, A. (1982). Horizontal eye position-related activity in neck muscles of the alert cat. *Experimental Brain Research*, **46**, 448–53.

4

A neurophysiological model for the directional coding of reaching movements

M. JEANNEROD

Introduction

The aim of this chapter is to present a model to account for directional coding of reaching movements. Several critical neural operations are needed for ultimately building up the appropriate motor commands that will steer the hand to its final position. First, the retinal map where the target projects must be transformed into a motor (or visuomotor) map of space in which target position is specified in a body-centred system of co-ordinates. Second, the position of the moving limb must be specified on a proprioceptive map using the same system of co-ordinates as the visuo-motor map, so that limb position and target position can coincide. Finally, error-correcting mechanisms must be available for ensuring accuracy.

One of the basic postulates of the model is that these operations cannot be carried out as a series of sequential steps. Instead, a hierarchical structure will be proposed, where the relevant signals (position of the target on the retinal map, eye position in the orbits, head position with respect to the body, relative positions of the limb segments, etc.) are simultaneously distributed at the different levels of representation of the goal of the movement.

A description of the different parts of the model, based on available neurophysiological data, will be given first. This description, as outlined in Fig. 4.1, will follow the main flow of information across the network, starting from the input level (visuomotor and proprioceptive maps), through the goal level, and finally the execution level. Subsequently, a few experiments will be described with the aim of validating specific and limited aspects of the model.

Neurophysiological background

The visuomotor map

At the input of the network, the function of the visuomotor map is to encode target position in a body-centred system of co-ordinates. This function implies the availability of a least two types of signals, namely,

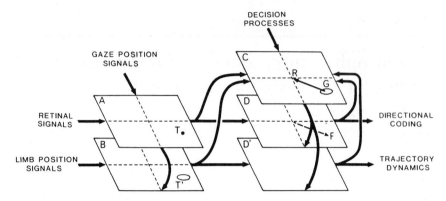

Fig. 4.1. A model for the central representation of goal-directed movements. Visuomotor map (A) encodes target position (T) in body-centred co-ordinates. Proprioceptive map (B) encodes limb position with respect to body and to target. Area T' represents the final position that the limb should reach in order to match target position. Goal level (C): the goal (G) of the action appears as a local activation of the network. This activation is assumed to propagate to execution levels (D–D'). Signals arising from execution levels and from the periphery deactivate the goal level and restore its resting activity (R). Execution level (D–D') generates execution commands for movement direction and kinematics in order to drive the limb at its final position. (From Jeannerod 1990a.)

retinal signals related to the location of the target, and extra-retinal signals related to gaze position. The reason for this distinction between retinal location and visuomotor localization of the target is two-fold. First, because the eyes move in the head, and the head moves with respect to the body, a single locus in space may correspond to a variety of retinal loci, according to the relative positions of the eye, head, and body axes. Second, because the arm movement originates from the body, the position of the target has to be reconstructed with respect to the body. This reconstruction is based on signals for eye and head position.

This role of a spatial encoder attributed to the visuomotor map leads to a number of predictions that may be verified experimentally. First, units that compose the map should be sensitive to the absolute position of visual targets, that is, they should be activated by objects appearing at a given location in body-centred space, irrespective of the actual eye position in the orbit. Second, stimulation of one of these units should produce orienting movements directed at a precise location in body-centred space, irrespective of the initial position of the eyes in the orbit. Third, destruction of one of these units should affect goal-directed movements toward a given spatial location. The neurophysiological record provides a large body of information for testing these predictions.

Neurons fulfilling the first prediction have been described in several structures and particularly in the superior colliculus (SC). Peck *et al.* (1980)

found in the posterior part of the cat SC a small number of neurons which responded to visual stimuli falling on an appropriate part of the retina (the classical definition of a receptive field), but only when these stimuli were situated within a given part of visual space. In other words, these neurons detected the absolute position of the stimulus in space, so that they fired when a given retinal zone was stimulated and when the gaze was fixated in a given direction. Neurons with similar responses were also found in the cat intralaminar thalamic nuclei (Schlag *et al.* 1974). The monkey SC seems to be organized in a different way. In the intermediate layers of the colliculus, Robinson and Wurtz (1976) found neurons that responded when a visual stimulus rapidly crossed their receptive field, but not when an eye movement in the corresponding direction swept their receptive field across the same but stationary stimulus. This finding clearly indicates that collicular neurons integrate retinal and extra-retinal position signals, but does not solve the question of whether this integration results in coding of the absolute spatial position of visual targets. The latter point was attacked by Sparks and his colleagues (Mays and Sparks 1980; Sparks and Mays 1983). They found two types of neurons related to the spatial position of visual targets. In the superficial layers, there were neurons signalling 'retinal position error', dependent on excitation of a particular region of the retina, and in which the receptive field moved in space with each change in gaze. In the intermediate layers, there were neurons signalling 'eye position error', that is, neurons discharging on stimulation of a particular region of the retina for as long as the gaze was not directed toward the corresponding location in space. This second type of neuron merely signals a discrepancy between stimulus position and eye position, but does not encode the absolute spatial position of the targets.

Monkey visual neurons sensitive to eye position with respect to the head, and therefore apt to signal the absolute spatial position of targets, are not found in primary visual areas, where stimulus position appears to be encoded in retinal co-ordinates. Area V2 has a few neurons (14 per cent) that encode orbital eye position during pursuit eye movements (Galletti *et al.* 1988). Neurons encoding target position with respect to eye position are found in visual area V3 (Galletti and Battaglini 1989). Yet the clearest evidence for neurons fulfilling my first prediction (that mapping units should be sensitive to the absolute position of targets), seems to have been found in the inferior parietal lobule (area 7). In this area, Lynch *et al.* (1977) found 'visual fixation neurons' in which activation depended upon stimulation of an appropriate retinal zone, and upon an appropriate eye position. Andersen *et al.* (1985) showed that the receptive field responses of these neurons to visual stimuli change by an amount proportional to the gaze angle, indicating that the interaction of the visual and eye position signals is multiplicative. This property is interesting, because it results in the fact that the neurons will respond best for visual stimuli located in restricted regions of head-centred space. An additional feature of the area 7 neurons receiving visual input is that they respond only when the stimulus, whether stationary or moving, is located within the monkey's reach. They stop firing whenever the target distance is increased by more than one metre or so.

The second prediction (above) concerning the function of the visuomotor map is fulfilled by experimental data showing the occurrence of 'goal-directed' eye movements on electrical stimulation of several neural structures, among which is the cat SC. Roucoux *et al.* 1980; see also McIlwain 1986) showed that, while eye movements elicited by stimulation of the anterior zone of the colliculus conformed with the collicular representation of the retina, those elicited by stimulation of the posterior zone were directed at a particular area of space without respect to eye position. Note that the collicular area from which goal-directed movements were elicited was the same as that in which Peck *et al.* (1980) recorded absolute-position neurons. Electrical stimulation of the intralaminar thalamic nuclei also produces goal-directed movements (Schlag and Schlag-Rey 1971). By contrast, there do not appear to be goal-directed eye movements on stimulation of the SC in the monkey (see Sparks and Mays 1983). Instead, stimulation elicits only movements, the amplitude and direction of which correspond to the position of the stimulating electrode on the retinal map within the colliculus. These findings appear congruent with the lack of neurons signalling the absolute position of targets in the monkey SC. Critical zones for eliciting goal-directed eye movements in this species have been discovered in the posterior parietal cortex (Shibutani *et al.* 1984) and in the pre-motor part of frontal cortex (Schlag and Schlag-Rey 1987).

Finally, the third prediction (that destruction of a unit should affect goal-directed movement) can be tested by studying the effects of lesions on spatial orienting in animals. In the monkey, a unilateral lesion of area 7 produces a clear deficit in reaching at visual objects with the arm contralateral to the lesion (Hartje and Ettlinger 1973; Faugier-Grimaud *et al.* 1978, 1985; Lamotte and Acuna 1978). In man, a similar deficit (termed optic ataxia) can be observed following lesions of the posterior part of the parietal lobe. Typically, subjects misreach for visual objects with their contra-lesional hand (for a complete description, see Jeannerod 1988; Perenin and Vighetto 1983, 1988).

The proprioceptive map

The above description of the visuomotor map stresses the similarity between the mechanism for encoding the spatial position of visual targets and that for generating eye movements directed toward those targets. In the cat

SC, spatially coded signals are transformed almost directly into oculomotor commands. In the monkey, stimulation of the parietal neurons encoding target position produces goal-directed eye movements. This mechanism, however, cannot apply to the generation of goal-directed *hand* movements. In order for the hand to be transported to a visual target located outside the body, its position with respect to the other body parts must be represented on a map distinct from the visuomotor map and connected to it.

This function is achieved by the proprioceptive map. One of its main inputs is signals of joint position arising from static and dynamic proprioceptive receptors. However, because proprioception is limited to personal space and cannot signal limb position with respect to the target, it is also necessary for the proprioceptive map to be fed by visual signals providing information about the relative positions of the limb and target. Among other possibilities, vision of the limb before and during the movement seems to play an important role in this mechanism of calibration of the proprioceptive map. This conclusion stems from a series of experiments by Prablanc and his colleagues. Accuracy of pointing movements in human subjects was compared in two different conditions. In one condition, the hand used by the subject for pointing remained invisible throughout the trial. In the other, the hand was visible only before the movement, that is, while it was stationary in its initial resting position (the light was turned off immediately at the onset of the movement). Large pointing errors were measured in the first condition, where no vision of the hand was provided. By contrast, in the second condition, which included visual information about the static position of the hand relative to the body and the target, the pointing performance was clearly improved, due to reduction of both the constant and the variable errors (Prablanc *et al.* 1979b). Finally, another experiment confirmed that vision of the limb and the target had to be available at the same time: if the target disappeared at the onset of the movement, even though vision of the limb remained available, accuracy of pointing also deteriorated (Prablanc *et al.* 1979a; see also Jeannerod and Prablanc 1983).

Calibration of the proprioceptive map by vision might be a possible function for a category of neurons identified by Leinonen *et al.* (1979), located in the posterior parietal zone (specially area 7b). These neurons receive somatosensory input (from skin, muscles, tendons, or joints) from localized zones of the body. In addition, a number of them also receive localized visual input. Convergence of these two functions (visual and somatosensory signals of limb position) on the same neurons would thus account for matching the limb position on the two maps. Furthermore, these neurons would also be able to signal contact of the hand with the target at the end of the intended movement, information that could be used by the whole system as a feedback device signalling completion of the task or possible reaching errors.

This cortical linkage, within the same neurons, of visual and somatosensory positional inputs is an essential aspect of visuomotor co-ordination. Its function is best demonstrated by the effects of lesions affecting posterior parietal areas in man. Whereas both visual localization of objects and limb position sense are normally preserved after such lesions (see Perenin and Vighetto 1983, 1988), visually directed movements with the contra-lesional hand appear to be profoundly changed. They are not only inaccurate (the typical misreaching already mentioned in the previous paragraph), but also kinematically abnormal: their peak velocity is lower, and their deceleration phase is longer than with the normal hand (Jeannerod 1986). This impairment might be an effect of disconnection between the visual and the proprioceptive signals documenting limb position. Indeed, both misreaching and alteration of kinematics become particularly apparent in the condition where visual feedback from the moving hand cannot be used. This suggests that, when the connection between the two maps is no longer possible, the whole system has to shift from the optimal, feed-forward, mode of motor programming and control to a much less efficient mode based on peripheral feedback.

Finally, the limb position has also to be matched to the position of the visual target in body space. In the proposed model (Fig. 4.1), the local activation of the visuomotor map by a visual stimulus also produces activation of an homologous area in the proprioceptive map; this area of the proprioceptive map would therefore represent the anticipated position that the limb has to reach in order to match the position of the visual target. Again, another class of neurons in the posterior parietal area of the monkey might fit this role. These neurons, which are selectively activated during visuomotor behaviour such as reaching or manipulation, were described by Hyvarinen and Poranen (1974) and by Mountcastle *et al.* (1975) in areas PE, PF and PG. In area PE, such cells comprise 10 per cent of the total sample (Mountcastle *et al.* 1975). They have no receptive field or other sensory properties in the visual or somatosensory modalities: instead, they discharge during active reaching for objects of motivational interest (a piece of food, for example), or during active manipulation of these objects. Hyvarinen and Poranen (1974) considered that activation of such neurons required association between a visual stimulus and a movement toward it. Neither presentation of the visual stimulus nor execution of the movement alone were sufficient conditions for firing them. Finally, another important property of these neurons is that they stop firing when the limb has reached the target; in other words, they signal the superimposition of the final limb position with target position.

The goal level

The visual and the proprioceptive maps jointly project to another part of the hierarchical structure, where the goal of the action of reaching is defined. This projection provides the goal level with signals about the relative spatial locations of the target, the body, and the moving limb. This goal level is also thought to receive information related to other aspects of the same action. In the case of reaching for an object, for example, the goal of the action may be not only to transport the hand to the position of that object but also to grasp it in view of using it. This implies that other input–output 'modules' (e.g. those specialized for coding hand movements related to the shape or size of the object), also involving visual and proprioceptive maps (see Arbib 1981; Jeannerod 1981), will project to the goal level in parallel with the module specialized for directional coding. Finally, the goal level should be connected to other parts of the system, where motivational and cognitive constraints on the action would be encoded.

The goal level is thus an area where the target loses its quality of mere visual stimulus and becomes represented as a goal for an action. For the purpose of the model, a neural representation may be described as a local activation of the network corresponding to the goal level. In turn, this activation will fire other levels, located dowstream of the goal level (the execution levels, see below), thus leading to execution of the movements. Finally, signals arising from activity of the execution levels, or from the movements themselves, will progressively deactivate the goal level, until it returns to its resting state. Assuming that the activation characteristics of the goal level reflect the content of the visual and the proprioceptive maps, this mechanism would make the motor commands compatible with the desired action. This tentative description of the goal level is very similar to that proposed by Robinson (1975) for the generation of saccadic eye movements. In Robinson's model, the spatio-temporal course of saccades was specified by signals related to the intended position of the eyes, from which signals related to the actual position of the eyes were subtracted, thereby driving the eyes at the target location until the difference between the two signals became zero.

It is of interest to look at the neurophysiological record for neuronal properties that could be relevant to the functioning of the goal level. According to the above description, the main criteria for assigning to neurons a role in encoding a target as a goal for a movement are that these neurons should fire in anticipation of the prescribed movement and that they should fire until completion of this movement. The second criterion is quite stringent, because it implies that the neurons should continue firing even though the target has disappeared. In other words, their activation should correspond to the represented goal, and not only to the perceived target. In addition, this activiation should persist in spite of the intervention of other movements before the prescribed movement has been executed. Such criteria are clearly not fulfilled by the already described sensorimotor neurons of the posterior parietal zone. Their discharge is strictly related to the presence in the visual field of a stimulus toward which the movement is being directed; they stop firing as soon as the target is turned off or hidden.

It is thus expected that goal neurons will integrate some of the temporal contingencies of the action (Fuster 1985). Neurons from the monkey prefrontal cortex have properties that may be relevant to this function. First, they fire in situations involving delays between presentation of a localized cue and selection of the corresponding target by a movement (delayed response or delayed alternation tasks: see Kubota and Niki 1971; Fuster, 1973). Second, their discharge during the delay bears some specificity either to the cue (e.g. position in the visual field) or to the movement (e.g. side of the arm, direction of the movement). Finally, their discharge is not influenced by the intervention of other target-oriented movements during the delay but unrelated to the cue. Barone and Joseph (1989) have described such cells in monkey area 8. In their experiments, animals were trained to watch for the temporal sequence of illumination of three targets. After a delay, the animals had to replicate the sequence by moving their eyes and their hand to the targets in the correct order. About 35 per cent of the recorded neurons fired while the monkey was fixating one given target and preparing to displacing its gaze toward the next in the sequence. During this period, activation of the neuron was sustained and was uninfluenced by the fact that, before moving the eyes to the next target, the monkey had to move its arm to press the fixated target. These neurons (context cells— Barone and Joseph 1989) thus encode both the target sequence and the completion of movements directed to those targets, hence fulfilling the requirements for a goal structure. Interestingly, the prefrontal areas where these neurons are located receive abundant projections from the posterior parietal cortex, particularly the inferior parietal lobule (see Petrides and Pandya 1984). It is thus possible for target-specific information available in the posterior parietal areas to be used for generating goal-specific information in the prefrontal areas.

Execution level

Completion of the movement involves activation of other categories of neurons that deal with detailed programming of the muscle contractions. In the present models, this function is assigned to the execution level (Fig. 4.1). The function of this level is to issue appropriate commands for directing the limb toward the target, for co-ordinating the displacements of the involved segments, and for specifying the dynamics of the trajectory.

This level is connected both with the input side of the network (the visual and proprioceptive maps), from which it receives signals related to the spatial location of the target, and with the goal level, from which it receives specifications concerning the constraints governing the action.

There are reasons to think that the execution level involves simultaneous processing of different aspects and different measures of the same movement. This point is illustrated by the fact that the amplitude and direction of reaching movements appear to be coded in parallel (see, for example, Favilla *et al.* 1989). Moreover, neurons dealing with different types of reaching area distributed in separate sub-areas. The distributed nature of executive motor functions has been postulated in several models of visuomotor co-ordination (see Paillard 1971; Paillard and Beaubaton 1978; Jeannerod and Biguer 1982). In the monkey pre-motor area, Gentillucci *et al.* (1988) described a population of neurons located in the lower part of area 6 (sector F4) that fired in relation to movements affecting the proximal joints, particularly during reaching for visual objects. These neurons can be passively activated by visual stimuli located within reaching distance. They also fire during arm movements directed to a particular zone of the working space, congruent with the location of the visual receptive field. Gentilucci *et al.* suggested that F4 neurons play a role in specifying the end-point area for reaching movements. Another population of neurons related to hand and finger movements was found in a distinct sub-area of area 6 (sector F5). These neurons are related to movements executed in response to visual stimuli with both the hand and the mouth or in the context of manipulation of small objects (Rizzolatti *et al.* 1988; see also Kurata and Tanji 1986).

In the primary motor area itself, Georgopoulos *et al.* (1982) found neurons whose activity changed in an orderly fashion with the direction of arm movements. Each of these neurons discharged preferentially before movements in a given direction and was therefore characterized by a preferred vector along which its discharge was maximum. By assuming that a movement in a particular direction involves the activation of a whole population of neurons, Georgopoulos *et al.* (1986) summated a large number of individual vectors measured during a reaching task. They found that the resulting population vector was a good predictor of the direction of movements.

A number of control signals are represented in the model (Fig. 4.1). First, intrinsic control signals, arising from the execution level, back-propagate to the goal level. There, these signals might provide information about the degree of execution of the action and contribute to deactivation of the goal level. Other control signals project from the input levels directly to the execution level. These signals are partly extrinsic in that they reflect changes occurring at the input as a consequence of movement execution.

Their role might be to provide information about possible errors arising during execution. One of the experiments reported below will illustrate this function.

Empirical validation of the model

A model like this generates predictions with different degrees of testability. Predictions related to the anatomical structure of the network (e.g. to which part of the brain can a given level be assigned) are hardly testable beyond the attempts described above; one has to wait for data based on further studies of neuronal activation in relevant behavioural situations. By contrast, predictions related to the nature of the signals used either at the input stage (e.g. for reconstructing target position), or at the output stage (for generating directional commands), are more accessible to empirical verification. In this section, two experiments will be reported, one about the role of signals of head position in the spatial representation of the target, the other about rapid corrections of movement trajectory.

The role of head position signals in target localization

Signals related to head position with respect to the trunk seem to play an important role in reconstructing the target position in space. In the monkey. Cohen (1961) showed that abolishing proprioceptive information from neck muscles (by sectioning the dorsal roots) rendered the animals unable to reach accurately for objects, even when their eyes were fixating them. In man, injection of local anaesthetics into the neck muscles produces a severe ataxia (De Jong *et al.* 1977). Other arguments in the same direction arise from the study of pointing or reaching accuracy in relation to head position. Marteniuk (1978) provided evidence that orienting the head toward a target consistently facilitated accurate localization of that target. However, determining precisely the contribution of signals of head position in the encoding of target location requires experiments where the accuracy of reaching movements is compared when subjects have their heads either fixed or free to move. Such an experiment was done by Biguer *et al.* (1984) and by Roll *et al.* (1986). Subjects were instructed to point at discrete visual targets appearing at various locations in the visual field. No visual re-afference from the hand movement was available at any time. One experimental session was run with the head free to move, and another with the head fixed straight ahead.

The latency data from the Biguer *et al.* experiment showed that the eyes moved first, followed by the head (in the head-free condition) and then the hand. Latencies and durations of movements were such that the head movement was always completed before the hand movement, i.e. the time interval between the end of the head movement and that of the hand movement was always positive (it ranged between 110 ms for targets located at 10° from the midline and 160 ms for targets located at 40°). Similarly, the time interval between the end of the gaze movement and the end of the hand movement was also largely positive. It ranged between 243 ms and 375 ms, on average, for targets located at 10° and 40°, respectively. These results indicate that time allows signals derived from head position to influence hand movements. Indeed, the pointing accuracy of hand movements was strongly affected by whether the head was fixed or free to move. In the head-fixed condition, large constant and variable errors were found. Both types of error tended to increase as a function of target distance from the midline. In the head-free condition, both constant and variable errors were consistently reduced.

The nature of the signals for head position involved in visuomotor behaviour has been demonstrated in an experiment by Biguer *et al.* (1986, 1988). They took advantage of the distortion of position sense produced by muscle vibration. It has been known since the work of Goodwin *et al.* (1972) that vibrating a muscle can induce an illusory movement of the corresponding segment. If the vibrated limb is prevented from moving, it is nevertheless felt to move. In their experiment, Goodwin *et al.* vibrated the biceps brachii of one arm in blindfolded subjects. The vibrated arm was immobilized, and the other arm was used to 'track' the illusory movement. With their tracking arm, subjects consistently indicated that they felt their vibrated arm more extended than it actually was. The explanation of this finding was that 'the Ia discharges set up by the vibration are interpreted by the sensorium as due to a stretch of the biceps muscle, and thus taken to indicate that the joint is more fully extended than it actually is. This might perhaps be through some higher centre recognizing a mismatch between the actual state of the muscle and that which was "intended" by the controlling centers'.

Biguer *et al.* applied vibrations at 100 Hz to the posterior neck muscles on one side. Their subjects were asked to maintain visual fixation on a dim luminous target which appeared directly ahead of them in an otherwise dark room. When vibration was applied, the subjects reported an apparent displacement of the fixation light. This illusory displacement was usually in the horizontal dimension and to the side opposite to the stimulation but, by altering the exact location of the vibrator, illusions of vertical or diagonal movement could also be produced. The target initially showed both motion and displacement; displacement ceased within a second or two. Afterwards the target appeared to continue in motion without further change in position. Apparent movement persisted as long as the vibratory stimulation was maintained. When vibration was discontinued, the light appeared to move in the reverse direction for a brief period of time. Control experiments showed that this effect was not due to either eye or head movements during vibration.

In accord with the explanation of Goodwin *et al.* (1972), vibration of the neck muscles on one side (e.g. the left) produces the same afferent spindle discharge as if the neck muscles were stretched by head rotation toward the opposite side (to the right in this example). This illusory change in head position is interpreted by the brain as an apparent displacement of visual objects to the right. Therefore, if a subject were asked to point at a visual object under this condition of vibration, the pointing should err in the direction of the apparent displacement. This is exactly what Biguer *et al.* reported. When their subjects had their left neck muscles stimulated, they systematically pointed to the right of the actual target position. In addition, the mean displacement of pointings increased as a function of magnitude of vibration (Fig. 4.2). Interestingly, De Jong *et al.* (1977) reported that, during inactivation of neck muscle spindles by local anaesthesia, pointings at visual targets were also displaced. But, whereas displacement due to stimulation of the spindles was in the direction opposite to the stimulated side, displacement during anaesthesia was in the direction of the anaesthetized side.

This experiment not only confirms the contribution of spindle afferents to position sense in general, it also demonstrates that perturbations in the sense of head position are directly referred to mislocation of objects in space and misdirection of visuomotor behaviour. In other words, the proprioceptive signal produced by the vibration was directly translated into a perceived visual displacement and centrally treated as such. As pointed out by Matthews (1988, p. 436), these experiments 'establish that spindles provide information not only for the creation of a subjective map of the body, but also for the orientation of the map in the external world'. In the present model, the latter function is attributed to the visuomotor map and its connection with the proprioceptive map.

Fast corrections in response to changes in target position

Visual feedback from the moving limb has often been invoked as an exception for the controlling of terminal accuracy in visually directed movements (e.g. Paillard 1971). This mechanism, however, has strong limitations, due to the relative slowness of the visuomotor loop used for corrections based on visual feedback, and to the inappropriateness of vision alone for controlling fine adjustments like co-ordination of finger movements during prehension, for example. The above model of motor representation allows for another mechanism whereby visual input, in conjunction with limb position sense, is proactive rather than retroactive in directing the limb

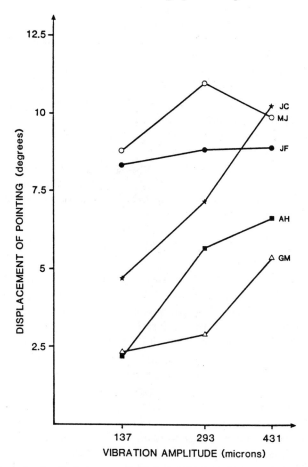

Fig. 4.2. Mean angular displacements, in degrees, of pointing movements towards a small visual target viewed in a dark surround. Results from five subjects (identified by initials) reflect the difference between pointings performed first without vibration of left neck muscles and then with vibration at 137, 293 and 431 microns. Displacement tends to increase with vibration amplitude. (From Biguer *et al.* 1988.)

at the target and in achieving co-ordination between the limb segments during target acquisition.

There are published data which show that accuracy of visually directed movements can be achieved, at least in part, in the absence of visual feedback (e.g. Prablanc *et al.* 1979b; see above). This was confirmed by Pélisson *et al.* (1986) in an experiment where subjects had to track by eye and by hand briefly presented visual targets; vision of the hand was prevented. Occasionally, the targets made double steps. In such cases, the first step (e.g. from 0° to 40°) was followed by a secondary step of a smaller amplitude (e.g. from 40° to 44°), triggered at the time of the maximum eye velocity. The results of this experiment showed that subjects consistently undershot the target position in both the single-step and the double-step trials. This was expected because of the lack of terminal visual feedback from the hand movement in the experimental setting (see Prablanc *et al.* 1979a). Nevertheless, the distribution of pointing positions for double-step trials was significantly shifted with respect to that of the corresponding single-step trials, indicating that the subjects did correct their hand trajectories in order to reach the final target positions. One might object that corrections were in fact new movements resulting from reprogramming but, Pélisson *et al.* clearly showed that this was not the case. Indeed, the durations of pointing movements toward the displaced targets followed the same linear relationship with amplitude as for movements toward single-step targets. In other words, the increased duration in double-step trials reflected only the additional distance that the hand had to move, indicating that there was no reprogramming of movements to accommodate the secondary target displacement. Another argument in favour of this point was given by the kinematic analysis of the pointing movements. If reprogramming had occurred, it should have became visible as a re-acceleration of the trajectory. No such re-accelerations were seen for the double-step trial movements, which therefore did not differ kinematically from the single-step movements. These findings suggest that, instead, corrections were generated in the feed-forward mode. Because the peripheral feedback loops were by-passed, and no reprogramming occurred, corrections took little extra time and were compatible with rapid adjustment of the responses.

Another experiment (Paulignan *et al.* 1990), which involved more complex movements, basically led to the same conclusion. Translucent graspable dowels were made to be displaced (by way of an optical method) at the onset of prehension movements. One dowel was first presented in a control position. In randomly occurring trials (perturbed trials), it was then suddenly displaced either to the right or to the left. Wrist movements (transport of the hand to the dowel) and movements of the index finger and thumb tips (preshaping of the hand) were monitored. The kinematics of the wrist marker showed that movements directed at the control position had the typical bell-shaped velocity profile with a single peak (Fig. 4.3A). By contrast, in perturbed trials, there were two peaks in the velocity profile (Fig. 4.3B and C). Quantitative analysis of the results showed that this pattern was in fact due to interruption of the initial acceleration in order to reorient the movement in the proper direction. Indeed, the first acceleration peak occurred about 30 ms earlier than in the control trials (about 100 ms after the onset of the movement in the perturbed trials compared

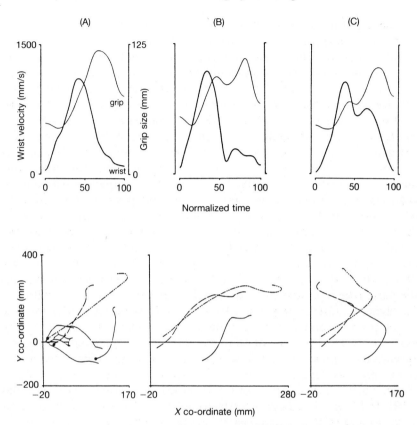

Fig. 4.3. *Upper row:* kinematic profile of prehension movements in the three conditions. (A): Control trial; (B): perturbed right; (C): perturbed left. In each diagram the thick line represents the instantaneous velocity of the wrist. Note single peak in the control trial, double peak in the perturbed trials. The thin line represents the change in size of the index finger–thumb grip. In (A), note maximum grip size occurring shortly after the maximum wrist velocity. In (B) and (C) note that peaks in grip size consistently follow peaks in wrist velocity. Duration of movements has been normalized for comparison. Actual movement duration, (A) 510 ms; (B): 549 ms; (C): 561 ms.

Lower row: Trajectories of wrist, index finger and thumb during prehension. In (A), the movement was directed at the central dowel, located 20° to the right of midline (control trial). In (B), the light was shifted to the dowel located at 30° (perturbed-right trial). In (C), the light was shifted to the dowel located at 10° (perturbed-left trial). Note sharp change in direction of movement, occurring 316 ms after movement onset in (B) and 266 ms in (C). The first change in acceleration of the wrist, which reflected the beginning of the correction, occurred 111 ms after movement onset in (B) and 159 ms in (C). In (A), where no perturbation occurred, the corresponding peak in acceleration of the wrist occurred at 175 ms. Subject's sagittal body axis approximately corresponds to the *Y* axis of the diagrams. (From Paulignan *et al.* 1990).

to about 130 ms in the control ones). Total movement time in the per-turbed trials increased by no more than 100 ms.

Taken together, the findings of Pélisson et al. (1986) and Paulignan et al. (1990) show that the change in the position of the object at the onset of an ongoing movement can elicit fast corrections and that the complex re-arrangement needed to reach and grasp the object can be achieved with no (Pélisson et al.) or little (Paulignan et al.) increase in movement time. These and other findings that stress rapid alteration of ongoing movements (Megaw 1974; Cook and Diggles 1984) therefore suggest an on-line control of execution based on a representation of the goal of the movement. This mechanism can be conceptualized as a continuous comparison between the represented goal and the instantaneous state and position of the effector, what Abbs (1982) has called an 'afferent-dependent feed-forward process'. Such a process implies that neural information about target position (the visual map in our model), and information about state and position of the effector (the proprioceptive map), are permanently accessible at the level of the representation of the goal of the movement. One has to assume that the part of the representation activated by perturbations will be sensitive to the 'dynamic' discrepancy arising between visual signals related to the new target position and in-coming proprioceptive signals generated by the movement. If so, any deviation in the target-limb configuration with re-spect to the represented action will produce a reorganization of the motor commands (see Jeannerod 1990b). This concept of movement 'correction' clearly fits into the definition of feed-forward mechanisms given by Arbib (1981, p. 1466). 'A strategy whereby a controller directly monitors disturb-ances to a system and immediately applies compensatory signals to the controlled system, rather than waiting for feedback on how the disturb-ances have affected the system.'

Conclusion

The representation of the goal of the movement, as postulated in this model, can be considered as a representation of the final state of the dynamic ensemble formed by the target, the gaze, the moving limb, and the body. In other words, the representation of the *executed* movement could be used as a reference to which the ongoing movement would be compared. Indeed, the experiments reported in the preceding section strongly suggest that the signals arising from the periphery are not used directly. In the neck vibration experiment, for example, the proprioceptive signals are not referred to as head–trunk position signals: instead, they appear to be directly related to the position of visual objects with respect to the head or the body. Similarly, the fact that responses to visual perturbations occur in much less than one reaction time suggests that they are not new movements based on reprogramming, but feed-forward corrections based on a stored representation.

Further experiments are obviously needed for testing the other aspects of motor representation. The behavioural approach used in the experiments reported here has obvious limitations. It can be of great potential importance, however, for bridging the gap between neurophysiological data in animals and clinical data in man. The study of pathological disorganization of goal-directed behaviour in humans might provide a unique insight into the neural mechanisms underlying mental representations and help in understanding many of the aspects of spatial representation and motor programming.

References

Abbs, J. H. (1982). A speech-motor-system perspective on nervous-system-control variables. *Behavioral Brain Science*, **5**, 541–2.

Andersen, R. A., Essik, G. K., and Siegel, R. M. (1985). Encoding of spatial location by posterior parietal neurons. *Science*, **230**, 456–8.

Arbib, M. A. (1981). Perceptual structures and distributed motor control. In *Handbook of physiology*. Section I, *The nervous system*. Vol. II, *Motor control*, part 2 (ed. V. B. Brooks), pp. 1449–80. Williams and Wilkins, Baltimore.

Barone, P. and Joseph, J. P. (1989). Prefrontal cortex and spatial sequencing in macaque monkey. *Experimental Brain Research*, **78**, 447–64.

Biguer, B., Prablanc, C., and Jeannerod, M. (1984). The contribution of coordinated eye and head movements in hand pointing accuracy. *Experimental Brain Research*, **55**, 462–9.

Biguer, B., Donaldson, I. M. L., Hein, A., and Jeannerod, M. (1986). La vibration des muscles de la nuque modifie la position apparente d'une cible visuelle. *Comptes-Rendus de l'Académie des Sciences (Paris)*, **303**, 43–8.

Biguer, B., Donaldson, I. M. L., Hein, A., and Jeannerod, M. (1988). Neck muscle vibration modifies the representation of visual motion and detection in man. *Brain*, **111**, 1405–24.

Cohen, L. A. (1961). Role of eye and neck proprioceptive mechanisms in body orientation and motor coordination. *Journal of Neurophysiology*, **24**, 1–11.

Cooke, J. D. and Diggles, V. A. (1984). Rapid error correction during human arm movements. Evidence for central monitoring. *Journal of Motor Behavior*, **16**, 348–63.

De Jong, P. T. V. M., Vianney de Jong, J. M. B., Cohen, B., and Jongkees, L. B. W. (1977). Ataxia and nystagmus induced by injection of local anesthetics in the neck. *Annals of Neurology*, **1**, 240–6.

Faugier-Grimaud, S., Frenois, C., and Stein, D. G. (1978). Effects of posterior parietal lesions on visually guided behavior in monkeys. *Neuropsychologia*, **16**, 151–68.

Faugier-Grimaud, S., Frenois, C., and Peronnet, F. (1985). Effects of posterior parietal lesions on visually guided movements in monkeys. *Experimental Brain Research*, **59**, 125–38.

Favilla, M., Henning, W., and Ghez, C. (1989). Trajectory control in targeted force impulses. VI. Independent specification of response amplitude and direction. *Experimental Brain Research*, **75**, 280.

Fuster, J. M. (1973). Unit activity in prefrontal cortex during delayed response performance. Neuronal correlates of transient memory. *Journal of Neurophysiology*, **36**, 61–78.

Fuster, J. M. (1985) The prefrontal cortex, mediator of cross-temporal contingencies. *Human Neurobiology*, **4**, 169–79.

Galletti, C. and Battaglini, P. P. (1989). Gaze-dependent visual neurons in area V3A of monkey prestriate cortex. *Journal of Neuroscience*, **9**, 1112–25.

Galletti, C., Battaglini, P. P., and Aicardi, G. (1988). 'Real-motion' cells in visual area V2 of behaving macaque monkeys. *Experimental Brain Research*, **69**, 279–88.

Gentilucci, M., Fogassi, L., Luppino, G., Matelli, M., Camarda, R., and Rizzolatti, G. (1988). Functional organization of inferior area 6 in the macaque monkey. I. Somatotopy and the control of proximal movements. *Experimental Brain Research*, **71**, 475–90.

Georgopoulos, A. P., Kalaska, J. F., Caminiti, R., and Massey, J. T. (1982). On the relations between the direction of two-dimensional arm movements and cell discharge in primate motor cortex. *Journal of Neuroscience*, **2**, 1527–37.

Georgopoulos, A. P., Schwartz, A. B., and Kettner, R. E. (1986). Neuronal population coding of movement direction. *Science*, **233**, 1416–19.

Goodwin, G. M., McCloskey, D. I., and Matthews, P. B. C. (1972). The contribution of muscle afferents to kinesthesia shown by vibration induced illusions of movements and by the effects of paralysing joint afferents. *Brain*, **95**, 705–48.

Hartje, W. and Ettlinger, G. (1973). Reaching in light and dark after unilateral posterior parietal ablations in the monkey. *Cortex*, **9**, 346–54.

Hyvarinen, J. and Poranen, A. (1974). Function of the parietal associative area 7 as revealed from cellular discharges in alert monkeys. *Brain*, **97**, 673–92.

Jeannerod, M. (1981). Intersegmental coordination during reaching at natural visual objects. In *Attention and performance* IX (ed. J. Long and A. Baddeley), pp. 153–68. Erlbaum, Hillsdale.

Jeannerod, M. (1986). The formation of finger grip during prehension. A cortically-mediated visuomotor pattern. *Behavioral Brain Research*, **19**, 99–116.

Jeannerod, M. (ed.) (1987). *Neurophysiological and neuropsychological aspects of spatial neglect*. North-Holland, Amsterdam.

Jeannerod, M. (1988). *The neural and behavioural organization of goal-directed movements*. Oxford University Press.

Jeannerod, M. (1990a). The representation of the goal of an action and its role in the control of goal-directed movements. In *Computational neuroscience* (ed. E. L. Schwartz), pp. 352–68. MIT Press, Cambridge, Mass.

Jeannerod, M. (1990b) The interaction of visual and proprioceptive cues in controlling reaching movements. In *Motor control: concepts and issues* (ed. D. R. Humphrey and H. J. Freund). Wiley, New York, (in press).

Jeannerod, M. and Biguer, B. (1982). Visuomotor mechanisms in reaching within extrapersonal space. In *Advances in the analysis of visual behaviour* (ed. D. Ingle, M. Goodale, and R. Mansfield), pp. 387–409. MIT Press, Boston, Mass.

Jeannerod, M. and Prablanc, C. (1983). The visual control of reaching movements. In *Motor control mechanisms in Man* (ed. J. Desmedt), pp. 13–29. Raven Press, New York.

Kubota, K. and Niki, H. (1971). Prefrontal cortical unit activity and delayed alternation performance in monkeys. *Journal of Neurophysiology*, **34**, 337–47.

Kurata, K. and Tanji, J. (1986). Premotor cortex neurons in macaques: activity before distal and proximal forelimb movements. *Journal of Neuroscience*, **6**, 403–11.

Lamotte, R. H. and Acuna, C. (1978). Defects in accuracy of reaching after removal of posterior parietal cortex in monkeys. *Brain Research*, **139**, 309–26.

Leinonen, L., Hyvarinen, J., Nyman, G., and Linnankoski, I. (1979). Functional properties of neurons in lateral part of associative area 7 in awake monkeys. *Experimental Brain Research*, **34**, 299–320.

Lynch, J. C., Mountcastle, V. B., Talbot, W. H., and Yin, T. C. T. (1977). Parietal lobe mechanism for detecting visual attention. *Journal of Neurophysiology*, **40**, 362–89.

Marteniuk, R. G. (1978). The role of eye and head positions in slow movement execution. In *Information processing in motor learning and control* (ed. G. E. Stelmach), pp. 267–88. Academic Press, New York.

Matthews, P. B. C. (1988). Proprioceptors and their contribution to somatosensory mapping: complex messages require complex processing. *Canadian Journal of Physiology and Pharmacology*, **66**, 430–8.

Mays, L. E. and Sparks, D. L. (1980). Saccades are spatially, not retinocentrically, coded. *Science*, **208**, 1163–5.

McIlwain, J. T. (1986). Effects of eye position on saccades evoked electrically from superior colliculus in alert cats. *Journal of Neurophysiology*, **55**, 97.

Megaw, E. D. (1974). Possible modification to a rapid on-going programmed manual response. *Brain Research*, **71**, 425–41.

Mountcastle, V. B., Lynch, J. C., Georgopoulos, A., Sakata, H., and Acuna, C. (1975). Posterior prietal association cortex of the monkey: command functions for operations within extra-personal space. *Journal of Neurophysiology*, **38**, 871–908.

Paillard, J. (1971). Les déterminants moteurs de l'organisation spatiale. *Cahiers de Psychologie*, **14**, 261–316.

Paillard, J. and Beaubaton, D. (1978). De la coordination visuo-motrice à l'organisation de la saisie manuelle. In *Du contrôle moteur à l'organisation du geste* (ed. H. Hécaen and M. Jeannerod), pp. 224–60. Masson, Paris.

Paulignan, Y., McKenzie, C., Marteniuk, R., and Jeannerod, M. (1990). The coupling of arm and finger movements during prehension. *Experimental Brain Research*, **79**, 431–6.

Peck, C. K., Schlag-Rey, M., and Schlag, J. (1980). Visuo-oculomotor properties of cells in the superior colliculus of the alert cat. *Journal of Comparative Neurology*, **194**, 97–116.

Pélisson, D., Prablanc, C., Goodale, M. A., and Jeannerod, M. (1986). Visual control of reaching movements without vision of the limb. II. Evidence for fast nonconscious processes correcting the trajectory of the hand to the final position of a double-step stimulus. *Experimental Brain Research*, **62**, 303–11.

Perenin, M. T. and Vighetto, A. (1983). Optic ataxia: a specific disorder in visuomotor coordination. In *Spatially oriented behavior* (ed. A. Hein and M. Jeannerod), pp. 305–26. Springer, New York.

Perenin, M. T. and Vighetto, A. (1988). Optic ataxia: a specific disruption in visuomotor mechanisms. I. Different aspects of the deficit in reaching for objects. *Brain*, **111**, 643–74.

Petrides, M. and Pandya, D. N. (1984). Projections to the frontal cortex from the posterior parietal region in the rhesus monkey. *Journal of Comparative Neurology*, **228**, 105–16.

Prablanc, C., Echallier, J. F., Jeannerod, M., and Komilis, E. (1979a). Optimal response of eye and hand motor systems in pointing at a visual target. II. Static and dynamic visual cues in the control of hand movements. *Biological Cybernetics*, **35**, 183–7.

Prablanc, C., Echallier, J. F., Komilis, E., and Jeannerod, M. (1979b). Optimal response of eye and hand motor systems in pointing at a visual target. I. Spatio-temporal characteristics of eye and hand movements and their relationships when varying the amount of visual information. *Biological Cybernetics*, **35**, 113–24.

Rizzolatti, G., Camarda, R., Fogassi, L., Gentilucci, M., Luppino, G., and Matelli, M. (1988). Functional organization of area 6 in the macaque monkey. II. Area F5 and the control of distal movements. *Experimental Brain Research*, **71**, 491–507.

Robinson, D. A. (1975). Oculomotor control signals. In *Basic mechanisms of ocular motility and their clinical implications* (ed. G. Lennerstrand and P. Bach-y-Rita), pp. 337–74. Pergamon, Oxford.

Robinson, D. L. and Wurtz, R. H. (1976). Use of an extra-retinal signal by monkey superior colliculus neurons to distinguish real from self-induced stimulus movement. *Journal of Neurophysiology*, **39**, 852–70.

Roll, R., Bard, C., and Paillard, J. (1986). Head orienting contributes to the directional accuracy of aiming at distant targets. *Human Movement Science*, **5**, 359–71.

Roucoux, A., Guitton, D., and Crommelinck, M. (1980). Stimulation of the superior colliculus in the alert cat. II. Eye and head movements evoked when the head is unrestrained. *Experimental Brain Research*, **39**, 75–85.

Schlag, J. and Schlag-Rey, M. (1971). Induction of oculomotor movements from thalamic internal medullary lamina in the cat. *Experimental Neurology*, **33**, 498–508.

Schlag, J. and Schlag-Rey, M. (1987). Evidence for a supplementary eye field. *Journal of Neurophysiology*, **57**, 179–200.

Schlag, J., Lehtinen, I., and Schlag-Rey, M. (1974). Neuronal activity before and during eye movements in thalamic internal medullary lamina of the cat. *Journal of Neurophysiology*, **37**, 982–95.

Shibutani, H., Sakata, H., and Hyvarinen, J. (1984). Saccade and blinking evoked by microstimulation of the posterior parietal association cortex of the monkey. *Experimental Brain Research*, **55**, 1–8.

Sparks, D. L. and Mays, L. E. (1983). Role of the monkey superior colliculus in the spatial localization of saccade targets. In *Spatially oriented behavior* (ed. A. Hein and M. Jeannerod), pp. 63–85. Springer-Verlag, New York.

5

Spatial programming of eye movements

JOHN SCHLAG, MADELEINE SCHLAG-REY, and
PAUL DASSONVILLE

To direct gaze on a visual target, the simplest solution for the brain would
be to derive the vector of the appropriate saccade directly from the retinal
error signal generated by the target. This signal represents a distance and a
direction from the centre of the fovea, and can be directly provided by the
retinal cells 'seeing' a single point on a blank background. There are good
reasons, however, to doubt that a scheme relying solely on a retinal error
signal is realistic. It does not explain how, in the dark, one can look
successively at two sites between which a photic target has jumped, remaining at each place for a very short time (double-step paradigm). Human
subjects can do this accurately even though the target is no longer visible
when the two eye movements are actually executed (Hallett and Lightstone
1976). As the trajectory from the first to the second location does not start
at the initial point from which the target has been seen, the vector of the
second saccade cannot be equal to the retinal error. The calculation of the
vector for the second saccade by the brain must take into account the
change in eye position. This implies a translation of co-ordinates, which in
fact remaps the visual image with respect to the head. Although changing
the frame of reference from eye to head seems to be an unnecessary com-
plication when targets are visual, a head-centred system of co-ordinates
intuitively makes sense. It is needed, for instance, to direct gaze towards
auditory stimuli, to combine eye and head turning in an orienting movement, or to reach for an object with the hand.

Hallett and Lightstone's observations were certainly influential in pro-
moting the view that saccades are not programmed in a retinal frame of
reference. The evidence they provided, however, is not foolproof because
correct target localization in the double-step situation can possibly be
performed using allocentric cues. Indeed, the task may be solved by taking
into account the configuration formed by two points visible in succession
(Hayhoe *et al.* 1990). An ingenious variation on Hallett and Lightstone's
paradigm, avoiding the presentation of more than one flash, uses an
electrical stimulation of the superior colliculus (SC) in the monkey to
evoke the initial saccade, the role of which is essentially to create a
perturbation (Sparks and Mays 1983). The electrical stimulation, applied

just after flashing a luminous target, abruptly displaces the eyes to a new position from which the targeting saccade starts. Subsequent acquisition of the target is nevertheless performed, which led the investigators to conclude that the programming of saccades is spatial not retinotopic.

New prospects arise if the order of the events is inverted in Sparks and Mays' experiment so that the electrically evoked movement occurs when a natural saccade is already launched. When the sequence is reversed, the electrically evoked saccade becomes the dependent variable (Schlag and Schlag-Rey 1987). As its particular trajectory is contingent upon the type of neural signal that is electrically triggered, the test (called the colliding saccade paradigm) can reveal the role played by the stimulated neurons. We shall argue that, by this method, one can distinguish a site eliciting a motor command from another carrying a retinal error signal. In the latter case, one can also determine whether or not the retinal error signal is corrected to take into account an intervening change of eye position. It is no longer the performance of the whole system of targeting which is tested but that of one of its components, the particular structure activated.

To carry out this colliding saccade paradigm, monkeys are trained to observe punctiform luminous targets in the dark and, on cue, to look at them. Their heads are fixed and their eye movements are recorded by a technique using a magnetic search coil (Schlag and Schlag-Rey 1987). Let us assume that an electrical stimulation is delivered at some place in the brain (which we shall specify later) and that it elicits the saccade A shown in Fig. 5.1. At most such places, the evoked response is an eye movement of specific amplitude and direction, and it is readily reproducible as a control. With no further information, how could one decide whether the movement itself is produced or whether it occurs as the consequence of imposing a goal (for instance, if the stimulus creates a phosphene)?

The difference between a command signal (e.g. move 10° rightward) and a goal signal (e.g. go to a point 10° to the right of this location) can be revealed by displacing the origin of the evoked movement. This is why the electrical stimulation is applied during an ongoing eye movement and, to be sure that this happens reliably, the movement itself serves to trigger the stimulus within a fixed delay. Three possible outcomes re conceivable and all three have been observed (Fig. 5.1; saccades B–D).

In B the trajectory of the evoked saccade is the same as in control A. No difference is expected if the signal issued at the site of stimulation is an instruction to move a certain amount in a given direction. The vector of the saccade is predetermined from wherever the eyes point at the end of the latency period. This outcome is typical of stimulation within the deep layers of the SC, at sites where cells do not respond to visual stimuli but where bursts of discharges accompanying saccades are recorded with the same micro-electrode used for electrical stimulation (Schlag-Rey

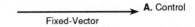

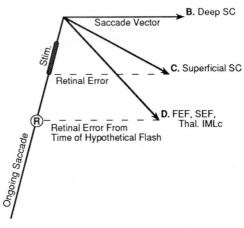

Fig. 5.1. The trajectory of electrically evoked saccades may or may not be altered when the stimulation is applied during an ongoing eye movement. Each of the outcomes (B)–(D) depends on the nature of the signal triggered at the stimulated site. (A) Control fixed-vector saccade elicited when the eyes are steady. (B) Unmodified trajectory by stimulation of deep layers of superior colliculus (SC). (C) Saccade compensating for eye displacement during latency period, elicited from superficial or intermediate layers of SC. (D) Compensation of part of the trajectory of the ongoing saccade, before onset of stimulation, obtained by forebrain stimulation (frontal eye field (FEF), supplementary eye field (SEF), or complex of thalamic–internal medullary lamina (IMLc)). Dash lines show retinal error vectors traced from stimulation onset in (C), and from reference point R in (D). Stimulation train indicated by thick line.

et al. 1989). Most likely, stimulation of the deep SC elicits a motor error signal.

The saccade evoked in C has neither the amplitude nor direction of the control A. In C, it is no longer the movement vector that is predetermined but the point where the movement terminates, which, we assume, corresponds to its intended goal. The location of the goal is specified in retinocentric co-ordinates from the eye position at stimulus onset or slightly afterwards. The goal is reached after a detour because the eyes continue to move during the latency period and, as in the work of Sparks and Mays (1983), there is compensation for the ongoing movement. The existence of such compensation suggests that the electrical stimulus plays the same role as a photic stimulus, namely, both point to a goal. The type of compensation shown in C (Fig. 5.1) is characteristic of saccades evoked from more superficial layers of the SC where visual responses are recorded by the micro-electrode before using it for stimulation (Schlag-Rey *et al.* 1989).

The deviation of the evoked saccade in D is similar to C but differs from it quantitatively. The compensation is larger as if the goal location were referred to an earlier eye position, before stimulus onset. This result is seen with stimulation of forebrain structures from which saccades of fixed dimensions are elicited when the eyes are steady (Schlag *et al.* 1989). Among these structures are the frontal eye field (FEF), supplementary eye field (SEF), and the complex centred on the thalamic internal medullary lamina (IMLc); the region of the inferior parietal lobule has not been tested yet.

Why and how would the brain refer a signal to some antecedent time? To deal with this apparent paradox, it is useful to visualize the sequence of events that would occur if the goal signal injected by stimulation were due instead to a real visual target. As the transmission through the retina and from there to the brain (afferent visual time) takes at least 40 ms, the target co-ordinates should be referred to an eye position (marked R, for reference position, in D of Fig. 5.1) some 40 ms or more before stimulus onset. Only thus can ocular aiming be correct whereas, in C, the saccade would miss the target, its co-ordinates being referred to a wrong origin.

Our interpretation of the compensatory trajectory illustrated in D assumes a transformation of target co-ordinates from retinal into spatial. This can be accomplished by algebraic summation of the retinal error with an eye position signal. One will note that, for spatial accuracy, the signal should be temporarily stored. The relevant value to be summed is not the current one, available at the time of summation with the retinal error, but one that precedes it by an interval equal to the afferent visual time, and can be retrieved only if a trace has been kept. As we pointed out, all this is theoretical and concerns the optimal case. There is little difficulty in accepting that movements are memorized as a whole; it is much more difficult to imagine that the timing of a particular event (e.g. a brief stimulus) can be recorded with precision during their course. However, were the system performing perfectly, the delay between R and stimulus onset in D should be constant whenever the stimulation is applied. We shall see that this is not what happens in reality. Perhaps it is impossible because the visual afferent time is variable: it depends on such factors as stimulus intensity or eccentricity, which the brain cannot estimate.

Measurements made in the FEF and IMLc indicate that intervals between the reference position R and stimulus onset become larger the later the stimulation is applied during a saccade (Schlag *et al.* 1989). The delay still continues to grow after the end of the saccade. At least 150 ms have to elapse after a saccade for ocular targeting to become accurate again, as if the brain were taking that long to realize that the eyes have reached their destination. In other words, the hypothetical signal of eye position used to determine the location of a target seems to proceed more slowly than the actual change of eye position. From this we conclude that the internal representation of eye position is probably a damped version of the movement itself, and we have sought to determine its temporal course from stimulation data (Dassonville *et al.* 1990a).

The experimental strategy outlined here may provide access to internal signals, to study their time course and observe their interactions. Although the approach is based on a number of assumptions, which are not all verified, one can check the findings against those obtained in a natural situation with natural stimuli. In this respect, it is comforting that the curves showing the time course of the eye position signal from experiments with stimulation are similar to those established with natural targets presented during saccades (Mateeff 1978; Dassonville *et al.* 1990b). This work is still in progress.

Let us digress a moment to comment on the implication of an imperfect signal of eye position. The anomaly may be in its shape or its timing, and these two cases are compared in Fig. 5.2. In each panel, the upper row includes a standard saccade (plain line) and its assumed internal representation, which, for convenience, is drawn twice. The broken line is the internal signal representing the saccade, traced in real time, presumably as it is generated in the brain. Being *internal*, this signal is not immediately accessible to observation. However, the observer can determine the position at which the visuo-oculomotor apparatus estimates the eyes to be for each target presentation before, during, and after a saccade. This estimate is shown by the dotted line; it represents the *external* manifestation of the internal signal. The dotted and broken lines have the same course but are separated by an interval equal to the visual afferent time. The lower row in Fig. 5.2 shows errors in ocular targeting of flashes presented around the time of a saccade. Errors are expressed as a fraction of saccade amplitude. The curves are related as follows: the representation of eye position (dotted curve) is the sum of the error curve with the trajectory of the actual saccade.

Ideally, as noted above, the internal eye position signal should be an exact replica of the saccade, but delayed by an amount equal to the afferent visual time. Only in this case would the error of targeting be nil (Fig. 5.2A). If there were no delay of the internal eye position signal, an error of the magnitude and duration schematically represented in B would occur. Cases shown in A and B are pure speculations because they have never been reported. The actual error of target localization, as observed by Dassonville *et al.* (1990b), is seen in C. It starts to grow before the saccade and reaches its peak around the onset of the saccade. The comparison illustrated in Fig. 5.2 suggests that the damping of the eye position signal attenuates to some extent the inaccuracy inherent in having no mechanism to delay such a signal.

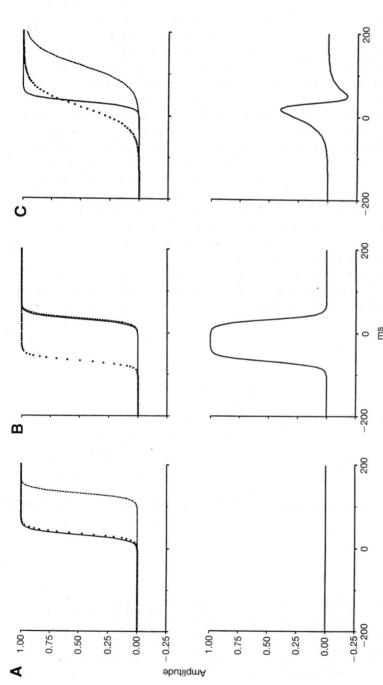

Fig. 5.2. Errors of targeting occur when targets are briefly flashed just before, during, or immediately after saccades. Errors are compared between the theoretical case in which the eye position is not delayed (B), the real case in which this signal is not delayed but damped (C), and the ideal condition of no error (A).

In upper row: actual saccade (plain line); *internal* eye position signal in real time (broken line); *external* manifestation of the effect of eye-position signal, plotted with respect to the instant of target presentations (dotted lines). *Lower row:* respective errors of targeting (calculated in (A) and (B), measured from actual data in (C)).

In the rest of this chapter, we shall be concerned more particularly with the results of forebrain stimulation and their implications regarding high-level mechanisms of ocular targeting. It may seem surprising that none of the forebrain stimulations produces the unmodified type of saccade expected if local neurons were sending true motor commands. We know that this unmodified type exists because it is obtained by stimulation of the SC. (see B in Fig. 5.1). Instead, saccades electrically evoked from the forebrain are always compensatory when the stimulation is applied during another saccade, and their trajectories can deviate considerably from those of controls. Under favourable circumstances, namely at sites of stimulation that yield small control saccades (e.g. no more than 10°), the conditions of collision can easily be set up such that the evoked saccade will have any chosen direction, even ipsiversive (Fig. 5.3). Ipsiversive saccades are readily evoked from forebrain sites where presaccadic cells recorded just before stimulation show the opposite preferred direction (Dassonville *et al.* 1989). This is evidence that local neurons do not inexorably impose a saccade vector; they seem, instead, to indicate a goal.

As in the case of the superficial and intermediate SC, the goal formed by forebrain stimulation is specified in retinocentric co-ordinates but, in contrast to the SC, the goal signal must be subsequently processed to compen-

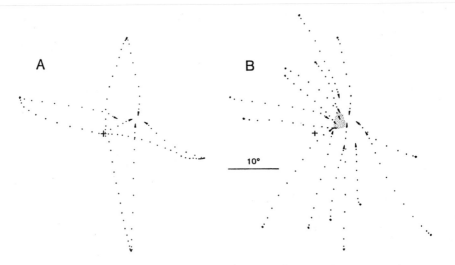

Fig. 5.3. Saccades electrically evoked from forebrain sites can be programmed, by collision, to have practically any desired direction, including ipsiversive. Example taken from a thalamic–internal medullary lamina stimulation, which produced the upward control saccade (less than 10°) shown in (B); dotted area in (B) encloses end-points of all control saccades. Four colliding saccades (ongoing followed by evoked) are shown in (A), starting from a common origin (+); (B) shows a larger sample of trials but, for clarity, only the evoked saccades (not the ongoing ones) are displayed. Sampling rate of traces—250 Hz.

sate for an eventual eye displacement produced since the presentation of the stimulus. This difference in handling the goal information implies that the site (or sites) where the eye position signal is combined with retinal error should lie downstream from the forebrain structures tested, but not from the SC (Schlag *et al.* 1989). The significance of this point is debatable with regard to the superficial and intermediate layers of the SC because inputs from elsewhere (including the forebrain) impinge there, thus obscuring the role of its own neuronal populations. With regard to forebrain structures, the implications are clearer, but they also challenge current views.

For instance, on the basis of unit recording, the FEF is often regarded as a source, possibly the primary one, of saccadic commands. Recently, Goldberg and Bruce (1990) found that many visuomovement and movement cells of the FEF discharge with any saccade terminating in their movement field, even if this saccade is the second one of the Hallett and Lightstone (1976) double-step paradigm described at the beginning of this chapter. If this means that the FEF output always specifies the actual dimensions of the saccade produced, the correction for intervening eye movements must take place upstream, in contradiction with the results of stimulation. However, signals recorded from single units may not be the outcomes of local processes; they can be retransmitted from elsewhere. In fact, the ubiquity of the same signals when a saccade is imminent is puzzling; such signals are found in many different structures which are interconnected. Conceivably, a natural movement is initiated and shaped through their co-operation. In recent years, single unit recording has been extremely successful in identifying the neuronal processes by which a saccade is programmed, but has given little information on where each processing step takes place. This may be the main reason for the present, conflicting views. We certainly need strategies for disclosing the contribution of individual structures, and microstimulation may be one of them.

Acknowledgement

This work was supported by USPHS grants EY 02305 and EY 05879, and NSF grant RCD87-58034.

References

Dassonville, P., Schlag, J., and Schlag-Rey, M. (1989). Microstimulation of primate frontal eye field specifies retinotopic goal of evoked saccade. *Society for Neuroscience Abstracts*, **15**, 1204.

Dassonville, P., Schlag, J., and Schlag-Rey, M. (1990a). Time course of internal representation of eye position as derived from microstimulation experiments. *Investigative Ophthalmology and Visual Science*, **31**, 84.

Dassonville, P., Schlag, J., and Schlag-Rey, M. (1990b). A damped representation of eye position is used in oculomotor localization. *Society for Neuroscience Abstracts*, **16**, 1.085.

Goldberg, M. E., and Bruce, C. J. (1990). Primate frontal eye fields: III. Maintenance of a spatially accurate saccade signal. *Journal of Neurophysiology*, **64**, 489–508.

Hallett, P. E. and Lightstone, D. A. (1976). Saccadic eye movements towards stimuli triggered by prior saccades. *Vision Research*, **16**, 99–106.

Hayhoe, M., Moeller, P., Ballard, D., and Albano, J. E. (1990). Guidance of saccades to remembered targets and the perception of spatial position. *Investigative Ophthalmology and Visual Science*, **31**, 603.

Mateeff, S. (1978). Saccadic eye movements and localization of visual stimuli. *Perception and Psychophysics*, **24**, 215–24.

Schlag, J. and Schlag-Rey, M. (1987). Does microstimulation evoke fixed-vector saccades by generating their vector or by specifying their goal? *Experimental Brain Research*, **68**, 442–4.

Schlag, J., Schlag-Rey, M., and Dassonville, P. (1989). Interactions between natural and electrically evoked saccades. II. At what time is eye position sampled as a reference for the localization of a target? *Experimental Brain Research*, **76**, 548–58.

Schlag-Rey, M., Schlag, J., and Shook, B. (1989). Interactions between natural and electrically evoked saccades. I. Differences between sites carrying retinal error and motor error signals in monkey superior colliculus. *Experimental Brain Research*, **76**, 537–47.

Sparks, D. L. and Mays, L. E. (1983). Spatial localization of saccade targets. I. Compensation for stimulus induced perturbations in eye position. *Journal of Neurophysiology*, **49**, 45–74.

PART 2

Reference frames and movement control

6

Reference frames for the perception and control of movement

A. BERTHOZ

Introduction

In order to build a coherent representation of the movement of limbs or the body in space, the brain must assemble the various messages from its sensors so as to select them according to the environment and to the task in which the subject is engaged, and must compare them with the expected values generated internally. An essential property of the processes underlying the construction of a coherent representation of movement is that it implies *multimodal* extraction of the important components of the movement (direction, position, velocity, acceleration, etc.). The discovery by Grüsser and his colleagues (Akbarian *et al.* 1988) of an area in the parieto-insular cortex in which head motion in space is reconstructed from visual, vestibular, and somatosensory information is a nice example of this fact.

All these operations require reference frames. By this I mean a set of values to which each neuronal variable can be referred. Reference frames can be formed in the physical world, in the sensors themselves, or in the effector system. They do not need to be 'frames'; they can be centres of rotation, for instance. They could also be virtual in the sense of being constructed internally by the brain to perform computations in a topological space, for instance, in which relative positions or motions are the variables that are processed.

In this chapter, I will review some aspects of the properties of the sensory systems that play a role as reference frames for spatial orientation, movement, and posture control in humans. It should be stressed that only vision and the vestibular system can contribute to the measure of head movement in space during complex movements in which a stable base is absent. They do this by a co-operative mechanism that implies visual–vestibular interaction at many levels of the brain (vestibular nuclei, cortex, etc.). Muscle and articular proprioception can only measure relative displacements of the limbs and therefore can only be used by the brain to reconstruct head movement when the body is standing on a fixed platform.

However, I would first like to put this review in a 'theoretical reference frame' by referring to ideas that have been developed recently (Droulez *et al.* 1985; Droulez and Berthoz 1986; Droulez and Darlot 1989).

We cannot consider the processes underlying the control of movement as simple 'sensorimotor loops' according to the current concepts of systems analysis and cybernetics. These kinds of concept do not account for the geometrical properties of the central transformation involved in sensorimotor integration; they have been unable to account for prediction, learning and, more generally, for adaptive mechanisms. We have to propose new ideas, even if they are only working hypotheses.

Most current models are based on the idea that signals given by the peripheral sensors are subjected to sensorimotor 'transformations' (Pellionisz and Llinas 1980, 1985) of the initial specific stimulus for each sensor. However the mechanisms underlying perception are much more subtle and complex than a simple 'transformation'. For example, Droulez and Darlot (1989) have proposed a model based on the notion of 'coherence constraint'. In this model, the movement of each body segment with respect to the stationary environment is coded (as it is in other models) by a central 'representation' (the state of a given set of neurons) that receives a direct input from a dedicated sensory transducer.

For instance, the central representations of head velocity with respect to the environment receive a direct input from the semicircular canals. But, in addition, the original idea of the model was that, in parallel to the measurement made by the dedicated sensors, so-called coherent copies of the velocity of each body segment with respect to the environment are estimated by combining the central representation of adjacent segmental velocities and the relative intersegmental velocity provided by proprioceptive signals and efferent copies of motor commands. These 'coherent copies' are then used as a complement to the direct estimate originating from the dedicated sensor, or even more, as a substitute when the dedicated sensor is temporarily or completely disabled.

In this model, the various central representations are fully interconnected and these interconnections ensure global coherence. Each neuronal activity acts as an operator to transform the other central representations in a coherent way. For instance, the oculomotor corollary discharge, which signals eye position in the orbit, or muscle length and velocity signals, measured by proprioception, can be used as operators that transform retinal slip (that is, eye velocity relative to the environment) into head velocity, and reciprocally can transform a head velocity signal (primarily originating from the vestibular organs) into a coherent estimate of the retinal slip.

This type of hypothesis is interesting because it modifies the perspective from which one may consider neural activity and the reference frames which are needed for central operations.

We have also to take into account the property of the brain to *simulate* movement without execution (Droulez *et al*. 1985; Droulez and Berthoz 1986). This internal simulation allows for the *prediction* of the movement in the future. All models must therefore have the capacity to operate without sensory input and provide some kind of storage or memory. This property of internal simulation must operate on *global* descriptions of movement and leave the *local* implementations to peripheral mechanisms: it determines *strategies* which are combinations of *synergies* or a repertoire of innate 'hereditary co-ordinations' (Lorenz 1975), and most important of all, simulation allows the selection of possible solutions for accomplishing a sensorimotor task from among the redundant possible solutions.

Secondly, there must be some mechanisms for active selection of configurations of expected sensory inputs that will be associated with each task. We can therefore expect active manipulation of reference frames depending upon the goal, and I will propose that gaze, for instance, is an important expression of this manipulation.

Thirdly, we have to consider the idea that perception and movement are not always servo-controlled, continuous processes but are highly discontinuous or intermittent. Recent experimental results concerning the segmentation of hand or arm movements (Lacquaniti *et al*. 1986; Viviani and Terzuolo 1988) are very much in accord with this theory.

We also have to accept the idea that, as Paillard (1982) and also Gurfinkel (Chapter 9) have advocated, there may be several reference frames, depending upon the speed of movement, the goal, the initial and final posture, and local as well as global factors related to the context of the movement (see also Chapter 7).

Multiplicity and hierarchy of reference frames

Reference frames have extensively been discussed in the writings of psychologists and neurophysiologists. The most classical distinction has been between *egocentric* and (exo-) or *allocentric* reference. A beautiful example of the ego–exocentric problem and the capacity for the brain to shift between these two references is provided by the perception of self-motion induced by moving visual scenes, known as linear (Berthoz *et al*. 1975; Berthoz and Droulez 1982) or circular (Dichgans and Brandt 1978) 'vection'. If a subject is surrounded by a moving visual scene the perception that is induced can be either of a movement of the visual scene around the fixed body, or of motion of the body itself in space that is perceived as immobile.

Direct demonstration that the brain can function in allocentric co-ordinates has been provided by the observation that some pyramidal slow-firing neurons in the hippocampus ('place cells') fire when an animal passes through a given location in the environment (O'Keefe and Nadel 1978; Fox and Ranck 1975) (see also Chapters 17 and 19). The proof that this type of neuron does code the location independently of any egocentric reference is given by the observation that the place cells fire when the animal crosses the location in any direction.

This distinction of two main types of reference frames is probably too restrictive. Paillard (1971) has proposed the idea that both the egocentric and the allocentric reference frames use a 'geocentric' frame based on the direction of gravity. A dependence between the two systems is also suggested by Ratcliff (Chapter 13), who shows that a deficit in the allocentric system can be without consequence on the egocentric system although the opposite has never been observed.

Another interesting idea is the importance of relative frames. Perret, for instance, when studying the neural basis of orienting movements in the monkey, proposed the distinction between viewer-centred, object-centred, goal-centred, and self-centred references. Arbib *et al.* (1986) have proposed the concept of 'opposition space', for reaching movements, which corresponds to a local, task-referred relative reference frame. An ethologist, Golani, following the work of Eshkol and Wachmann (1958), has described the movements of animals that were engaged in various social activities in co-ordinates which he called subjectwise, environment-wise and partnerwise. This last co-ordinate system was used to describe the movements of a given animal with reference to its partner. Using this triple description he could demonstrate, for instance, that during a fight between two dogs there is an absolutely fixed, invariant geometrical relation, like a set of rigid metal rods, linking the eyes of the dogs, and that the 'dominant' dog could induce a loss of equilibrium in the other by merely rotating his head. In other words, the relation between the eyes and heads had become a fixed reference frame.

The findings of Soechting and Flanders (1989a, b), that aiming movements of the arm are performed around a shoulder-centred reference, also suggest that the brain may choose an *ad hoc* centre of rotation as a reference for various tasks, depending upon the segment and the relation between the body and the environment.

A crucial property of reference frames is to be *hierarchically* organized. A most instructive example of this hierarchy is the demonstration that, during adaptation to visual prisms in a mono-articular, visuomotor pointing task, if the subject is trained only to do the task with the wrist, adaptation to the modified visual environment does not induce the capacity to perform the movement with the arm (Hay and Brouchon 1972). More generally, if the wrist, the arm, or the shoulder are respectively used to perform the task, the adaptation follows a proximo-distal hierarchy.

However, if the subject can use the head, the adaptation extends to the hand. This also indicates that the head is a fundamental element as a reference in the hierarchy.

In the space of this chapter I cannot review all the aspects of this fascinating problem. I will insist upon the properties of the vestibular system as an egocentric (and possibly 'geocentric') reference frame and its role in perceptual and motor *stabilization*, but also its possible role in *navigation*. I will not deal with the question of visual–vestibular interactions, which have been reviewed by Cohen and Henn (1988). It is well known that the vestibular system co-operates with the visual system for the elaboration of central estimates of head motion and position in space (Berthoz *et al.* 1975; Berthoz *et al.* 1979; Berthoz and Droulez 1982; Dichgans and Brandt 1978; Grüsser *et al.* 1982).

I will then review some questions relative to orienting, and describe a model which can generate orienting movements of eye, head, and body, based only on retinotopic (or more generally 'sensoritopic') and not 'craniotopic' (or 'spatiotopic') representations of target position in space. The first idea of this model is that it is eventually not necessary to reconstruct the target in space in spatiotopic co-ordinates; in other words, it is not necessary to work in absolute co-ordinates to perform a reaching or orienting movement. The second idea is that, during movement, computation of sensorimotor transformations uses a channel in which only dynamic representations of motor error (in the form of velocities, or derivatives of displacement) are used. This concept has some common points with the proposals of Paillard (1980) and Paillard *et al.* (1980, 1981) concerning the existence of two distinct processing algorithms: one dealing with 'l'espace des positions' and the other with 'l'espace du mouvement'.

With these remarks in mind let us now consider the remarkable properties of the egocentric reference frame provided by the vestibular system.

The vestibular system: A goal-dependent Euclidean egocentric reference frame

Canal planes: an Euclidean reference frame under gaze control

Planes, geometry, and flexibility by rearrangement of connectivity

The semicircular canals are involved in stabilizing reactions. They are important either in reducing retinal slip, or in maintaining upright posture. They constitute an Euclidean reference frame for the measurement of the angular accelerations of the head. This reference frame follows three interconnected principles of (a) bilateral symmetry, (b) push-pull operation, and (c) mutual orthogonality of the canals. It has some interesting, parallel features with motor systems such as the oculomotor system, as described in the review by Cohen and Henn (1988). Simpson and Graf (1985) have shown that, throughout phylogeny, in spite of the migration of the eye from a lateral position in the fish or in the rabbit to the frontal position in primates, some invariants have been retained between the geometry of the canals and the pulling directions of the oculomotor system.

The vestibulo-ocular reflex (VOR), which allows the stabilization of gaze in space, is a very interesting example for understanding their properties. Figure 6.1 recapitulates the main historical steps in the study of the VOR. After the pioneering studies by Szentagothai (1950) (Fig. 6.1A), and Lorente de Nó (1933) (Fig. 6.1C), the synaptic organization and connectivity of the 'three neuron arc' were described for the horizontal (Baker *et al.* 1969; Precht 1978) (Fig. 6.1B) and the vertical eye muscles (Berthoz and Baker 1972; Baker *et al.* 1973; Berthoz *et al.* 1973; Baker and Berthoz, 1974). Subsequently, the dynamic properties of signal transmission were examined using the concepts and models of system analysis (Robinson 1975; Fig. 6.1D). The most recent step has been the use of the tensor theory (Fig. 6.1E) to describe the geometrical transformations which are necessary between the Euclidian sensory frame of the vestibular receptors and the complex motor frames of the six extra-ocular muscles (Pellionisz and Llinas 1980; Pellionisz 1985; Pellionisz and Graf 1987).

A most fascinating discovery has come, however, from the observation of the anatomy of the pattern of axonal connectivity in vestibular second-order neurons, which are the intermediate 'leg' in the VOR. The main finding is that the geometry of the actions of each individual canal on the extra-ocular muscles is organized through the connectivity of the second order neurons by the pattern of their axonal branching.

An illustration of this property has been provided by a comparative study of the neuronal organization of the VOR in the shark and in the mammal (Graf and Brunken 1984). The optic axes in these two species are at right angles to each other and because the canals have a similar orientation in the head, and in spite of an invariance of the position of the eye muscles with respect to the canal planes, the connectivity has to be different.

Fig. 6.1. The recent history of the study of the vestibulo-ocular reflex. (A) The discovery of the one to one projection from the semicircular canals to the extra-ocular muscles by Szentagothai (1950). (B) The description of the synaptic connections in the reciprocally organized, disynaptic, horizontal, vestibulo-ocular reflex arc and the inhibitory feed-forward action of the vestibulo-cerebellum by Baker *et al.* (1969); Highstein and Baker (1978); Ito (1982). Similar descriptions were made by Baker *et al.* (1973); Berthoz *et al.* (1973); Baker and Berthoz, (1974) for the oblique system. (C) The basic scheme proposed by Lorente de No (1933) to explain the generation of nystagmus in the brain stem vestibulo-ocular and

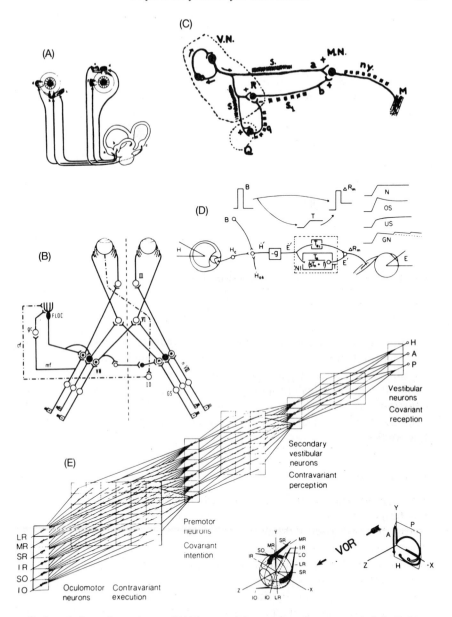

vestibulo-reticulo-ocular pathways. (D) The use of the concepts of system analysis by Robinson (1968) for the description of the dynamics of neuronal operations made in the brain stem to transform head acceleration detected by the semicircular canals into compensatory eye position. This description led to the concept of neural integrator. (E) The use of the tensor theory by Pellionisz (1985) to describe the geometrical transformations necessary to proceed from the Euclidian vestibular reference frame into the motor space of the extra-ocular muscles.

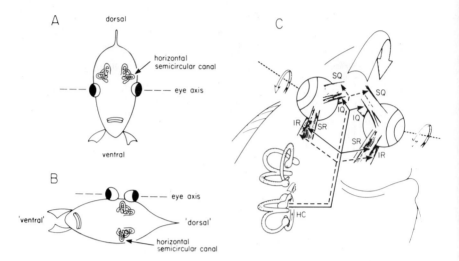

Fig. 6.2. Transformation of the connectivity pattern of second-order, vestibulo-ocular neurons in the flounder during metamorphosis (from Graf and Baker 1983; Simpson and Graf 1985).

An even more interesting feature of this organization is that it has some plastic properties. In the flat-fish, for instance, the eyes migrate during metamorphosis and the axonal connectivity is reorganized (Fig. 6.2) to adopt the geometrical properties of the reflex to the new geometrical constraints (Graf and Baker 1983; Simpson and Graf 1985). What phylogeny has performed over millions of years, metamorphosis performs in a few weeks.

Common preferred directions for visual motion detection

The vestibulo-ocular reflex does not operate in isolation. It constitutes a functional unit together with vision, which also detects head movement in space. Recent studies (Simpson 1984; Hoffman 1988; Hoffmann 1989; Magnin *et al.* 1989) have revealed a neural network of several parallel pathways, converging on the vestibular nuclei, which is specialized in the measurement of visual motion. This network involves the pretectum, the accessory optic system, the inferior olive, the flocculus of the cerebellum, the nucleus reticularis tegmenti pontis, and the nucleus prepositus hypoglossi, whose role in eye movement control was discovered by Baker and Berthoz (Baker and Berthoz 1975; Lopez-Barneo *et al.* 1982). The neurons that process the visual motion information are direction-selective and their preferred directions of activation are aligned with the planes of the semicircular canals (review in Cohen and Henn 1988).

The reference frame of the three semi-circular canals therefore has a fundamental role as a kind of template for the geometry of the sensory systems involved in the representation of movement. Among other advantages of this property I would like to stress the fact that it could reduce complexity of computation because what appears to be a three-dimensional problem is reduced, by the projection on three orthogonal planes, to a two-dimensional problem. In other words, the brain has found a way to simplify the extraordinary difficulty of matching several sensory and motor spaces by adopting an intrinsic Euclidian common frame of reference.

Active modification of the vestibular reference by internally generated gaze signals

The preceding considerations imply a high degree of rigidity in the organization of the vestibular system (although the reorganization of connectivity, as discussed above, provides an elegant form of plasticity to the geometrical organization of the reference frame). I will now show that this reference frame can be modified from moment to moment by internally generated signals dependent upon the motor goal, and particularly the signals related to gaze. Figure 6.3 shows an example of an identified second-order vestibular neuron which is involved in the VOR in the cat. This neuron receives monosynaptic activation from the labyrinth. It subserves the horizontal VOR but also the vestibulo-nuccal reflex (VCR) because of its axonal branching to both the abducens nucleus and the neck. During head oscillation in the horizontal plane at about 0.1 Hz, the firing rate of this neuron is modulated in phase with head angular velocity at the frequency of the sinusoidal oscillation. However, if the head is fixed, the firing rate is modulated in parallel to horizontal eye angular displacement. The firing rate–eye position curve for this neuron is very similar to that of abducens motoneurons, as shown by Berthoz *et al.* (1989a). This so-called vestibular neuron is therefore actively modulated by gaze direction. There is a motor dependence of sensory input, which indicates that perception is intimately blended with movement.

This gaze dependence of central neurons has been now shown in several brain centres implicated in the representation of space: the dorsal and ventro-lateral geniculate nucleus (Magnin *et al.* 1974), the visual cortex (Vanni-Mercier and Magnin 1982; Galetti and Battaglini 1989), the Clare–Bishop area (Kennedy and Magnin 1977), the intralaminar nucleus of the thalamus (Schlag-Rey and Schlag 1984), the posterior parietal cortex (Andersen and Mountcastle 1983), the superior colliculus (Jay and Sparks 1984) and the hippocampus (Chapter 19). The reorganization of the auditory maps in the superior colliculus which occurs during shifts of gaze (Jay

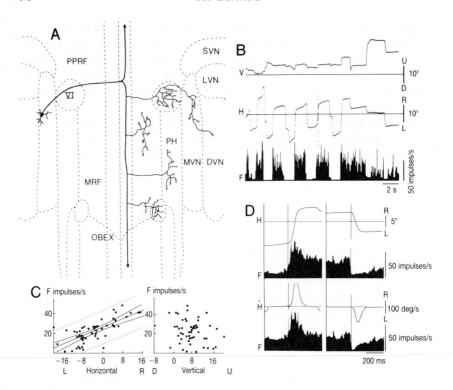

Fig. 6.3. The modulation of second-order, 'vestibular' neurons by gaze signals. Morphological and physiological properties of a second-order, excitatory, vestibular neuron. (A) Reconstruction of the cell body and axonal terminations of the neuron. Abbreviations: VI, abducens nucleus; PH, prepositus nucleus; PPRF, paramedian pontine reticular formation; MRF, medial reticular formation; MVN, SVN, LVN, DVN, respectively medial, superior, lateral, and descending vestibular nuclei. (B) Firing of the neuron during spontaneous saccades in the light. Same notations: H, horizontal and V, vertical components of eye position; Ḣ, horizontal eye velocity; F, neuron firing rate; U, up; D, down; R, right; L, left. (C) Rate position relationship for the horizontal (left) and vertical (right) components of eye position. (D) Extraction of the saccadic eye velocity sensitivity during horizontal saccades. (From Berthoz *et al.* 1989a.)

and Sparks 1984) is another spectacular example of this active internal manipulation of the so-called sensory representations. It demonstrates the tight interdependence between perception and movement. But it is very important to see that in the vestibular system, gaze dependence is already occurring at the very first relay in the brain stem. The consequence is that the so-called vestibular nuclei, which are now well known to receive visual, cervical, and gaze signals, are not a simple relay for the processing of vestibular information but a basic processor for the elaboration of a central estimate of head movement in space referred to a gaze-dependent goal.

Otoliths

Setting a horizontal postural preferred plane for movement

The otolithic organs (sacculus and utriculus) are inertial detectors of the linear acceleration of the head in the plane of their maculae. They also detect the angular displacement of the head with respect to gravity: when the head is tilted the otoliths are stimulated by the component of gravity in the plane of each macula. They are 'tiltmeters', not only 'accelerometers'. They constitute, therefore, a very important reference frame (see review by Berthoz and Droulez 1982). Can we show that they are actually used as a reference for the detection of head tilt?

Let us first consider a recent observation concerning the posture of the head–neck system. The investigation of the spatial organization of the cervical column in various species (Vidal *et al.* 1986) has shown (Fig. 6.4) that the cervical vertebral column at rest is kept parallel to gravitational force lines, even in total darkness. This is accomplished by the particular S-shape of the cervical vertebral column in quadrupeds: this resting position in cats, rabbits, or rodents in general is maintained such that their cervical column has a posture very similar to that of birds. The relevance of this finding for our discussion on reference frames is two-fold. Firstly, animals can only maintain this posture if a sensor detects the angle of the head with respect to gravity (in order to give a 'set point'), and the otolith is well suited for this purpose. Secondly, this posture has allowed the organization of a neuronal network specialized for orienting movements in the plane of the horizontal canal which is maintained (by this posture) perpendicular to gravity.

Through this discussion I have introduced the idea that biomechanics is an essential aspect of the problem of reference frames—a point of view which is sometimes forgotten by those who concentrate on the neuronal organization of movement.

The perception of the vertical

The role of the otoliths in the perception of the vertical can also be shown by an experiment which provides a selective stimulation of the otoliths by gravity through off-vertical axis rotation (OVAR; Darlot *et al.* 1988a, b). With this method the subjects are rotated at constant velocity around an axis that is inclined with respect to gravity. This condition induces, after the disappearance of the transient canal response, a set of pure otolithic stimuli. The important role of the otolithic system in the perception of the vertical is demonstrated by the fact that, although the rotation is around a fixed axis, the perceived movement is distributed around a cone whose summit is either above or below the subject.

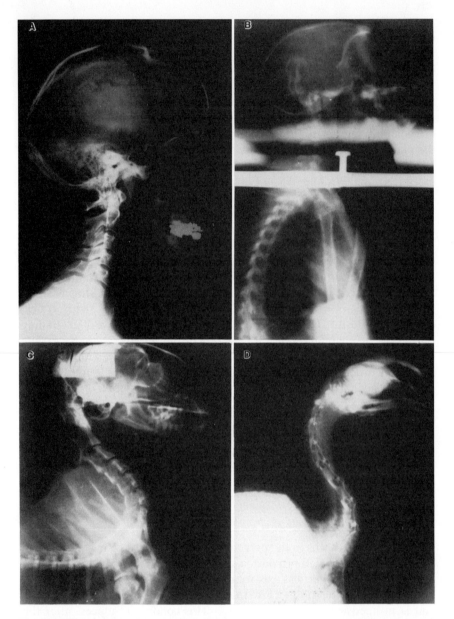

Fig. 6.4. The resting position of the head–neck system of several species (A) man; (B) monkey; (C) cat; (D) pigeon, studied by radiography (from Vidal *et al.* 1986).

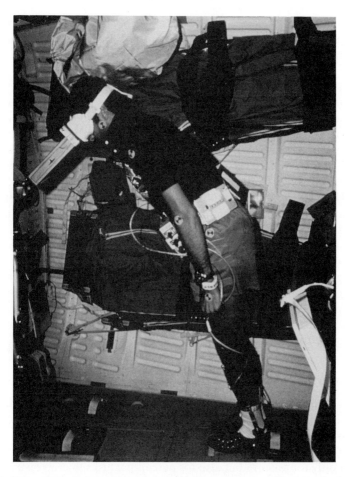

Fig. 6.5. The posture of an astronaut who was asked to stand perpendicular to the floor of the space station. This subject reported that he was perfectly perpendicular to the platform. This photograph was taken on the first day of flight. The visual world was stabilized: the subject wore a small box fixed to the head which was illuminated inside providing him with a visual world stable with respect to his head (from Clement *et al.* 1987).

What happens when the otoliths do not provide this reference? Such a condition is met in microgravity. Figure 6.5 illustrates the posture of an astronaut who is in space for the first time and who has been instructed to keep his body perpendicular to the floor of the space station. His vision is restricted to the inside of a small box that provides a visual world moving with him. We have called this condition 'visual stabilization' (Nashner and Berthoz 1978; Vidal *et al.* 1982). In this condition the body is leaning forward by near 20° although the astronaut perceives himself as perfectly perpendicular to the floor. This result is interesting because it shows that the somatosensory information from the ankle joints, etc., is not enough to allow precise localization of the angle of the body with respect to the ground. Some calibration, or error detection, is necessary. After a few days in space some adaptation occurs.

The otoliths are, of course, not the only sensors that contribute to this multimodal reconstruction of the vertical; several reviews have dealt with this question (Howard and Templeton 1966; Howard 1982; Amblard *et al.* 1988; Berthoz *et al.* 1990). For instance, it is well known that vision also provides the so-called visusal vertical, and that the visual vertical has reciprocal influences on the perception of forms (Rock 1973; Mittelstaedt 1989). The tactile retina formed by the sole of the feet also constitutes an important array for the detection of differential pressure which may be involved in these processes (see also a recent study by Ohlman 1988). However, in the absence of vision, or if vision is blurred by a high retinal slip, or during complex movements in which the ground reference is not available any more, the otoliths are indeed essential for the subjective estimation of the vertical. But rather than analyse these rather well-documented properties, I would like now to discuss another point of view which is underestimated in most contemporary analyses of brain mechanisms relative to space.

Non-sensory, internal reference frames

It is not totally correct to speak only about sensors when trying to describe reference frames. It is well established that in normal gravity conditions, although the perceived gravitational vertical does deviate from the objective vertical by a few degress (Aubert 1967), gravitational reference is used not only for posture but also for perceptual tasks that involve orientation in space, including mental rotation (Corballis *et al.* 1978; Hock and Tromley 1978; Attneave and Olson 1990).

However, Mittelstaedt (1983, 1986) has repeatedly proposed that their are *internal* egocentric references. The 'ideotropic' vector of Mittelstaedt is probably related to the trunk main axis and not to the head. We do not know the mechanism of formation and the exact role of these putative reference frames, which are part of what has also been called the body scheme (Head 1920; Gurfinkel *et al.* 1986).

Switching from one reference to another

A very important avenue of research for the future is to study the switching from one reference frame to another. For instance, it is known that subjects performing a spatial assignment task use the gravity reference when upright but a body-centred reference when lying on their side or supine (Rock 1973). Frederici and Levelt (1990) have now established that, during exposure to microgravity, human subjects tend to assign the position in space of visual objects using a body-centred reference frame.

When a sequence of complex movements is performed it is possible that the movements will be broken down into segments for which different reference frames will be used. However, it still remains probable that the vestibular system will be used in many cases because of its marked dynamic capacity and the independence of its information from retinal slip or from the physical characteristics of the visual environment.

The head as an inertial guidance platform

Most of the studies of sensorimotor systems have been made under labora-tory conditions or in conditions in which the animal or the subject was standing on a fixed platform or seated and restrained. I have tried to study what may be the reference frames used during complex natural motor tasks such as locomotion, running, and jumping in which the stable reference of the ground is no longer available.

In order to assess the movements of the head I first took some of the beautiful pictures of Muybridge (1957), which show humans performing various tasks in the sagittal plane. I translated each picture in order to superimpose the meatus of the ear without modifying the rotation of the head with respect to gravity. The main qualitative observation that stem-med from this exercise was that the head is intermittently stabilized in space for rotation.

These qualitative data have been further confirmed by a quantitative analysis (Berthoz and Pozzo 1988; Pozzo *et al.* 1989, 1990a) using a two-dimensional video computerized system of measurement (Elite System) developed by Pedotti in Milan. The results are illustrated on Figs. 6.6 and 6.7. This analysis also holds true during trampoline jumps. The angle of the head with respect to gravity during each period of stabilization seems to be dependent upon the direction of gaze and, for this reason, I have proposed the hypothesis that there is an *intermittent, gaze-dependent stabilization of the head in space during these complex natural tasks*. In other words, here again man is like a pigeon: in flight the head of birds is remarkably stabilized! The difference is that in humans we not only have stabilization in a plane perpendicular to gravity (the resting position described above) but each complex task is *segmented* in time and space into portions during which the head is stabilized around a given, probably gaze-dependent, angle. This stabilization is disorganized in patients with vestibular deficits (Pozzo *et al.* 1990b).

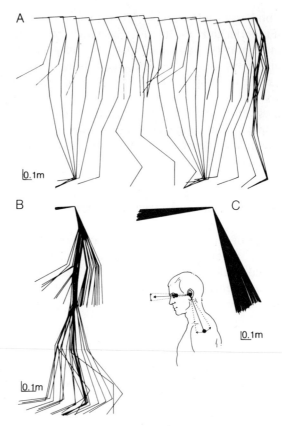

Fig. 6.6. The stabilization of head motion during locomotion (from Berthoz and Pozzo 1988). (A) Stick figures reconstructed by computer during locomotion. Nine markers have been placed on body segments. At the head level, as indicated in the insert, these markers were placed on the outer canthus of the eye and near the auditory meatus. (B) Same stick figures as in (A) but moved by translation so as to superimpose the markers on the auditory meatus. Note the very small variations of the head angular position. (C) Enlarged view of the lines in (B) corresponding to the head and trunk markers.

We may have studied posture in the past 50 years from the wrong point of view. We have considered that posture is organized with the feet as a reference platform. This may be true in a rather limited series of cases—quiet stance or small-amplitude perturbations—and Nashner (1985) has described such a strategy of head stabilization in a particular case. However, when posture is combined with movements in which the stable platform of the feet is absent, the head is used as a reference platform.

What is the advantage of this stabilization of the head?

The hypothesis could be formulated in this way: during complex movements, the brain uses the head as a *stabilized inertial guidance platform*.

A   B

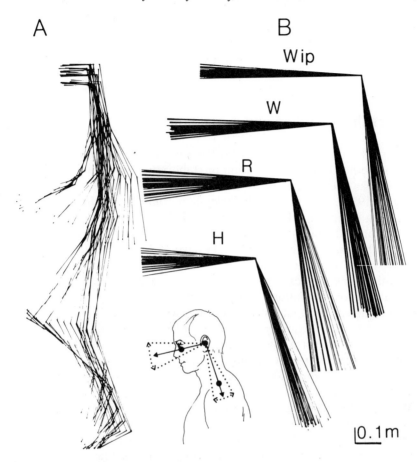

Fig. 6.7 Head stabilization during various locomotory tasks (insert as in Fig. 6.6). (A) Stick figures of human subjects during running on the spot. Note, in spite of the vertical oscillations of the head, the stable orientation of the head with the Frankfurt plane near to the earth horizontal. (B) Enlarged view of the two links defined by the three markers indicated in the insert (canthus of the eye, meatus of the ear, trapezius at the level of C7) during walking on the spot (WIP), free walking (W), running on the spot (R), and hopping (H). (From Pozzo *et al.* 1990a,b.)

This principle is used by engineers as an elegant way of controlling a heavy mass during three-dimensional motion. This platform contains the sensors that will serve both for stabilizing the platform and controlling the movements of the heavy mass.

Head rotational stabilization may simplify the task of the brain in performing the 'fusion of sensors'. For instance, having only translations may simplify the fusion between the two-dimensional detection of movement by the optic flow on the retina (Warren *et al.* 1988), and the three-dimensional gravito-inertial measurement given by the vestibular organs. Such a strategy of stabilization may also be very advantageous in simplifying the transformations necessary to build a coherent internal representation of space.

The vestibular system and navigation

Let us now consider what may be the role of the vestibular system in functions other than the regulation or stabilization of posture and movement. It has been suggested by Beritashvili (1965), and more recently by Potegal (1982), that the vestibular system could be used as an inertial navigation device in animals for the calculation of head trajectory during locomotion and would therefore contribute to the so-called path integration. In this case the trajectory would have to be calculated by a double integration of head acceleration measured by the receptors. This path integration function has been confirmed by Etienne *et al.* (1988) for rotation but not for translations in the golden hamster. In humans, Thomson (1983) demonstrated that a subject can reach by walking (without vision) a target that he has previously seen visually. This result could imply that the subject can construct a map of space, memorize it and update it while walking. However, recent findings in insects suggest the need for great caution in the interpretation of behaviours such as path integration in term of cognitive maps.

We have studied this property with a paradigm proposed by Bloomberg *et al.* (1988) to test the ability of the brain to derive angular head displacement from head acceleration measured by the semicircular canals. The subject is first asked to fixate two superimposed, small lights of different diameters in front of him in the horizontal plane. The smaller light is fixed to the head and the larger to the ground. The larger light is turned off and the subject is then rotated horizontally (random amplitude) in total darkness while looking at the head-fixed light, which he is asked to continue fixating in order to suppress the VOR. When the rotation is completed the head-fixed light is turned off and, after a small delay (10 s) to allow for the disappearance of any canal-induced eye movements, the subject is asked to make a saccade to the original location of the ground-fixed target as he imagines it. This saccade to the remembered target is very accurate in normal subjects.

We have applied a similar paradigm during linear translation and shown that the subject could keep the target location in memory (Berthoz *et al.* 1987b; Berthoz *et al.* 1989b; Israel and Berthoz 1989). Figure 6.8 shows the recordings of horizontal eye movements during linear acceleration in the frontal plane either on line (A, B, C) or with a delayed response (D, E). The

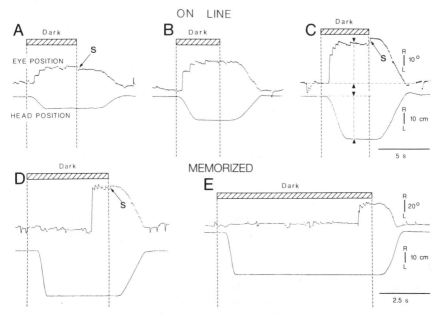

Fig. 6.8. The brain can derive linear displacement from vestibular information and store this information to produce a saccade to an imagined, memorized target (R, right; L; left). (A–C) Records of horizontal components of eye position (upper trace) and horizontal, cart (or head) translation. Before darkness the subject views the target. During darkness he is asked to keep his eye directed towards the imagined, earth-fixed target. S indicates the corrective saccade, which is made when the light is turned on and the subject redirects his eye to the now visible target. (D, E) Same notations, but in darkness the subject is asked to keep the eye immobile until some time after the end of cart motion. Note the excellent amplitude of the saccade made in darkness to the imagined and memorized target. (From Israel and Berthoz 1989.)

subject is seated on a moving cart. He is first asked to look at a target close to him (60 cm). Then, in complete darkness, he is asked to keep the eye directed to the imagined target. Instead of a VOR the brain generates a sequence of saccades which produce a pseudo-reflex with adequate amplitude. The remarkable thing is that when the subject is asked to wait after the cessation of the cart motion, he can still produce a saccade of adequate amplitude to the memorized target. The brain has therefore indeed been capable of deriving displacement with the adequate metrics from the acceleration and of feeding this information into the saccadic system. This experiment suggests that vestibular information is sent either directly, or indirectly through the parieto-insular cortex, to the parietal cortex and possibly to the prefrontal cortex, where Goldman-Rakic (1987) has found areas involved in 'visual representational memory'. Little is known yet concerning the exact pathways for these saccades to remembered targets, although there is evidence that the caudate nucleus (Hikosaka *et al.* 1989a, b) is involved in their generation.

For this reason we have attempted to see if patients with cortical lesions show an impairment in this task. Preliminary results indicate a strong deficit in patients with prefrontal lesions.

We may suppose that these vestibular signals are essential for co-ordinate transformations when a reconstruction of targets in spatiotopic co-ordinates is required. We can then predict that most probably, in addition to an orbital dependence of firing rate, further studies of central structures involved in the representation of space will reveal a head position (vestibular) dependence, because what has to be finally controlled is gaze (eye plus head) and not only eye movements.

Reference frames in orienting movements: spatiotopic movements can be accomplished with only retinotopic or sensoritopic representations of target location

I would like now to approach the problem of reference frames in orienting movements. The detailed mechanisms of the generation of eye saccades and of eye head co-ordination are described in Chapters 1, 2 and 3. However, they have all supposed explicitly or implicitly that, in order to perform an orienting movement to a visual target, the brain reconstructs the position of the visual target in space (in so-called spatiotopic co-ordinates). Generally this idea is supported by findings mentioned in the first part of this chapter, namely that a number of structures are influenced by signals related to eye position in the orbit. This 'orbital' dependence of firing rate provides a putative neural substrate for co-ordinate transformation. However, coding of neural activity in spatiotopic co-ordinates has not really been found in any of these structures (parietal or frontal cortex, superior colliculus, etc.).

We have studied the tectoreticulo-spinal system, which is involved in the generation of saccades (Grantyn and Berthoz 1985, 1987). By recording from identified tectoreticulo-spinal neurons in the alert cat we could show that, in most cases, the firing of these descending neurons was in phasic bursts whose firing rate could be considered as close to the tangential (or 'vectorial') velocity profile of the subsequent saccade, if the saccade occurred at all. This led us to propose, in contrast to what was thought at that time, that there could be some dynamic coding of the desired saccade parameters in superior colliculus neurons (Berthoz *et al.* 1987a). This finding was confirmed later by Sparks and his group (Rohrer *et al.* 1987) and by Munoz and Guitton (1988). However, Waitzman *et al.* (1988) introduced the idea that what was coded at the level of the superior colliculus was in fact 'dynamic motor error', in other words the instantaneous error between the direction of gaze and the direction of the target.

Whatever the final word will be on this matter, these findings encouraged us to develop a model in which only dynamic signals would be present and no specification of the desired eye position would be necessary. I shall now describe a theory (Berthoz and Droulez 1989), which states that eventually the brain does not have to perform a spatiotopic reconstruction in order to reach a target; in addition, the theory tries to hint at mechanisms that allow the reaching of a target when the target has disappeared or is blurred by excessive retinal slip.

In order to try to meet at least some of these requirements, Droulez has proposed a mechanism called 'dynamic memory'. This is a neural map whose architecture is close to those described in the brain as sensorimotor maps. The main feature of these dynamic memory maps is that their content would be updated permanently by sensory afference and by copies of the motor commands during the execution of the movement. Obviously, the dynamic memory model does not satisfy all the theoretical requirements listed above. This model was developed to explain mainly two features: the ability to memorize visually guided goals, and the spatial constancy of the goal in spite of a retinoptic representation.

Current models concerning eye movement control have been described in other chapters. The most recent feature has been the introduction by Goldberg of the idea of 'vector coding' (see the recent review by Andersen, 1989).

The model developed by Droulez, called the 'dynamic memory' model is summarized on Fig. 6.9 (for more detailed descriptions see Berthoz and Droulez 1990).

Four main ideas form the basis of the dynamic memory concept:

1. Their main substrate is two-dimensional maps and not circuits.
2. The activity of a neuron on the map is (spatially) dependent upon the activity of its neighbours.
3. The activity on the map is updated by both sensory inputs and by corollary activity from motor commands. In the absence of sensory activity, the copy of the motor command can be used by the memory as a dynamic equivalent of the sensory input. In other words the motor command is used as a surrogate sensory signal.
4. The main signal which updates the map is a velocity signal (either from the target or from the eye).

In essence, the role of the dynamic memory is to maintain the stored information stable with respect to space. In a 'static' memory, the information is maintained at the same place it has been stored. In such a map, the stability of the information with respect to space requires the use of spatiotopic co-ordinates. In contrast, the information stored in a dynamic memory is permanently refreshed according to the movements of the eye

A. Berthoz

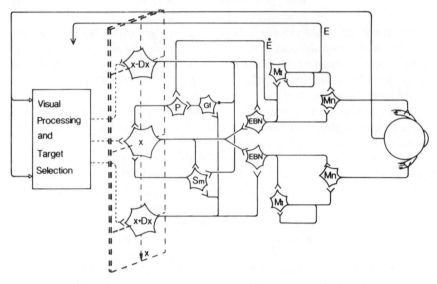

Fig. 6.9. The dynamic memory model: a mechanism for generation of orienting movements based on retinotopic maps (from Droulez and Berthoz 1990). (E: eye position; EBN: excitatory burst neuron; Mn: motor neuron; P: neuron producing the product of the gradient of activity on the map (Gf) multiplied by a feedback of eye velocity ($\dot{E}$); S_m: neuron summating feedback from neighbouring cells; x: co-ordinate of neuron on the map.)

with respect to space: the activity in such a map changes when the eye moves, so that the stability of the visual environment is maintained in spite of the retinoptic organization.

We thought that an adequate model has to allow the orienting movement to be performed indifferently with the eyes, the head, or the body, or with a combination of these. The central mechanisms responsible for orienting have therefore to express the movement in a way which is general enough to be implemented by any of these very different effector systems.

The basic idea of the model is that the visual target, when it appears, activates a population of neurons on a sensoritopic (or retinotopic if it is only visual) map. The activity of each neuron on the map is the product of the *gradient of activity* of the neighbouring neurons on the map (Gf), multiplied by a re-afferent copy of eye velocity feedback from the periphery (E). The advantage of this device is that when a light appears and then subsequently disappears the network will keep a memory of the activity and, as soon as the eye moves and generates a velocity signal, the activity will shift on the map and the eye movement will be made, so bringing the eye onto target without any reconstruction of its position in retinotopic co-ordinates.

Let us give an example of the process in such a bi-dimensional map. At time *t*1 there is a mountain of activity on the map (this mountain represents a population of active cells with a peak of firing rate) which is centred on the initial position of the target $x1$. Each neuron of the map receives the scalar product of this gradient and eye velocity. This product predicts exactly the temporal variation of firing rate that would be observed if visual information was still available. Therefore, the temporal integration of this scalar product yields the resultant activity at time $t2=t1+DT$.

The maximum activity on the map has slightly shifted at $t2$ and has moved in the direction opposite to the eye movement: if the eyes move towards the target, the maximum of activity shifts towards the area which corresponds to the fovea. This process can be repeated until the maximum activity reaches the foveal region: at this time, the dynamic memory may indicate that the target has been 'foveated' and that the eyes have to stop.

The prediction from this theory is therefore that the activity on some of the maps involved in orienting will shift. No such evidence is yet available; however, the experiments may not have been made with the right paradigm.

Let us imagine that the first saccade is not directed towards the target but in the opposite direction. At the beginning of the saccade the target is in the position $x1$. The activity and its gradient are unchanged. However, $\dot{E}$ (eye velocity) has changed sign. Therefore the product $\dot{E}Gf$ is reversed (it is now negative on the left of $x1$ and positive on the right). The activity at time $t1$ is now decreased, on the left for instance, of $x1$ and increased on the right of $x1$ compared with activity at time $t1$. The mountain moves to the right, away from the fovea. At the end of the saccade, the activity has shifted on the retinotopic map by an amount equal to the amplitude of the first saccade. Therefore, when the animal makes a second saccade based on the information stored in the dynamic memory map, the amplitude (and direction) of the second saccade will be exactly the same as if the target was still visible, just as it has been shown to be the case by Mays and Sparks (1980).

The interesting property of this mechanism is that it will give the appearance of a saccade coded in spatiotopic co-ordinates although the whole process has been made entirely in retinotopic co-ordinates. To the proposal of Mays and Sparks (1980) that 'saccades are coded in spatiotopic and not retinotopic co-ordinates', we would add that spatiotopic saccades could also be made by retinotopic dynamic memory mechanisms.

Conclusion

In the present state of knowledge of this question I can only conclude with several questions and a few hypotheses.

We are faced with the challenging problem that the brain obviously has several types of reference frames within which the neural mechanisms of perception and action are operating. An open question, for instance, is the way in which the three-dimensional properties of the physical world are embedded in the neural mechanisms of sensorimotor processing. I personally like the idea, proposed by Llinas (1988, 1990), that the internal organization of the central networks is matched with the properties of the motor system, and to the 'affordance' (as Gibson 1977 would say) or 'resistance' of the outside physical world, by active internally generated oscillatory or resonant processes during development. But such mechanisms need a common reference frame. I would propose that the vestibular system is the fundamental egocentric (and geocentric) reference frame to which many if not all motor frames and the part of the visual system that deals with motion are spatially tuned. In spite of the fundamental ambiguities which I have described and which require co-operation with the other sensors, the vestibular system provides two important types of information:

1. A *relative* estimation of motion measured by basic functions of Newtonian mechanics (acceleration, velocity) which are available to the brain and, because they are derivatives of position, allow *anticipation* of movement. It is a very general property of mechanoreceptors to detect the first or second derivatives of the mechanical factors they measure (velocity, force, pressure). The reference frame of the vestibular system is therefore not a static one but a really *dynamic* reference; in addition, we have shown that it can be goal-referenced through the action of gaze.

2. It can contribute to head-centred allocentric estimation of head displacement in space for such tasks as navigation. We know that such allocentric signals exist in the hippocampus (see Chapters 17 and 19). This latter function may only be useful during rather slow movements: if the movement is slow, as during locomotion, there may be time to reconstruct target or goal position in space, but if the movement if fast (prey catching, avoidance, etc.) it may be better to use a velocity coding.

We should also consider the proposal by Paillard (1987) that there are two simultaneously operating reference systems: one dealing with positions (velocity being calculated as the derivative of displacement), and another operating on velocities (and positions being calculated by integration of velocities). These two estimates could yield two independent assessments of movement in space; this concept is in accord with the idea of Droulez and Darlot (1989) of a 'coherence copy'. More experimental evidence is obviously needed to verify these ideas.

References

Akbarin, S., Berndl, K., Grüsser, O. J., Guldin, W. O., Pause, M., and Schreiter, U. (1988). Responses of single neurons in the parietoinsular vestibular cortex of primates. *Annals of the New York Academy of Sciences*, **545**, 187–202.

Amblard, B., Berthoz, A., and Clarac, F. (ed.) (1988). *Posture and gait. Development, adaptation and modulation*. Excerpta Medica, Amsterdam.

Andersen, R. A. (1989). Visual and oculomotor functions of the posterior parietal cortex. *Annual Review of Neurosciences* **12**, 377–403.

Andersen, R. A., and Mountcastle, V. B. (1983). The influence of the angle of gaze upon the excitability of the light sensitive neurons of the posterior parietal cortex. *Journal of Neuroscience*, **3**, 532–48.

Arbib, M., Iberall, T., and Bingham, G. (1986). Opposition space as a structuring concept for the analysis of skilled hand movements. *Experimental Brain Research*, **15**, 158–73.

Attneave, F. and Olson, R. K. (1990). Discriminability of stimuli, varying in physical and retinal orientation. *Journal of Experimental Psychology*, **74**, 149–57.

Aubert, H. (1967). Über eine scheinebare Drehung von Objecten bei Neigung des Kopfes nach rechts oder links. *Virchows Archiv*, **20**, 381–93.

Baker, R. and Berthoz, A. (1974). Organisation of vestibular nystagmus in the oblique oculomoteur system. *Journal of Neurophysiology*, **37**, 195–217.

Baker, R. and Berthoz, A. (1975). Is the prepositus hypoglossi nucleus the source of another vestibular ocular pathway? *Brain Research*, **86**, 121–7.

Baker, R., Mano, N., and Shimazu, H. (1969). Postsynaptic potentials in abducens motoneurons induced by vestibular stimulation. *Brain Research*, **15**, 577–80.

Baker, R., Precht, W., and Berthoz, A. (1973). Synaptic connections to trochear motoneurons determined by individual vestibular nerve branch stimulation in the cat. *Brain Research*, **64**, 178–88.

Beritashvili, J. S. (1965). *Neural mechanisms of higher vertebrates behaviour*. Little Brown, Boston.

Berthoz, A. and Baker, R. (1972). Localisation électrophysiologique des motoneurons du noyau oculomotor innervant le petit oblique, et nature des influences d'origine labyrinthique sur ces motoneurones. *C R de l'Academie des Sciences*, **275**, (serie D), 425–8.

Berthoz, A., Baker, R., and Precht, W. (1973). Laybrinthine control of inferior oblique motoneurons. *Experimental Brain Research*, **18**, 225–41.

Berthoz, A. and Droulez, J. (1982). Linear motion perception. In *Tutorials on motion perception* (ed. A. H. Wertheim, W. A. Wagenaar, and H. W. Leibowitz), pp. 157–99. Plenum Press, London.

Berthoz, A. and Pozzo, T. (1988) Intermittent head stabilisation during postural and locomotory tasks in humans. In *Posture and gait: development, adaptation and modulation* (ed. B. Amblard, A. Berthoz and F. Clarac), pp. 189–98. Elsevier, Amsterdam.

Berthoz, A. Pavard, B. and Young, L. (1975). Perception of linear horizontal self *motion induced by peripheral vision (linear-vection). Experimental Brain Research, **23,** 471–89.*

Berthoz, A., Lacour, M., Soechting, J., and Vidal, P. P. (1979). The role of vision in the control of posture during linear motion. In *Reflex control of movement of posture* (ed. O. Pompeiano and R. Granit), pp. 197–209. Elsevier, Amsterdam.

Berthoz, A., Grantyn, A., and Droulez, J. (1987a). Some collicular neurons code saccadic eye velocity. *Neuroscience Letters,* **72,** 289–94.

Berthoz, A., Israel, I., Vieville, T., and Zee, D. S. (1987b). Linear head displacement measured by the otoliths can be reproduced through the saccadic system. *Neuroscience Letters,* **82,** 285–90.

Berthoz, A., Droulez, J., Vidal, P. P., and Yosida, K. (1989a). Neural correlates of horizontal vestibulo-ocular reflex cancellation during rapid eye movements in the cat. *Journal of Physiology,* **419,** 717–51.

Berthoz, A., Israel, I., Zee, D. S., and Vitte, E. (1989b). Linear displacement can be derived from otholic information and stored on spatial maps controlling the saccadic system. *Advances in Oto-rhino-laryngology,* **41,** 76–81.

Berthoz, A., Graf, W., and Vidal, P. P. (1990). *The head–neck sensorimotor system.* Wiley, Chichester.

Bloomberg, J., Melvill Jones, G., Segal, B., McFarlane, S., and Soul, J. (1988). Vestibular contingent voluntary saccades based on cognitive estimates of remembered vestibular information. In *Advances in Otorhinolaryngology* (ed. E. Pirroda and O. Pompeiano), pp. 71–5. Karger, Basel.

Clement, G., Vieville, T., Lestienne, F., and Berthoz, A. (1987). Adaptive modifications of posture and oculomotor reflexes in microgravity. In *Three decades of life science research,* pp. 216–17. NASA Life Sciences, Washington.

Cohen, B. and Henn, V. (ed.) (1988). *Representation of three-dimensional space in the vestibular, oculomotor, and visual systems.* The New York Academy of Sciences.

Corballis, M. C., Nagourney, B. A., Shetzer, L. I., and Stefanatos, G. (1978). Mental rotation under head tilt: factors influencing the location of the subjective reference frame. *Perception and Psychophysics,* **24,** 263–73.

Darlot, C., Denise, P., Droulez, J., Cohen, B., and Berthoz, A. (1988a). Eye movements induced by off-vertical axis rotation (OVAR) at small angles of tilt. *Experimental Brain Research,* **73,** 91–105.

Darlot, C., Denise, P., Droulez, J., Cohen, B., and Berthoz, A. (1988b). Motion perceptions induced by off-vertical axis rotation (OVAR) at small angles of tilt. *Experimental Brain Research,* **73,** 106–14.

Dichgans, J. and Brandt, T. (1978). Visual-vestibular interactions: Effects on self-motion perception and postural control. In *Handbook of sensory physiology,* Vol. V, (ed. H. Leibowitz and H. L. Teuber), pp. 755–804. Springer, Berlin.

Droulez, J. and Berthoz, A. (1986). Servo-controlled conservative versus topological (projective) mode of sensory motor control. In *Disorders of posture and gait* (ed. W. Bles and T. Brandt), pp. 83–97. Elsevier, Amsterdam.

Droulez, J. and Berthoz, A. (1990). The concept of dynamic memory in sensorimotor control. In *Motor control: concepts and issues* (ed. D. R. Humphrey and H. J. Freund), Dahlem Conference, Berlin. Wiley, Chichester.

Droulez, J. and Darlot, C. (1989). The geometric and dynamic implications of the coherence constraints in three dimensional sensorimotor coordinates. In *Attention and performance, XIII* (ed. M. Jeannerod), pp. 495–526. Erlbaum, Hillsdale, NJ.

Droulez, J. Berthoz, A., and Vidal, P. P. (1985). Use and limits of visual vestibular interaction in the control of posture. Are there two modes of sensorimotor control? In *Vestibular and visual control on posture and locomotor equilibrium* (ed. M. Igarishi and O. Black), pp. 14–21. Karger, Basel.

Eshkol, N. and Wachmann, A. (1958). *Movement notation*. Weidenfeld and Nicolson, London.

Etienne, A. S., Mowrer, R., and Saucy, F. 1988). Limitations in the assessment of path dependent integration. *Behaviour*, **106**, 81–111.

Fox, S. E., and Ranck, J. B., (1975). *Experimental Neurology*, **49**, 299–313.

Frederici, A. D. and Levelt, W. J. M. (1990). Spatial reference in weightlessness: perceptual factors and mental representations. *Perception and Psychophysics*, **47**, 253–66.

Galetti, C. and Battaglini, P. P. (1989). Gaze dependent visual neurons in area V3A of monkey prestriate cortex. *Journal of Neuroscience*, **9**, 1112–25.

Gibson, J. J. (1977). The theory of affordances. In *Perceiving, acting and knowing* (ed. R. E. Shaw and J. Bransford). Erlbaum, Hillsdale, NJ.

Goldman-Rakic, P. (1987). Circuitry of primate prefrontal cortex and regulation of behaviour by representational memory. In *Handbook of physiology. The nervous system V* (ed. V. B. Mountcastle, F. Plkum and S. R. Geiger), pp. 373–417. American Physiological Society.

Graf, W. and Baker, R. (1983). Adaptive changes in the vestibulo-ocular reflex of the flatfish are achieved by reorganisation of central neurons pathways. *Science*, **221**, 777–9.

Graf, W. and Brunken, W. J. (1984). Elasmobranch oculomotor organisation. *Journal of Comparative Neurology*, **227**, 569–81.

Grantyn, A. and Berthoz, A. (1985). Burst activity identified tecto-reticulo-spinal neurons in the alert cat. *Experimental Brain Research*, **57**, 417–21.

Grantyn, A. and Berthoz, A. (1987). The role of the tecto-reticulo-spinal-system in control of head movement. In *Control of head movement* (ed. B. W. Peterson and F. J. Richmond), pp. 224–44. Oxford University Press.

Grüsser, O. J., Pause, M., and Schreiter, U. (1982). Neuronal responses in the parieto-insular vestibular cortex of alert Java monkeys (*Macaca fascicularis*). In *Physiological and pathological aspects of eye movements* (ed. A. Roucoux and M. Crommelinck), pp. 251–70. Junk, The Hague.

Gurfinkel, V., Debreva, E. E. and Levik, Y. S. (1986). The role of internal model in the position perception and planning of arm movement. *Fiziologiya Chelova*, **12–5**, 769–76.

Hay, L. and Brouchon, M. (1972). Analyse de la réorganisation des coordinations visuo-motrices. *Annee Psychologique*, **1**, 25–38.

Head, H. (1920) *Studies in neurology*. Hodder and Stoughton, London.

Highstein, S. M. and Baker, R. (1978). Excitatory termination of abducens internuclear neurons on medial rectus motoneurons:relationship to syndrome of internuclear ophthalmoplegia. *Journal of Neurophysiology*, **41**, 1647–61.

Hikosaka, O., Sakamoto, M., and Usui, S. (1989a). Functional properties of monkey caudate neurons. III. Activities related to expectation of target and reward. *Journal of Neurophysiology,* **61,** 814–32.

Hikosaka, O., Sakamoto, M., and Usui, S. (1989b). Functional properties of monkey caudate neurons. I. Activities related to saccadic eye movements. *Journal of Neurophysiology,* **61,** 780–98.

Hock, H. S. and Tromley, C. L. (1978). Mental rotation and perceptual uprightness. *Perception and Psychophysics,* **24,** 529–33.

Hoffman, K. P. (1988). Responses of single neurons in the pretectum of monkeys to visual stimuli in three dimensional space. In *Representation of three-dimensional space in the vestibular, oculomotor and visual systems* (ed. B. Cohen and V. Henn), pp. 1–261. Annals of New York Academy of Sciences.

Hoffman, K. P. (1989). Visual inputs relevant for the optokinetic nystagmus in mammals. In *The oculomotor and skeletamotor systems: differences and similarities. Progress in Brain Research,* Vol. 64 (ed. H. J. Freund, U. Buttner, B. Cohen and J. North), pp. 75–84. Elsevier, Amsterdam.

Howard, I. P. (1982). *Human visual orientation.* Wiley, London.

Howard, I. P. and Templeton, W. B. (1966). *Human spatial orientation.* Wiley, London.

Israel, I. and Berthoz, A. (1989). Calculation of head displacement by the otoliths in humans. *Journal of Neurophysiology,* **82,** 285–90.

Ito, M. (1982). Cerebellar control of the vestibulo-ocular reflex around the flocculus hypothesis. *Annual Review of Neuroscience,* **5,** 275–96.

Jay, M. F. and Sparks, D. L. (1984). Auditory receptive fields in primate superior colliculus shift with changes in eye position. *Nature,* **309,** 345–7.

Kennedy, H. and Magnin, M. (1977). Saccadic influences on single neuron activity in the medial bank of the cat's suprasylvian sulcus (Clare Bishop area). *Experimental Brain Research,* **27,** 315–17.

Lacquaniti, F., Soechting, J., and Terzuolo, C. (1986). Path constraints on point to point arm movements in three dimensional space. *Neuroscience,* **17,** 313–24.

Llinas, R. (1988). Possible role of tremor in the organisation of the nervous system. In *Movement disorders* (ed. L. J. Findley, R. Capildeo, and A. Tremor), pp. 475–7. Macmillan, London.

Llinas, R. (1990). The non continuous nature of movement execution. In *Dahlem Conference* (ed. H. J. Freund and D. Humphrey). Dahlem Conferences, Berlin (in press).

Lopez-Barneo, J., Darlot, C., Berthoz, A., and Baker, R. (1982). Neuronal activity in prepositus nucleus correlated with eye movement in the alert cat. *Journal of Neurophysiology,* **47,** 329–52.

Lorente de Nó, R. (1933). Vestibulo-ocular reflex arc. *Archives of Neurological Psychiatry, Chicago,* **30,** 245–91.

Lorenz, K. (1975). *L'envers du miroir.* Flammarion, Paris.

Magnin, M., Jeannerod, M., and Putkonen, P. T. S. (1974). Vestibular and saccadic influences on dorsal and ventral nuclei of the lateral geniculate body. *Experimental Brain Research,* **21,** 1–18.

Magnin, M., Kennedy, H., and Hoffman, P. (1989). A double labeling investigation of the pretactal visuo-vestibular pathways. *Visual Neuroscience,* (in press).

Mays, L. E. and Sparks, D. L. (1980). Saccades are spatially, not retinocentrically, coded. *Science*, **208**, 1163–5.

Mittelstaedt, H. (1983). A new solution to the problem of the subjective vertical. *Naturwissenschaften*, **70**, 272–81.

Mittelstaedt, H. (1986). The subjective vertical as a function of visual and extra-retinal cues. *Acta Psychologica*, **63**, 63–85.

Mittelstaedt, H. (1989). Interactions of form and orientation. In *Spatial displays and spatial instruments*, NASA Conference Publications 10032 (ed. S. R. Ellis and M. K. Kayser), pp. 42–1–14. NASA, Moffet Field.

Munoz, D. P. and Guitton, D. (1988). Tecto-reticulo-spinal neurons have discharges coding the velocity profiles of eye and head orienting movements. *Society for Neuroscience Abstracts*, **13**, 112.9.

Muybridge, E. (1957). *The human figure in motion*. Dover, New York.

Nashner, L. M. (1985). Strategies for organization of human posture. In *Vestibular and visual control of posture and locomotor equilibrium* (ed. M. Igarashi and O. Black), pp. 1–8. Karger, Basel.

Nashner, L. M. and Berthoz, A. (1978). Visual contribution to rapid motor responses during postural control. *Brain Research*, **150**, 403–7.

O'Keefe, J. and Nadel, L. (1978). *The hippocampus as a cognitive map*. Clarendon Press, Oxford.

Ohlman, T. (1988). La perception de la verticale. Variabilité interindividuelle dans la dépendance à l'égard des référentiels spatiaux. Thesis, Université de Paris VIII.

Paillard, J. (1971). Les déterminants moteurs de l'organisation spatiale. *Cahiers de Psychologie*, **14**, 261–316.

Paillard, J. (1980). The multichanneling of visual cues and the organisation of a visually guided response. In *Tutorials in motor behaviour* (ed. G. E. Stelmach and J. Requin), pp. 259–79. North Holland, Amsterdam.

Paillard, J. (1982). Le corps et ses langages d'espace. In *Le corps en psychiatrie* (ed. E. Jeddi), pp. 53–69. Masson, Paris.

Paillard, J. (1987). Cognitive versus sensorimotor encoding of spatial information. In *Cognitive processes and spatial orientation in animals and man* (ed. P. Ellen and C. Blanc Thinus), pp. 43–77. Martinus Nijhoff, Dordrecht.

Paillard, J., Jordan, P. L., and Brouchon, M. (1981). Visual motion cues in prismatic adaptation: evidence for two separate and additive processes. *Acta Psychologica*, **48**, 253–70.

Pellionisz, A. J. (1985). Tensorial aspects of the multidimensional approach to the vestibulo-oculomotor reflex and gaze. In *Reviews of oculomotor research. I. Adaptive mechanisms in gaze control* (ed. A. Berthoz and G. Melvill Jones), pp. 281–96. Elsevier, Amsterdam.

Pellionisz, A. J. and Graf, W. (1987). Tensor network model of the 'three-neuron vestibulo-ocular reflex-arc' in cat. *Journal of Theoretical Neurobiology*, **5**, 127–51.

Pellionisz, A. J. and Llinas, R. (1980). Tensorial approach to the geometry of brain function. Cerebellar coordination via a metric tensor. *Neuroscience*, **5**, 1761–70.

Pellionisz, A. J. and Llinas, R. (1985). Tensor network theory of the metaorganization of functional geometries in the CNS. *Neuroscience*, **16**, 245–74.

Potegal, M. (1982). Vestibular and neostriatal contribution to spatial orientation. In *Spatial abilities. Development and physiological foundations* (ed. M. Potegal), pp. 361–87. Academic Press, New York.

Pozzo, T., Berthoz, A., and Lefort, L. (1989). Head kinematics during various motor tasks in humans. In *Progress in brain research*, Vol. 30 (ed. J. Allum and M. Hulliger), pp. 377–83. Elsevier, Amsterdam.

Pozzo, T., Berthoz, A., and Lefort, L. (1990a). Head stabilisation during various locomotory tasks in humans. *Experimental Brain Research*, (in press).

Pozzo, T., Berthoz, A., Lefort, L., and Vitte, E. (1990b), Head stabilisation during various locomotor tasks in normals and patients with peripheral vestibular lesions. *Acta Otolaryngologica*, (in press).

Precht, W. (1978). *Neuronal operations in the vestibular system*. Springer, Berlin.

Robinson, D. A. (1968). The oculomotor control system: A review. *Proceedings IEEE*, **56**, 1032–49.

Robinson, D. A. (1975). Oculomotor control signals. In *Basic mechanisms of ocular mobility and their clinical implications* (ed. G. Lennerstrand, Y. Bach, and P. Rita), pp. 337–74. Pergamon, Oxford.

Rock, I. (1973). *Orientation and form*. Academic Press, New York.

Rohrer, W. H., White, J. M., and Sparks, D. L. (1987). Saccade-related burst cells in the superior colliculus: relationship of activity with saccadic velocity. *Society for Neurosciences Abstracts*, **13**, 1092.

Schlag-Rey, M. and Schlag, J. (1984). Visuomotor functions of the central thalamus in monkey: I. Unit activity related to spontaneous eye movements. *Journal of Neurophysiology*, **51**, 1159–74.

Simpson, J. (1984). The accessory optic system. *Annual Review of Neuroscience*, **7**, 13–14.

Simpson, J. I. and Graf, W. (1985). The selection of reference frames by nature and its investigators. In *Adaptative mechanisms in gaze control. Facts and theories*, Vol. 1, *Review of oculomotor research* (ed. A. Berthoz and G. Melvill-Jones), pp. 3–20. Elsevier, Amsterdam.

Soechting, J. F. and Flanders, M. (1989a). Errors in pointing are due to approximations in sensorimotor transformations. *Journal of Neurophysiology*, **62**, 595–608.

Soechting, J. F. and Flanders, M. (1989b). Sensorimotor representations for pointing to targets in three-dimensional space. *Journal of Neurophysiology*, **62**, 582–94.

Szentagothai, J. (1950). The elementary vestibulo-ocular reflex arc. *Journal of Neurophysiology*, **13**, 395–407.

Thomson, J. (1983). Is continuous visual monitoring necessary in visually guided locomotion? *Journal of Experimental Psychology*, **9**, 427–43.

Vanni-Mercier, G. and Magnin, M. (1982). Single neuron activity related to natural vestibular stimulation in the cat's visual cortex. *Experimental Brain Research*, **45**, 451–5.

Vidal, P. P., Berthoz, A., and Milanvoye, M. (1982). Difference between eye closure and visual stabilization in the control of the posture in man. *Aerospace Medicine*, **2**, 1966–7.

Vidal, P. P., Graf, W., and Berthoz, A. (1986). The orientation of the cervical vertebral column in unrestrained awake animals. I. Resting position. *Experimental Brain Research*, **61**, 549–59.

Reference frames for movement 111

Vivani, P. and Terzuolo, C. (1988). Trajectory determines movement dynamics. *Neuroscience,* **7,** 431–7.
Waitzman, D., Optican, L. M., and Wurtz, R. E. (1988). Superior colliculus neurons provide the saccadic motor error signal. *Experimental Brain Research,* **112,** 1–4.
Warren, W. H. Jr., Morris, M. W., and Kalish, M. (1988). Perception of translational heading from optical flow. *Journal of Experimental Psychology and Human Perception Performance*, **4,** 646–60.

7

Proprioception as a link between body space and extra-personal space

JEAN PIERRE ROLL, RÉGINE ROLL, and
JEAN-LUC VELAY

Introduction

In order to perform actions successfully, it is necessary to interrelate two spaces, both of which are known to the subject: these have been classically termed body space and extra-personal space. The key to adapting action to goals lies in the specificity of the nervous processes responsible for coding and then representing each of these two spaces. But over and above this processing, it is the mechanisms dealing with the integration of these two spaces into a single entity encompassing both the subject and his environment that are worth elucidating. We are far from having a complete picture of the nervous mechanisms underlying the specific coding of each of these spaces, but the biggest gap in our knowledge probably concerns how a common reference system for body and external space is built up (Gurfinkel *et al.* 1988; Paillard 1988 and Chapter 10, this volume; Roll *et al.* 1990).

In this chapter, we would like to put forward some experimental arguments supporting the assumption that whole-body, spatially oriented behaviour might be based on a body reference frame which results mainly from the common processing of various sensory feedbacks arising in the muscles that are stretched together during body postures and movements, from the eyes down to the supporting sole. Furthermore, we propose that this type of kinaesthetic body representation might also be used in the spatial coding of retinal information in terms of egocentric co-ordinates (Roll and Roll 1988).

In fact, this proposition relies directly on one of the oldest questions in the study of human motor activities as to the respective roles played by central signals arising from the motor command, the so-called efferent copy or corollary discharge (Von Holst and Mittelstaedt 1950), and the peripheral messages elicited by ongoing motor activities. In this context, we would suggest that a large proportion of body awareness in terms of posture and movement is based on sensory feedback, especially feedback of muscle proprioceptive origin, elicited by ongoing actions.

We propose to show that it is possible by experimentally stimulating this proprioceptive sensory channel in humans using tendon vibration:

(1) to induce illusory sensations of movement which can be said to be 'experimental asomatognosia', attesting to the fact that muscle proprioception contributes to motor representation;

(2) to elicit spatially oriented postural reactions, particularly by activating extra-ocular proprioception—these motor effects point to the fact that extra-ocular proprioception associated with the direction of gaze is of major importance in the organization of whole-body posture and orientation;

(3) to change visual perception, which suggests that the spatial processing of retinal information takes place on the basis of the proprioceptive reference frame that functionally links the eye to the foot support, and consequently to alter visually guided behaviour, which seems to indicate that muscle proprioception is involved in unifying body space with the visually perceived external space.

Modifying body-space representation by means of muscular vibration

The controversy about the contribution of muscular feedback to motor representation dates back to Sherrington (1900), who postulated the existence of muscular sense. This debate has been thoroughly documented in reviews by McCloskey (1978), Roll (1981), and Matthews (1982). The final proof that muscular feedback contributes to the awareness of movement and posture was provided by the very simple observation that in humans it is possible to induce kinaesthetic illusions by vibrating the tendons of an immobilized body segment (Eklund 1972; Goodwin *et al.* 1972; Bonnet *et al.* 1973; Roll *et al.* 1980). The characteristics of these illusions, such as the direction, speed, or duration, crucially depend on the location of the vibrators, the parameters of the stimulus, and the environmental context in which they are induced (Roll 1987).

In our research, we have analysed the characteristics of these illusory sensations of movement in human subjects and attempted to establish their neurophysiological substrate. In particular, we have determined the exact nature of the underlying sensory modalities involved and have described the patterns of the vibration-induced afferent messages in terms of space and frequency. We then correlated these data with the perceived characteristics of the illusory sensations of movement. By applying mechanical vibration to one, two, or several muscles simultaneously, it is therefore possible to induce complex kinaesthetic sensations with specific and predictable spatio-temporal characteristics (Gilhodes *et al.* 1986; Roll *et al.* 1990). This suggests that each movement, or postural pattern, is closely associated with a specific proprioceptive set that is clearly linked to the features of the movement execution themselves. The fact that artificially vibration-induced afferent feedback suffices to evoke the corresponding sensations of movement supports the idea that the former at least partly mediates the awareness of the latter. This suggests that there may exist at the cortical level a 'motor memory', the contents of which may be partly proprioceptive, consisting of a repertoire of afferent patterns, each of which is associated with a specific learned movement performed in a definite context.

Figure 7.1 illustrates the fact that in the absence of visual control, muscle

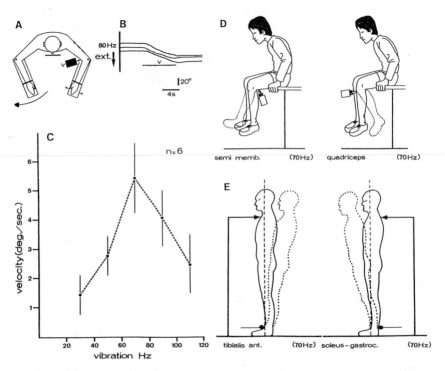

Fig. 7.1. Main characteristics of kinaesthetic illusions induced by muscular vibration. (A–C) Illusory extension of forearm perceived by the subject during tendon vibration of biceps brachii (BB) at various frequencies; (A) experimental conditions—vibration (v) is applied to the left arm with the elbow joint immobilized; the perceived movements are reproduced by the right arm and recorded using a potentiometer; (B) characteristics of the illusory movements (reproduced by the tracking arm) perceived during BB vibration (v) at 80 Hz —vibration trains (dotted line) were applied three times in the same experiment; (C) relationship between vibration frequency and velocity of the illusory movement—the curve illustrates the mean results obtained from six subjects; each point represents 18 trials and the confidence limits were calculated at 5 per cent; (D–E) Illusory movements perceived according to the postural conditions and the tendons vibrated (from Roll and Vedel 1982; Roll 1987).

vibration can induce segmental or postural kinaesthetic sensations, depending on the position of the vibrators. In all cases, the direction of these illusions corresponds to that of an actual movement in which the vibrated muscle is stretched. These vibration-induced illusory movements can be quantitatively analysed by asking the subjects to track with the unvibrated arm what they feel in the vibrated arm when performing an active movement. The velocity of the illusory movements was always within a low range from a few degrees to 15–20° per second. Using simple vibration, that is vibrating only one muscle with a constant frequency, resulted, in all subjects, in an illusion the velocity of which was frequently dependent with a sharp maximum occurring at about 80 Hz.

While confirming that muscle proprioceptive information subserves kinaesthetic sensibility, these findings point to the major sensory role played by spindle messages originating in muscles stretched during a given movement, that is, in antagonists. As the execution of a movement is associated with an increase in spindle activity in the stretched muscles, micro-neurography reveals in man that this activity decreases or falls silent, despite alpha–gamma co-activation, in the shortened muscle (Vallbo 1973; Roll and Vedel 1982). In order to investigate how the peripheral sensory codes are organized in terms of agonist and antagonist proprioceptive information, we simultaneously vibrated two or several muscles. Fig. 7.2A summarizes the results we obtained (Gilhodes *et al.* 1986) by applying two vibrators to the biceps and triceps muscles. The illusion was always one of forearm flexion when the frequency of triceps vibration was higher than that of biceps vibration, and one of extension in the opposite case. Two main facts emerged from these findings: the first was that when the vibration frequencies applied to the two antagonist muscles were equal, no illusory movements occurred; the second was that the perceived velocity increased when the difference between the biceps and triceps frequencies increased. This means that a sensation of movement can only arise from a dynamic Ia afferent imbalance between stretched and shortened muscles acting at a particular joint. The proprioceptive sensory codes may therefore have to take into account all the feedbacks originating in all the muscles associated with the performance of a given movement.

Moreover, as the vibration frequency seems to be a determining factor for defining the velocity of movement illusions, it was decided to use spindle-like vibration frequency modulation. The data we obtained (Roll *et al.* 1989) clearly indicate that the resulting illusions reflected the variations (increase or decrease) in the vibration frequency. In brief, it seems that by applying vibratory stimuli to specific muscles with given frequencies and durations, it is possible to induce complex kinaesthetic illusions, the parameters of which are predictable for each motor shape. This means that in man, the body reference frame, which is something like the body

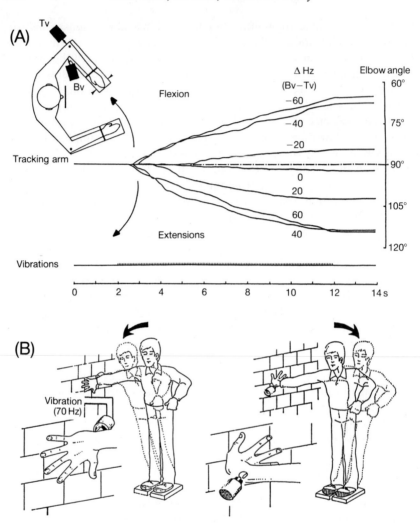

Fig. 7.2. Kinaesthetic illusions induced by vibration of a pair of antagonist muscles and switching effect of context. (A) Schematic diagram of experimental situation and recordings illustrating kinaesthetic sensations (from Gilhodes *et al.* 1986). Vibrators Bv and Tv were applied to the distal tendons of the left biceps brachii and triceps brachii, respectively. The left arm was resting on a fixed, horizontal bracket. The contralateral arm (tracking arm) was placed on a movable bracket connected to the recording system (goniometer). Traces reproducing movement sensations in one subject have been superimposed; above each trace is marked the difference in vibration frequency between Bv and Tv. (B) Postural illusions induced by vibration of hand flexor muscles in an erect subject. Note that a simple change of the orientation of the subject's hand on the wall suffice to reverse the direction of the whole-body illusion (from Roll 1987).

scheme, may be at least partly specified in terms of the muscular proprioceptive cues associated with a given posture, attitude, or movement.

Furthermore, it is possible to induce either whole-body or segmental illusions, depending on the functional role of the muscles stimulated, i.e., depending on whether or not they are involved in the posture adopted by the subject. A single stimulation can, however, induce various illusory sensations of movement, depending on the sensory, postural, or cognitive context (Roll 1987; Quoniam *et al.* 1990).

The following experiment shows what a crucial role the postural configuration of the body can play in the central decoding of a vibration-induced afferent pattern (Fig. 7.2B). A vibration applied to the flexor muscles of the hand induced an illusion of hand extension alone when the hand was free; whereas when the subject was leaning on a wall with his hand the same flexor vibration, inducing the same peripheral afferent message, gave rise to a whole-body illusion. It was even more striking that a simple change in the orientation of the subject's hand on the wall (from fingers forward to fingers backward) sufficed to reverse the whole-body illusion from forward to backward. This result points to the surprising plasticity of the central processing of a particular afferent feedback, in terms of its kinaesthetic content, and suggests that one sensory message can give rise to multiple central interpretations, depending on the posture and more generally on the environmental context.

What is the sensory substrate of kinaesthetic illusions?

If the occurrence of conscious sensations of movement in humans subjected to vibration is to be used as evidence for the central use of muscular feedback in motor representation, it is first necessary to elucidate the exact nature and the spatio-temporal organization of the sensory messages involved. With this aim in mind, and in an attempt to extend to man findings previously obtained in animals concerning the sensory effects of vibrations (Brown *et al.* 1967; Clark *et al.* 1981; Matthews and Watson 1981), the activity of single proprioceptive fibres was recorded from the peroneus lateralis nerve using tungsten micro-electrodes. Unitary discharges originating from primary and secondary endings of muscle spindles and from Golgi tendon organs were identified by classical physiological tests (see Burke *et al.* 1976a, b; Vallbo 1973). The sensitivity of these various kinds of proprioceptors to low-amplitude mechanical vibration was then studied (amplitude 0.2 to 0.5, peak to peak; Roll *et al.* 1989). The results we obtained are shown in Fig. 7.3. Primary endings of muscle spindles (left histogram) were found to be the most sensitive to this mechanical stimulus ($n=36$). The discharge of some of them could be driven in a one-to-one

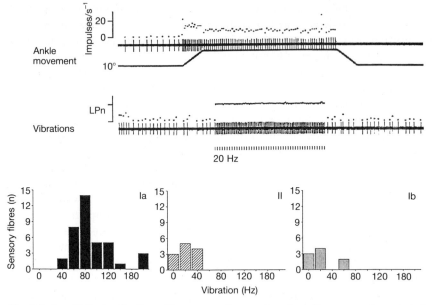

Fig. 7.3. Sensitivity to vibration of human muscle proprioceptors. *Upper recordings:* typical response of a muscle-spindle primary ending to ramp stretch and release of tibialis anterior muscle in man (passive ankle movement). *Lower recordings:* one-to-one driving response to vibration (20 Hz) of the same Ia fibre from the lateral peroneal nerve LPn. *Histograms:* distribution of (from the left to the right) muscle-spindle primary endings (Ia) secondary endings (II) and Golgi tendon organs (Ib) in terms of their maximal sensitivity (one-to-one driving mode) to tendon vibration (from Roll *et al.* 1989).

manner up to 180 Hz. Most of them fired harmonically with the vibration up to 80 Hz and then discharged in a sub-harmonic manner with increasing vibration frequency. Secondary endings (*n*=12; central histogram) and Golgi tendon organs (*n*=8; right histogram) were found to be either insensitive or only slightly sensitive to tendon vibration. Most of them did not follow the stimulus up to 20–30 Hz.

These findings are consistent with those of Burke *et al.* (1976a, b) and with the conclusion reached by Brown *et al.* (1967) that in man 'vibration applied to tendon, in the absence of muscle contraction, can be presumed to be a specific stimulus for primary endings'. Moreover, the fact that, in man, most primary endings respond in phase to vibratory stimuli up to 80–100 Hz suggests that within this frequency range the stimulus frequency is more or less proportional to the responses of the majority of the primary endings. The existence of a one-to-one linkage within this frequency range means that by modulating the vibration frequency, it is possible to induce a proportional modulation in the discharge frequency of the primary endings. This makes it possible to predict the activity level of the Ia afferent messages induced in man when muscle tendons are vibrated. This predictability makes tendon vibration a useful tool for experimentally eliciting kinaesthetic illusions based on previously known afferent messages.

Eye muscle proprioception contributes to postural regulation

All in all, both the experimental findings and the hypotheses presented above clearly show that skeletal muscle proprioception may constitute one of the main sources of awareness of body position and movement.

Surprisingly, the existence and functional role of the proprioceptive afferents arising in extra-ocular muscles have only recently been recognized (see review by Steinbach 1987), although it has been well known for many years that, both in man (Cooper and Daniel 1949; Ludvigh 1952; Cooper *et al.* 1955) and animals (Cooper *et al.* 1951; Lennerstrand and Bach y Rita 1974), these muscles are richly endowed with spindle-like stretch receptors.

In fact, numerous recent studies have focused on the functional role of eye proprioceptive afferents in animals. In particular, Buisseret and Gary-Bobo (1979), and Buisseret (1990), have demonstrated that in the kitten's early development, the acquisition of orientation selectivity by cortical neurons no longer occurred in the absence of proprioceptive inputs from both eye and neck. Likewise, reports by Fiorentini *et al.* (1982), Graves *et al.* (1987), and Fiorentini *et al.* (1985) show that depth perception was largely impaired in cats with extra-ocular de-afferentation.

Furthermore, the sequential organization of visually guided behaviour, which requires that the kitten should be able to see its self-produced limb movements, was found to be dramatically impaired after suppression of proprioceptive afferents from eye muscles (Hein and Diamond 1982).

For man, there exists a body of indirect data about eye muscle proprioception consisting of clinical observations and reports describing rehabilitation methods used on postural deficiencies (Gagey 1987; Martins Da Cunha 1987). In particular, Gagey *et al.* (1973, 1975) have explained the influence of extra-ocular afferents in stance regulation by assuming that this kind of message might act as an 'endo-input to the postural system' (Gagey 1987).

In fact, these investigators demonstrated that in subjects seated with their legs relaxed, a sustained ocular version induced a progressive tonic change in specific leg muscles, which varied with the direction of the version.

Interestingly, others have described a body rotation around the vertical axis in standing subjects undergoing the tramping test (Fukuda 1959) while maintaining an ocular version (Gagey and Baron 1983), or after wearing a prism for 3 s (Ushio *et al.* 1975). In all cases the direction of the observed body deviation corresponded to that of the eye version or prism displacement. The most noteworthy item is the prism-induced body rotation because it constitutes a strong argument in favour of the proprioceptive origin of this effect. Prism wearing corresponds in fact to passive eye stretching in the direction opposite to the prism basis. The possibility that an eye position signal of central origin may be involved can therefore be ruled out.

Likewise, as described in the above section, a muscle tendon vibration elicits a stretching-like afferent pattern in the vibrated muscle, which induces an illusory sensation of limb movement. As we have a means of activating muscle stretch receptors, and in view of the density of muscle spindles in extra-ocular muscles, we attempted to activate specifically the eye muscle proprioceptors in man, bearing in mind that no clear sensations of eye displacement have yet been reported.

In fact, vibrations applied to extra-ocular muscles were found to elicit directional kinaesthetic illusion and involuntary motor responses of the head, trunk, and whole body which depended strictly on the postural context and the position of the vibrator around the eyeball. Illusory and/or actual movements were produced, depending on the postural constraints: seated or standing subjects, head free or fixed (Roll and Roll 1987). Taking into account the clinical and experimental data mentioned above and given the fact that the gaze is known to play a major role in body and limb orientation, we then investigated to what extent eye muscle proprioception might influence the regulation of stance.

Vibrations were applied to the periphery of the eyeball by means of mini-vibrators mounted on a helmet fixed on the subject's head. The contacting surface of the vibrator probe was polished and its length and shape could be varied depending on the shape of the subject's eye and on which eye muscle was to be vibrated. Either one eye or both eyes were vibrated. When both eyes were stimulated, vibrations were applied to the same muscle of each eye: two inferior and two superior recti, or to the synergist muscles, i.e. the lateral rectus of one eye together with the medial rectus of the other. The duration of the vibration train was 5 s; the frequency could vary from 1 to 100 Hz, but was usually 70 Hz. Subjects' postural sways were recorded from four strain gauges which were enclosed in the stabilometer set under each subject's foot.

Application of mechanical vibration to the extra-ocular muscles of a standing subject with his eyes closed elicited, with a lag of 1–2 s, whole-body shifts, the direction of which was found to depend strictly on which muscle was vibrated. Simultaneous vibration of the two superior recti resulted in a whole-body forward displacement, whereas a backward shift was observed during vibration of the two inferior recti. When the stimulation was applied simultaneously to the lateral rectus of the right eye and to

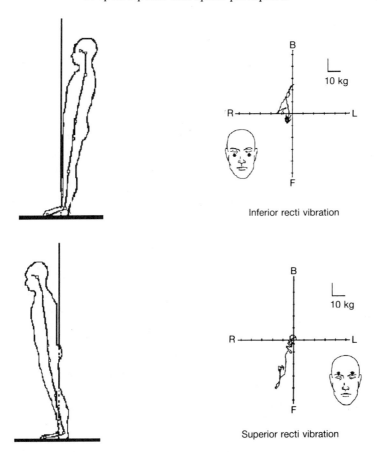

Fig. 7.4. Directional, postural effects of high-frequency vibrations (70 Hz, 5 s) applied to homonymous extra-ocular muscles of both eyes as illustrated by posturograms and the corresponding whole-body shifts. The arrows indicate the muscle stimulated (inferior and superior rectil)—R, right; L, left; B, back; F, front.

the medial rectus of the left eye, a leftward displacement was elicited, and vice versa. As an example, the posturograms in Fig. 7.4 give two-dimensional plots of the lateral (x) and antero-posterior (y) components of postural forces recorded during simultaneous vibration of the two inferior and posterior recti.

These effects clearly suggest the existence of a close linkage between 'eye posture' and the spatial organization of whole-body posture. Moreover, they furnish proof of the proprioceptive origin of this linkage, thanks to the fact that the direction of body shifts varies with the site of stimulation. Another major proof is provided by the fact that, as in the case of skeletal muscles (see Fig. 7.1), the mean amplitude of the postural displacement changes as a function of the frequency from 20 Hz up to 100 Hz, with a maximum at 70 Hz.

The last point we would like to discuss is the fact that, as with extra-ocular proprioception, vibration of both the neck and ankle muscles was capable of giving rise to similar body sways when a relevant site for the stimulus was chosen. For instance, vibrations applied separately to the inferior recti, the sternocleidomastoid, or the soleus muscles induced analogous postural effects, i.e. a backward whole-body displacement. Moreover, it was possible to combine these stimulations in different ways. In all cases, co-stimulation of two muscle groups had a more powerful influence on body posture than isolated vibrations applied separately to each muscle group. The findings did not clearly point to the existence of any particular predominant proprioceptive input. However, whilst the effects of combined vibrations of 'synergistic' muscle groups were additive, the summation was not linear, as the combined effects were clearly smaller than the sums of the individual effects (Roll and Roll 1988).

The postural effects of eye muscle vibration clearly suggest that the extra-ocular proprioceptive input—and not merely retinal cues as classically assumed—contributes to the control of human stance.

Proprioception: a link between body and external space

The egocentric localization of objects in extra-personal space requires the simultaneous processing of both retinal and extra-retinal signals. The question as to whether this extra-retinal signal is of central or peripheral origin is still a matter of controversy, however. It therefore seemed to be worth investigating whether the proprioceptive feedback originating in eye and neck muscles might provide the central nervous system (CNS) with some information about the gaze direction.

The role of eye and neck proprioception was studied in an open-loop, visuo-manual pointing task during which vibration was applied to eye and/or neck muscles. The subjects were asked to localize visually and try to touch a luminous target placed on a vertical panel facing them (Fig. 7.5A). Under most of the experimental conditions the left eye was covered with a patch. The subjects were required to gaze at the target from its onset until it was turned off and then to point with their right hand to the place from which it had just disappeared. The duration of both target illumination and vibration was 3 s; target and vibrator started and stopped simultaneously. As regards the eye, only the inferior rectus muscle of the subjects' right eye was vibrated. In the first experiment, the frequency range was between 20 and 100 Hz; in the subsequent fixed-frequency experiments, vibrations had

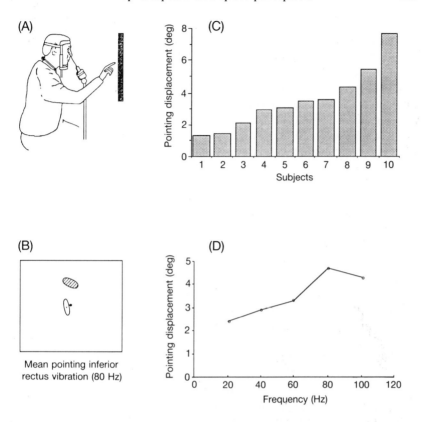

Fig. 7.5. (A) Schematic representation of the experimental set-up including pointing grid and both neck (eccentric DC motor) and eye (electro-magnetic) vibrators; (B) upward pointing displacement induced by right eye inferior rectus; (C) individual mean scores all frequencies combined; (D) mean upward shift as a function of vibration frequency.

a 80 Hz frequency. As regards the neck, the vibrator was placed on the back of the neck (trapezius and splenius muscles); a constant vibration frequency of 80 Hz was applied. An initial series of pointings was carried out under monocular vision, without any muscle vibration. The mean error recorded in this control session served as a baseline for the computation of vibration-induced error in the subsequent tests.

Vibration of the inferior rectus alone

Vibration of the inferior rectus of the subjects' right eye induced in all of them the illusion that the target was moving slowly in the upward direction. The extent of the illusory movement was measured directly in terms of the subjects' degree of inaccuracy in pointing at the perceived target position

(Fig. 7.5B). Each subjects' performance showed an upward displacement of the pointing area as compared to that obtained in the control situation. The amplitude of the pointing displacement varied from 1.3° to 7.7° from one subject to another, all frequencies combined (Fig. 7.5C). This means that, as the vibration was for 3 s, the mean perceived velocity of the illusory movement of the target was approximately one degree per second. The pointing displacement increased, however, as a function of the vibration frequency between 20 Hz, where it was 2.5°, and 80 Hz, where it reached 4.5°. The corresponding computed target velocities were 0.8° and 1.5° per second, respectively.

Similar results, but in different directions, were obtained on vibrating the external rectus muscle. Here, vibration of the right external rectus induced illusory movements of the target towards the left, whereas that of the left external rectus induced illusions towards the right.

It is worth noting that the illusion of target displacement did not result from an actual eye movement. This was put to the test by inducing a post-image on the retina of the vibrated eye. In this case, as the retinal locus of the target could not change, the persistence of the visual illusion was not attributable to any eye movement.

The low velocity of the illusory movement and its increase within the 20–80 Hz frequency range provides the main argument in favour of the proprioceptive origin of this visual illusion. The curve showing the error as a function of the vibration frequency (Fig. 7.5D) is similar to that obtained when somatic muscles were vibrated (Fig. 7.1).

These findings suggest that proprioceptive messages arising in extra-ocular muscles constitute an important component of the extra-retinal signal that attributes spatial bearings to the target first coded in terms of retinal co-ordinates. As we already know, however, the eye-in-head position is necessary but not sufficient to assign a locality in extra-personal space to a given retinal input. A signal informing about head-on-trunk position has to be taken into account. Although the possibility that the signal of head position may be of central origin cannot be totally ruled out (Berthoz 1974), the contribution of neck proprioception has been suspected for many years (Cohen 1961). Furthermore, illusory displacements of a visual target during vibration of neck muscles have been described before (Biguer *et al.* 1988; Roll and Roll 1988). Roll and Roll reported that upward illusory displacements of a visual target were elicited by vibrating the tendon of the sternocleidomastoid muscle located in the anterior part of the neck, whereas downward displacements were obtained when posterior neck muscles (including the splenius and trapezius) were stimulated. In both cases, the direction of these perceptual effects corresponded to the direction of the actual head movements that would have stretched the vibrated muscle; that is, a raising and a lowering of the head, respectively.

As eye and neck proprioception seem to contribute independently to ego-centric localization, we were interested in testing their functional synergy.

Vibrations of neck muscles alone

The vibratory stimulation of the neck muscles, including both splenius and trapezius muscles, induced in all subjects an illusory downward displacement of the target that resulted in a 5.4° downward shift of the mean pointing score as compared with the control level (Fig. 7.6A).

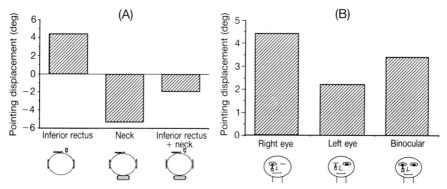

Fig. 7.6. (A) Mean pointing displacement induced by single or combined vibration of eye and neck muscles; (B) variation of mean pointing displacement induced by vibration of right eye inferior rectus as a function of the target viewing conditions, i.e. right eye, left or both eyes.

Effects of combined stimulation of inferior rectus and neck muscles

As separate stimulation of the inferior rectus and neck muscles induced effects in opposite directions, the resulting effects were manifold: depending on whether the subjects were more sensitive to vibration of eye or neck muscles, the direction of the perceived displacement could either be upward or downward; in some subjects in whom the vibration-induced effects were approximately equivalent whether the eye or neck muscles were stimulated, the target was perceived as being immobile. In all the subjects, these combined effects resulted in a mean pointing score that did not differ significantly from zero (Fig. 7.6A). In the majority of subjects the errors obtained with combined vibrations were clearly a summation of the errors observed with a single vibration. The vibratory stimulation of neck and eye was assumed to simulate roughly the proprioceptive signals emitted when the eye is tracking a target while the head is moving in the opposite direction. In this case, the velocity signals that arise simultaneously in eye and neck muscles have to be somehow summed or compared, the result of this operation then determining the perceived direction and speed of the target.

One question raised by these experimental effects of eye vibration concerns the functional coupling between the retinal and the proprioceptive extra-retinal messages, depending on whether they were of binocular or monocular origin. In general, visual localization is accomplished with both eyes and it involves the binocular processing of retinal and extra-retinal signals. If the retinal input to one eye is solely associated with the proprioceptive signals from the same eye, then vibration applied to one eye while the target is seen by the other should not generate any illusory movement. On the contrary, if the two extra-retinal signals are equivalent, that is if both eyes are treated as if they were a single (cyclopean) eye, then vibration of one closed eye should induce the same illusory movement of a target as that perceived by the other eye. We therefore attempted to dissociate the origins of the retinal and proprioceptive extraretinal messages by sharing out information among the two eyes. The outcome of this experiment is shown in Fig. 7.6B. We shall use the terms 'retinal eye' for the eye receiving visual input and 'proprioceptive eye' for the vibrated eye.

When the same eye was both *retinal* and *proprioceptive*, we obtained the same results as previously described. The mean upward displacement was 4.5°. When the *proprioceptive eye* (right) and the *retinal eye* (left) were dissociated, an upward apparent movement of the target was still reported, but the resultant pointing errors dropped significantly by half (2.20°). The latter value differed significantly from zero, however. When both eyes were open, there were two *retinal eyes* and one *proprioceptive eye* (right eye) and subjects again reported a target shift in the upward direction with an amplitude of 3.46°. This mean value was slightly below those obtained under monocular conditions of vision, but the difference was not statistically significant.

The fact that subjects always reported an apparent movement of the target when the right vibrated eye was closed and the left one open seems to indicate that if the CNS has to know the exact position of a target in extra-personal space, the proprioceptive messages arising in both eyes are jointly processed as if they were a single cyclopean eye. This is in agreement with many experimental data, particularly those of Ono and Weber (1981), who have demonstrated by comparing subjects' pointing performances under monocular and binocular viewing conditions that the visual direction was specified from both eye positions if one eye was occluded.

The question arises, however, as to why the amplitude of the pointing displacement was reduced by half when the target was viewed with the left eye while the right eye was vibrated. In fact, it is not possible to draw any definite conclusions on this point from our findings. We can assume, however, that the effect of eye muscle vibration is maximized when a retinal input arises simultaneously in the same eye. This suggests that a proprioceptive signal may somehow be potentiated if accompanied by a retinal input to the same eye. The movement illusion may result from the comparison between an erroneous movement signal arising in the vibrated eye and a stabilized position signal coming from the other, closed, eye. When one eye is simultaneously open and vibrated, the movement signal may be maximized due to the presence of a retinal input. If the vibrated eye is closed, the retinal input is associated with the stabilized position signal, which will be stronger and therefore reduce the illusory movement. Likewise, the intermediate error amplitude observed when both eyes were open and only the right one vibrated might also be interpreted along these lines. If this is so, it is to be expected that applying vibration to both eyes when they are open will result in the greatest illusion. This is probably the optimal condition for the CNS, which thus simultaneously receives congruent proprioceptive and retinal information from both eyes.

One important point to be considered is the fact that all the subjects had a dominant right eye. A further control needs to be effected by investigating whether or not vibration of subjects' closed left eye while their right eye is open results in an identical perceived target velocity.

Finally, neither the mechanisms nor the neural structures involved in the common processing of retinal and extra-retinal proprioceptive inputs from one or both eyes have yet been fully elucidated. In the monkey, the proprioceptive afferent projections are known to be ipsilateral up to the two first relays (Gasserian ganglia and trigeminal nucleus) where there are no visual projections (Porter 1986). On the other hand, Donaldson and Long (1980) have reported that activity was induced in cat collicular units by delivering visual stimulation to one eye while the extrinsic eye muscles of either eye were stretched.

Taken as a whole, these findings seem to demonstrate clearly that eye and neck muscle proprioception contributes to the specification of gaze direction in visually oriented activities. The question remains, however, as to whether this proprioceptive information is directly available to the CNS for use as a directional reference in the egocentric localization of objects in space. Some investigators, such as Mittelstaedt (1989), have suggested that this proprioceptive influence acts by means of a sub-loop controlling gaze stabilization. Our general interpretation of the visual effects of the eye and/ or neck muscle vibration is based on the assumption that by this means one can artificially reproduce a natural orienting reaction of the gaze when the eye alone, or both eye and head, move in a given direction. This is typically the case when a subject is looking at a moving target with his head free. It is noteworthy that both our results and assumptions are strongly supported by numerous recent studies, in particular the clinical data of Campos *et al.* (1986), who have shown that subjects with pathological de-afferentation of the ophthalmic branch of the trigeminal nerve made target mislocations in an open-loop pointing task. Pointing errors were also reported by Gauthier *et al.* (1988) in normal subjects whose one covered eye was abducted by means of a suction lens. Likewise, experimental de-afferentation in cats was found to result in localization errors in a whole-body ballistic task

(Fiorentini *et al.* 1982). We propose that the proprioceptive feedback arising in eye and neck muscles might be included in a larger process, involving all the body proprioceptive feedbacks liable to build up a directional reference that takes into account the whole-body posture. This directional body reference might constitute the prerequisite for any action to be performed in extra-personal space.

Conclusions

The experimental data given here suggest the existence of a close linkage between eye and foot, via muscular proprioceptive messages, and support the idea that this chain makes a decisive contribution to the control of human stance. In this chain, extra-ocular proprioception seems to have a dominant role. This fact is of major importance because it means that the direction of gaze plays a leading role in postural regulation. This is not surprising because the relationship between body and environment is, in most cases, first organized on the basis of gaze orientation and grasping.

Another point concerns the fact that the extra-ocular proprioceptive input might add its postural regulatory influence to that of other inputs coming from various body segments. This is easy to imagine by simply remembering that the legs, like the trunk and head, are also *carriers* of the eyes in space. This suggests that a common processing of all these muscular feedbacks subserves postural adjustment and that these feedbacks participate together in the elaboration of a body reference frame. This proposition may contribute to further specifying the body scheme concept in terms of proprioceptive content. Moreover, the centrally elaborated postural scheme, built up from simultaneously collected proprioceptive cues, might be used in the spatial processing of retinal information, as shown by the fact that vibration of eye, neck, or leg muscles gives rise to apparent movement of a visual target in a specific direction.

In addition, the finding that vibratory manipulation of proprioceptive pathways from the eye, and neck affects the visually guided behaviours suggests, in conclusion, the existence of an eye-to-foot muscular proprioceptive chain which is used by the brain to specify the spatial coordinates of objects in relation to the body. This kind of proprioceptive reference frame may be of major importance in interrelating body space with extra-personal space.

Acknowledgements

This work was supported by grants from CNRS and Fondation pour la Recherche Médicale.

References

Berthoz, A. (1974). Oculomotricité et proprioception. *Review of EEG Neurophysiology*, **4**, 569–86.

Biguer, B., Donaldson, I. M. L., Hein, A., and Jeannerod, M. (1988). Neck muscle vibration modifies the representation of visual motion and direction in man. *Brain*, **111**, 1405–24.

Bonnet, M., Roll, J. P., and Lacour, M. (1973). High frequency activation of myotatic pathway in man and illusion of movement. *Electroencephalography and Clinical Neurophysiology*, **34**, 810.

Brown, M. C., Engberg, I., and Matthews, P. B. C. (1967). The relative sensitivity to vibration of muscle receptors in the cat. *Journal of Physiology*, **192**, 773–800.

Buisseret, P. (1990). Suppression of cervical afferents impairs visual cortical cells development. In *The head–neck sensory motor system* (ed. A. Berthoz, W. Graf, and P. P. Vidal). Oxford University Press (in press).

Buisseret, P. and Gary-Bobo, E. (1979). Development of visual cortical orientation specificity after dark-rearing: role of extraocular proprioception. *Neuroscience Letters*, **13**, 259–63.

Burke, D., Hagbarth, K. E., Lofstedt, L., and Wallin, B. G. (1976a). The responses of human muscle spindle endings to vibration of non-contracting muscles. *Journal of Physiology*, **261**, 673–93.

Burke, D., Hagbarth, K. E., Lofstedt, L., and Wallin, B. G. (1976b). The responses of human muscle spindle endings to vibration during isometric contraction. *Journal of Physiology*, **261**, 695–711.

Campos, E. C., Chiesi, C., and Bolzani, R. (1986). Abnormal spatial localization in patients with herpes zoster ophthalmicus. *Archive of Ophthalmology*, **104**, 1176–7.

Clark, F. J., Matthews, P. B. C., and Muir, R. B. (1981). Response of soleus Ia afferents to vibration in the presence of the tonic vibration reflex in the decerebrate cat. *Journal of Physiology*, **311**, 97–112.

Cohen, L. A. (1961). Role of eye and neck proprioceptive mechanisms in body orientation and motor coordination. *Journal of Neurophysiology*, **24**, 1–11.

Cooper, S. and Daniel, P. M. (1949). Muscle spindles in human extrinsic eye muscles. *Brain*, **72**, 1–24.

Cooper, S., Daniel, P. M., and Whitteridge, D. (1951). Afferent impulses in the oculomotor nerve from the extrinsic eye muscles. *Journal of Physiology*, **113**, 463–74.

Cooper, S., Daniel, P. M., and Whitteridge, D. (1955). Muscle spindles and other sensory endings in the extrinsic eye muscles. *Brain*, **78**, 564–83.

Donaldson, I. M. L. and Long, A. C. (1980). Interactions between extraocular proprioceptive and visual signals in the superior colliculus of the cat. *Journal of Physiology*, **298**, 85–110.

Eklund, G. (1972). Position sense and state of contraction; the effects of vibration. *Journal of Neurology and Neurosurgical Psychiatry*, **35**, 606–11.

Fiorentini, A., Berardi, N., and Maffei, L. (1982). Role of extraocular proprioception in the orienting behavior of cats. *Experimental Brain Research*, **48**, 113–20.

Fiorentini, A., Maffei, L., Cenni, M. C., and Tacchi, A. (1985). Deafferentation of oculomotor proprioception affects depth discrimination in adult cats. *Experimental Brain Research*, **59**, 296–301.

Fukuda, T. (1959). The stepping test. Two phases of the laryrinthine reflex. *Acta Otolaryngologica*, **50**, 95–108.

Gagey, P. M. (1987). L'oculomotricité comme endo-entrée du système postural. *Agressologie*, **28**, 899–903.

Gagey, P. M. and Baron, J. B. (1983). Influence des mouvements oculaires volontaires sur le test de piétinement. *Agressologie*, **24**, 117–18.

Gagey, P. M., Baron, J. B., Lespargot, J., and Poli, J. P. (1973). Variations de l'activité tonique posturale et activité des muscles oculocéphalogyres en cathédrostatisme. *Agressologie*, **14B**, 87–96.

Gagey, P. M., Baron, J. B., Amphoux, M., Blaizot, M., Gentaz, R., and Goumot, H. (1975). Perturbations de l'activité tonique posturale des membres inférieurs en cathédrostatisme au cours des mouvements ocularies horizontaux recontrées dans certains syndrome post-commotionnels d'origine tronculaire. *Agressologie*, **16D**, 77–82.

Gauthier, G., Nommay, D., and Vercher, J. L. (1988). Ocular muscle proprioception and visual localization in man. *Journal of Physiology*, **406**, 24P.

Gilhodes, J. C., Roll, J. P., and Tardy-Gervet, M. F. (1986). Perceptual and motor effects of agonist–antagonist muscle vibration in man. *Experimental Brain Research*, **61**, 395–402.

Goodwin, G. M., McCloskey, D. I., and Matthews, P. B. C. (1972). The contribution of muscle afferents to kinaesthesia shown by vibration induced illusions of movement and by the effects of paralysing joint afferents. *Brain*, **95**, 705–48.

Graves, A. L., Trotter, Y., and Fregnac, Y. (1987). Role of extraocular muscle proprioception in the development of depth perception in cats. *Journal of Neurophysiology*, **58**, 816–31.

Gurfinkel, V. S., Levik Yu S., Popov, E. E., Smetanin, B. N., and Shlikov, V. Y. (1988). Body scheme in the control of postural activity. In *Stance and motion, facts and concepts* (ed. V. S. Gurfinkel, M. E. Ioffe, J. Massion, and J. P. Roll), pp. 185–93. Plenum Press, New York.

Hein, A. and Diamond, R. (1982). Contribution of eye movement to representation of space. In *Spatially oriented behaviour* (ed. A. Hein and M. Jeannerod), pp. 119–33. Springer-Verlag, New York.

Lennerstrand, G. and Bach y Rita, P. (1974). Spindle responses in pig eye muscles. *Acta Physiologica Scandinavica*, **90**, 795–7.

Ludvigh, E. (1952). Possible role of proprioception in the extraocular muscles. *Archives of Ophthalmology*, **48**, 436–41.

Martins Da Cunha, H. M. (1987). Le syndrome de deficience posturale (SDP). *Agressologie*, **28**, 941–3.

Matthews, P. B. C. (1982). Where does Sherrington's 'muscular sense' originate? Muscles, joints, corollary discharges? *Annual Review of Neuroscience*, **5**, 198–218.

Matthews, P. B. C. and Watson, J. D. G. (1981). Action of vibration on the response of cat muscle spindle Ia afferents to low frequency sinusoidal stretching. *Journal of Physiology*, **317**, 365–81.

McCloskey, D. I. (1978). Kinaesthetic sensibility. *Physiological Review*, **58**, 763–820.

Mittelstaedt, H. (1989). Basic solutions to the problem of head-centric visual localization. In *The perception and control of self-motion* (ed. R. Warren and A. H. Wertheim), pp. 3–23. Erlbaum, Hillsdale, NJ.

Ono, H. and Weber, E. U. (1981). Nonveridical visual direction produced by monocular viewing. *Journal of Experimental Psychology*, **7**, 937–47.

Paillard, J. (1988). Posture and locomotion: old problems and new concepts. In *Posture and gait, development adaptation and modulation* (ed. B. Amblard, A. Berthoz, and F. Clarac), pp. v–xi. Elsevier, North Holland, Amsterdam.

Porter, J. D. (1986). Brainstem terminations of extraocular muscle primary afferent neurons in the monkey. *Journal of Comparative Neurology*, **247**, 133–43.

Quoniam, C., Roll, J. P., Deat, A., and Massion, J. (1990). Proprioceptive induced interactions between segmental and whole body posture. In *Disorders of posture and gait* (ed. T. Brandt), pp. 194–7. Georg Thieme Verlag. Stuttgart.

Roll, J. P. (1981). Contribution de la proprioception musculaire à la perception et au contrôle du mouvement chez l'homme. Thèse Faculté des Sciences, Marseille.

Roll, J. P. (1987). Les bases physiologiques des conduites: fonctions de prises d'informations et d'exploration. In *Encyclopédie de la Pléiade*, pp. 1476–535. Editions Gallimard, Paris.

Roll, J. P. and Roll, R. (1987). Kinaesthetic and motor effects of extraocular vibration in Man. In *Eye movements: from physiology to cognition* (ed. J. K. O. Regan and A. Levy-Schoen), pp. 57–68. Elsevier, North Holland, Amsterdam.

Roll, J. P. and Roll, R. (1988). From eye to foot: a proprioceptive chain involved in postural control. In *Posture and gait, development adaptation and modulation* (ed. B. Amblard, A. Berthoz, and F. Clarac), pp. 155–64. Elsevier, North Holland, Amsterdam.

Roll, J. P. and Vedel, J. P. (1982). Kinaesthetic role of muscle afferents in man studied by tendon vibration and microneurography. *Experimental Brain Research*, **47**, 177–90.

Roll, J. P., Gilhodes, J. C., and Tardy-Gervet, M. F. (1980). Effets perceptifs et moteurs des vibrations musculaires chez l'homme normal: Mise en évidence d'une réponse des muscles antagonistes. *Archives of Italian Biology*, **118**, 51–71.

Roll, J. P., Gilhodes, J. C., Roll, R., and Velay, J. L. (1990). Contribution of skeletal and extraocular proprioception to kinaesthetic representation. In *Attention and performance XIII* (ed. M. Jeannerod), pp. 549–66. Erlbaum, Hillsdale, NJ.

Roll, J. P., Vedel, J. P., and Ribot, E. (1989). Alteration of proprioceptive messages induced by tendon vibration in man: A microneurographic study. *Experimental Brain Research*, **76**, 213–22.

Sherrington, C. S. (1900). The muscular sense. In *Textbook of physiology*, Vol. 2 (ed. E. A. Schäfer), pp. 1002–25. Pentland, Edinburgh and London.

Steinbach, M. J. (1987). Proprioceptive knowledge of eye position. *Vision Research*, **27**, 1737–44.

Ushio, N., Matsuura, K., Hinoki, M., Baron, J. B., and Gagey, P. M. (1975).

Deux phases de réflexe dans l'équilibre provoquées par les propriocepteurs des muscles oculaires. Analyse à l'aide du test de piétinement de Fukuda et du test de réflexe orthostatique. *Agressologie*, **16D**, 39–52.

Vallbo, A. B. (1973). Muscle spindle afferent discharge from resting and contracting muscles in normal human subjects. In *New developments in EMG and clinical neurophysiology 3*, (ed. J. E. Desmedt), pp. 251–62. Karger, Basle.

Von Holst, E. and Mittelstaedt, H. (1950). The reafference principle. Interaction between the central nervous system and the periphery. In *Selected papers of Erich von Holst: 1. The behavioural physiology of animals and Man*, pp. 139–73. Methuen, London.

8

Parietal cortex area 5: a neuronal representation of movement kinematics for kinaesthetic perception and movement control?

JOHN F. KALASKA

The original title of this section of the symposium was 'Interfacing body and environmental space'. In this chapter, I will examine cortical mechanisms of the representation of internal (somatic) space. This representation is essential for successful interaction with the environment (Hyvarinen 1982; Stein 1989; Soechting and Flanders 1990). I will briefly review evidence that cortical area 5 is an important component of the central representation of body posture and movement. Moreover, I will argue that area 5 represents movement in a co-ordinate system encoding kinematic parameters. Movement kinematics refers to all the externally measurable spatio-temporal parameters of movement, such as direction, velocity, and joint angle changes, that describe motion through space. These are distinct from the parameters of movement dynamics, such as the internal forces, joint torques, and patterns of muscle activity required to perform the movement.

Anatomical considerations

The superior parietal cortex area 5 of primates is located immediately posterior to the primary somatosensory cortex, SI. Much of it lies buried in the anterior bank of the intraparietal sulcus, which conceals its greatly expanded antero-posterior extent at a point corresponding to the representation of the contralateral arm and hand (Shanks *et al.* 1985).

The major ascending thalamic input to area 5 arises in the lateral posterior and anterior pulvinar nuclei (Pearson *et al.* 1978; Jones *et al.* 1979; Pons and Kaas 1985). Area 5 may also receive a weak input from the ventro-posterior nuclei (Pons and Kaas 1985). It receives a major cortico-cortical input from SI, in particular from area 2 (Jones *et al.* 1978; Künzle 1978; Pearson and Powell 1985; Pons and Kaas 1986). It is reciprocally connected with the primary motor and pre-motor cortex (Jones and Powell

1970; Künzle 1978; Strick and Kim 1978; Petrides and Pandya 1984; Caminiti *et al.* 1985; Johnson *et al.* 1989). Other output targets include area 7b, the basal ganglia, pontine nuclei, and the spinal cord (Wiesendanger *et al.* 1979; Hyvarinen 1982).

This brief review of area 5 connectivity indicates that this area is a critical cortical link between the somatosensory and motor systems. While a major cortico-cortical input is from SI, its principal thalamic input is from nuclei not normally associated with primary sensory pathways, and it is also reciprocally connected with cortical and sub-cortical motor areas. Therefore, description of area 5 only as a somatosensory association area, hierarchically superior to SI (Jones and Powell 1970; Sakata *et al.* 1973), probably fails to capture the full complexity of its role.

Some pertinent response properties of area 5 neurons

Many, but not all, area 5 cells respond to passive somaesthetic stimuli, particularly those evoked by joint movement (Duffy and Burchfiel 1971; Sakata *et al.* 1973; Mountcastle *et al.* 1975; Seal *et al.* 1982; Kalaska *et al.* 1983). Early studies (Duffy and Burchfiel 1971; Sakata *et al.* 1973) emphasized the high degree of convergence and complexity of the passive receptive fields of area 5 neurons compared to that in SI. Consistent with a successive association model of cortical function, Sakata *et al.* (1973) proposed that area 5 was a site of intramodal and intermodal sensory convergence to generate a representation of the posture, form, and orientation of body segments for kinaesthetic perception.

Two other important features of area 5 activity, first reported by Mountcastle *et al.* (1975), are that the discharge of many cells is more intense during active arm movements than in response to similar passive movements, and that it precedes the onset of active movement. These properties of the response have been interpreted in different ways. Mountcastle *et al.* (1975) proposed that the parietal cortex contained a high-order 'command apparatus' for arm movement. Seal and his colleagues have supported this conclusion (Seal *et al.* 1982, 1983; Seal and Commenges 1985). Others have suggested that these properties are due to a selective pre-movement enhancement of important sensory input, as part of a mechanism controlling the direction of spatial attention (Robinson *et al.* 1978; Bushnell *et al.* 1981; Stein 1989). Thus, enhanced discharge in area 5 could reflect a selective amplification of input from parts of the body before and during active movement (Chapman *et al.* 1984; Stein 1989).

Another question concerns the capacity of area 5 cells to encode spatial parameters of somatomotor behaviour, such as arm posture and movement direction. Sakata *et al.* (1973) stressed the graded responses of area 5 cells to different static joint angles, and the selective responses to complex postures and movements, indicating a strong spatial component to area 5 activity. In contrast, Mountcastle *et al.* (1975) reported that area 5 cells were not strongly related to movement direction during whole-arm, reaching movements. However, when area 5 cells were studied in a task exploiting a much broader range of reaching directions, most cells were directionally tuned for movement, centred on a particular preferred direction of movement which differed from cell to cell (Kalaska *et al.* 1983). The pattern of population activity reliably signalled the direction of arm movement between targets (Kalaska *et al.* 1983). Likewise, the tonic activity of many area 5 cells co-varied with actively maintained arm postures (Georgopoulos *et al.* 1984). These findings confirmed that area 5 activity encoded detailed information about spatial parameters of active somatomotor behaviour. We proposed that area 5 processes a combination of peripheral and centrally generated inputs to synthesize a neuronal representation of body posture, movement, and spatial orientation during active movement (Kalaska *et al.* 1983; Kalaska 1988; see also MacKay *et al.* 1978; Hyvarinen 1982; Stein 1989). A parallel study of the motor cortex found that area 4 cells had similar directional tuning properties (Georgopoulos *et al.* 1982).

Neuronal representations of movement kinematics and dynamics

In the reaching task used to study areas 5 and 4, parameters of movement kinematics and movement dynamics were confounded. As a result, one could not determine whether the directional tuning curves observed in both areas encoded the co-variation of parameters of movement kinematics or of dynamics with movement direction (Georgopoulos *et al.* 1982). Many previous experiments had demonstrated that the discharge of certain motor cortex cells varied with changes in output force and muscle activity during movement, and in isometric tasks (Thach 1978; Cheney and Fetz 1980; Evarts *et al.* 1983). In contrast, only one brief report had studied this question in area 5, and it suggested that area 5 cells were less sensitive to changes in movement dynamics than were motor cortex cells (MacKay *et al.* 1978).

Confirmation of this difference between the two areas would provide an important insight into their relative roles in motor control. Therefore, we made a new series of experiments, using a modified task apparatus to permit a partial dissociation of kinematic and dynamic parameters (Kalaska and Hyde 1985; Kalaska *et al.* 1989, 1990). The modification allowed us to apply loads to the handle in eight directions, corresponding to the eight directions of movement in the task. For each direction, we could alter the dynamics by varying the direction of the applied loads. Biomechanical studies confirmed that the monkeys compensated for the external loads by altering the levels of muscle activity, particularly at the shoulder joint, while kinematics for each direction of movement (hand paths between targets, joint angle changes, etc.) remained essentially unaltered (Kalaska *et al.* 1989, 1990).

This new study reconfirmed that area 5 cells related to movements of the proximal arm showed broad directional tuning in response to normal, unloaded arm movements (Fig. 8.1). When external loads were applied to the handle, most area 5 cells were only modestly affected by the change in movement dynamics, or showed no significant change in activity at all (Kalaska and Hyde 1985; Kalaska *et al.* 1990). Furthermore, there was no consistent relation within the cell sample between the preferred direction of movement of each cell and the direction of load that produced the largest increase of the cell's activity (its 'load axis'). Because there was no consistent spatial relation between the preferred direction and load axis, the modest variations in single-cell response induced by the loads cancelled out when summed across the active population. The resulting pattern of population activity unambiguously encoded the movement of the limb through space under a broad range of external loads (Fig. 8.1; Kalaska 1990; Kalaska *et al.* 1990).

In contrast, the discharge of many motor cortex cells was strongly modulated by changes in load direction (Fig. 8.1; Kalaska and Hyde 1985; Kalaska *et al.* 1989). These load-related variations in discharge showed the same pattern of broad directional tuning as with movement direction. For most motor cortex cells, loads which pulled the arm in directions opposite to that of the preferred direction of movement of the cell produced a large increase in cell discharge, while loads which pulled the arm in directions corresponding to the preferred direction reduced cell activity (Kalaska *et al.* 1989). Because of this consistent spatial relation between the preferred direction of movement and the load axis of motor cortex cells, load-related changes in single cell activity summed across the sample population (Fig. 8.1), rather than cancelling out as in area 5. As a result, the changes in population activity caused by the loads represented an appropriate signal to compensate for the loads. Not all cells in the motor cortex were sensitive to external loads, however. Some shoulder-related motor cortex cells were as unaffected by the loads as were area 5 neurons (Kalaska *et al.* 1989).

This study demonstrated that area 5 cells encode arm movement in a kinematic co-ordinate system. However, the experiments did not identify which specific parameters were encoded. For instance, the neurons could be signalling purely abstract kinematic signals concerned with direction

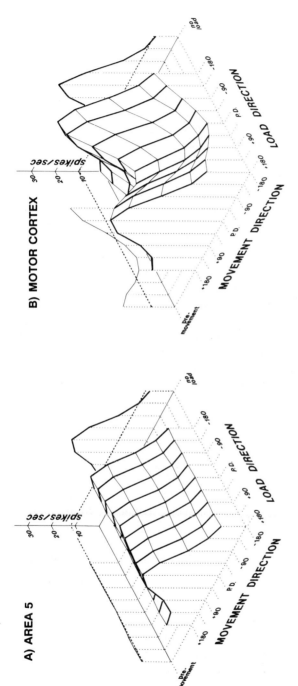

Fig. 8.1. (A) Mean response of 100 area 5 cells to different directions of movement and load. Each thick curve illustrates the variation of activity with movement direction, centred on the preferred movement direction (P.D.) of each cell. The isolated curve on the right is the population response during arm movements without external loads. The other eight thick curves (at P.D. along the 'Load direction' dimension) illustrates the response when the load pulls the limb with loads. The central curve (at P.D. along the 'Load direction' dimension) illustrates the response when the load pulls the arm in the direction corresponding to the P.D. of the cells (i.e. 'assisting' load). The curve at ±180° is the response when the load pulls the arm in the direction opposite to the P.D. ('opposing' load). The similarity of the curves demonstrates that external loads have little effect on total population activity in area 5. (From Kalaska *et al.* 1990; reproduced with permission of the publisher.) (B) Mean response of 73 phasic–tonic motor cortex cells (same display format as (A)). Assisting loads reduce cell discharge and opposing loads enhance it, relative to movement without external loads.

and velocity of movement, or the path of the hand through space. Alternatively, the neurons could be representing arm movement in more 'biological' co-ordinates of joint angle changes, muscle lengths, etc. The latter seems more likely than the former (Kalaska 1990; Kalaska *et al.* 1990), but definitive experiments have yet to be done. Moreover, the design of the task controlled the spatial parameters of movement but not the temporal parameters such as velocity. A complete description of the spatio-temporal representation of movement kinematics in area 5 awaits further study.

The motor cortex population was more heterogeneous in this task than that of area 5, in that a broad range of sensitivities to external loads was evident within area 4. The discharge of an important population of motor cortex cells co-varied with changes in movement dynamics. The presence of cells that were insensitive to loads suggests that a representation of movement kinematics may also coexist in area 4 (Kalaska *et al.* 1989). Therefore, the cortical representation of movement kinematics is not necessarily confined to area 5.

These findings are also pertinent to the question of the origin of the enhanced discharge of many area 5 cells during active movement. One explanation is that it is caused by a more effective activation of peripheral receptors during active muscle contractions. As the loads produced large changes in the level of muscle contraction, but produced minor changes in area 5 activity, our observations argue against this peripheral mechanism. Combined with the continued discharge of some area 5 cells after peripheral de-afferentation (Bioulac and Lamarre 1979; Seal *et al.* 1982; Burbaud *et al.* 1985), this provides compelling evidence in favour of a central origin for this behavioural enhancement.

Movement planning as a hierarchical process

William Hughlings-Jackson was the first to propose that the processes controlling movement in the central nervous system (CNS) are organized into a sequential hierarchical series of steps, beginning with more general or global aspects of the movement, and proceeding to more specific parameters (Mountcastle *et al.* 1975; Thach 1978; Seal *et al.* 1982, 1983; Lamarre and Chapman 1986; Kalaska 1990; Soechting and Flanders 1990; Wiesendanger 1990). Many models state that movements are first planned in kinematic co-ordinates, before dynamics and patterns of muscle activity can be determined (Soechting and Flanders 1990; Kalaska 1990). These models predict that there should be separate neuronal populations, encoding movement in various kinematic, dynamic, and muscle-centred co-ordinate frameworks, which are sequentially activated during the planning of movement.

By using a task paradigm that manipulated spatial parameters of movement kinematics and dynamics, we had been able to confirm the existence of sub-populations of cells representing arm movement in kinematic and dynamic/muscle co-ordinates. The kinematic representation in area 5 implied that it occupies a position hierarchically superior to the representation of movement dynamics in the motor cortex (Mountcastle *et al.* 1975; Seal *et al.* 1982, 1983). However, the task was a reaction-time paradigm, in which the monkey responded to the target stimulus as soon as it appeared. As the behavioural reaction times were short, all stages of the planning hierarchy were compressed into a very brief period of time, making it difficult to show a sequential activation of the different sub-populations.

We are currently investigating this aspect of the hierarchical model, using a new task that allows us to manipulate the temporal coupling between cell activity and the ensuing movement. In the new design, we have introduced an instructed delay into the trial. Two stimuli are presented to the monkey in series, separated by a delay interval of 1–3 s. The first stimulus (CUE) instructs the monkey which of the eight directions of movement to make. However, the monkey cannot perform the movement until the second stimulus (GO) is presented. During the 'instructed-delay' period between the two stimuli, the monkey has knowledge of the intended movement, and can pre-plan many of its parameters. However, the monkey is not permitted to make any overt peripheral response (movements or changes in muscle activity) until the GO signal appears.

The assumption in this paradigm is that any changes in neuronal activity observed during the instructed-delay period are implicated in the early planning stages of the movement, that is, at higher levels of the planning hierarchy. Cell discharge occurring only after the GO signal must be more tightly coupled to the actual production of the response and so must represent the final stages of the planning hierarchy.

Preliminary findings from one monkey indicate that changes in cell activity can be seen in area 5 less than 200 ms after the presentation of the CUE stimulus (Fig. 8.2; Crammond and Kalaska 1989a). This activity takes the form of step or ramp changes in the rate of tonic discharge, which are sustained throughout the instructed-delay period. The sign (increase or decrease) and intensity of the change in tonic rate vary with the direction of impending movement (Fig. 8.2). About one half of the proximal, arm-related cells of area 5 showed this property of differential activation as a function of impending direction of movement during the instructed-delay period. The majority of these cells were also active before the onset of movement in a reaction-time task without CUE stimuli (Crammond and Kalaska 1989a). In contrast, the majority of area 5 cells that did not show changes in activity during the instructed-delay period were only activated after the onset of movement in a reaction-time task.

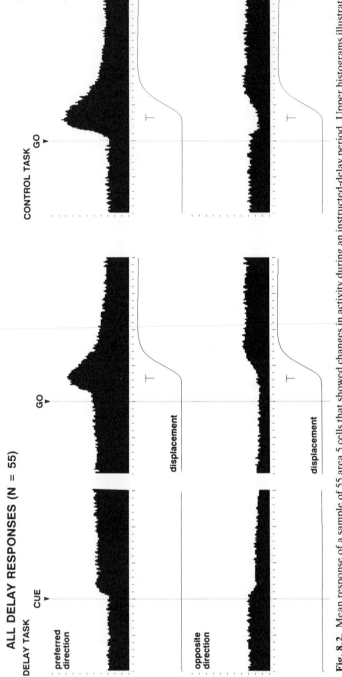

Fig. 8.2. Mean response of a sample of 55 area 5 cells that showed changes in activity during an instructed-delay period. Upper histograms illustrate the activity at the preferred direction of each cell and the lower histograms that for the opposite movement direction. Curves below the histograms represent the displacement of the handle away from the start position. The histograms at the right show the activity during a reaction-time task, aligned to the appearance of the GO signal (vertical line). The activity of the sample population was reciprocally related to the two opposite directions of movement. The histograms on the left illustrate the response of the same cells in an instructed-delay task, aligned to the presentation of the CUE and GO signals, respectively. Note the sustained and directionally tuned changes in tonic activity, beginning shortly after the appearance of the CUE signal. Each division of the time scales below the histograms indicates 100 msec.

Recordings were also made in the primary motor and premotor cortex of the same monkey (Crammond and Kalaska 1989b). Cells located in the central sulcus, where most of the load-sensitive area 4 neurons are concentrated (Kalaska *et al.* 1989), rarely showed changes in discharge during the instructed-delay period, even though most of the cells were active before the onset of movement. Thus, their discharge was almost exclusively related to movement execution. Changes in delay-period activity were common in neurons located more anteriorly, in area 6 of the premotor cortex. A similar antero-posterior gradient has been described by Weinrich *et al.* (1984).

Movement planning, perception, or both?

These preliminary observations indicate that, during an instructed-delay period, a pattern of neuronal activity arises in area 5 that co-varies with the direction of an impending movement. This finding, and the coding of arm movements in kinematic co-ordinates, are both consistent with the idea that area 5 functions at a higher level in the planning hierarchy than does the primary motor cortex. For instance, the instructed-delay activity may signal the trajectory of the intended movement, well in advance of the recruitment of the motor cortex. This interpretation would be reinforced if area 5 cells are also active before motor cortex neurons in reaction-time tasks. However, evidence for this is contradictory. Some studies have concluded that the earliest area 5 cells preceded the discharge of area 4 cells, and so functioned 'upstream' of the motor cortex (Seal *et al.* 1982, 1983; Burbaud *et al.* 1985). Others have found that area 5 discharge preceded movement but consistently lagged behind that in area 4 in reaction-time tasks (Bioulac and Lamarre 1979; Kalaska *et al.* 1983; Chapman *et al.* 1984; Lamarre and Chapman 1986). If the latter findings are correct, one must question whether area 5 is generating, under all circumstances, an arm-trajectory signal needed by area 4 to execute the movement.

The delay-period activity can also be interpreted in terms of a perceptual role for area 5. Kinaesthetic perception during active movement is thought to involve both peripheral and centrally generated signals (Kalaska 1988; Matthews 1988), and activity from both sources appears to coexist in area 5. Thus, the delay-period activity could be generated within area 5, or be a response to a corollary discharge about intended movement generated elsewhere in the CNS (Tanji *et al.* 1980; Weinrich *et al.* 1984; Alexander 1987) and relayed into area 5 (Mountcastle *et al.* 1975; Bioulac and Lamarre 1979; Kalaska 1988). This central signal about motor intention, and the convergent proprioceptive input about actual peripheral events, would generate a representation of body posture and movement for kinasethetic perception (Kalaska *et al.* 1983; Kalaska 1988; Stein 1989). This interpretation of area 5 activity is reminiscent of the concept of 'morphosynthesis'—the formation and maintenance of an adequate body image—proposed by Denny-Brown and Chambers (1958) as an important function of the superior parietal lobule of humans. The studies with external loads in area 5 demonstrated that the kinaesthetic representation in area 5 provides an unambiguous signal about arm posture and movement in kinematic co-ordinates, irrespective of the muscle activity required to produce the behaviour. Paradoxically, however, the directionally tuned changes in activity during the instructed-delay period (while the arm is motionless in a specific posture) would appear to introduce a source of ambiguity, reflecting motor intention before the onset of movement, to this representation of body form and movement.

Other interpretations of the delay-period activity are that it results from central mechanisms which enhance sensory input from the body during active movement (Mountcastle *et al.* 1975; Robinson *et al.* 1978; Bushnell *et al.* 1981), or might even be a form of selective attention directed toward the parts of the body that will move (Bushnell *et al.* 1981; Chapman *et al.* 1984; Stein 1989).

These alternative interpretations do not preclude a role for area 5 in motor planning. For instance, some models require a signal about the current (i.e. starting) position of the limb in order to plan a movement (Soechting and Flanders 1990). This information is already embedded in the ongoing pattern of activity within area 5 at the time the target appears (Kalaska *et al.* 1983; Georgopoulos *et al.* 1984), and so could be furnished by area 5 without necessitating any precocious change in activity after the presentation of a target stimulus. The area 5 somatomotor representation, continually updated before and during the movement by signals of central and peripheral origin, could contribute to the guidance of movement throughout its course. The central component of this updating mechanism would account for the pre-movement activity in area 5 in reaction-time tasks, and the activity in the instructed-delay period. In this way, area 5 can be seen to be simultaneously 'upstream' and 'downstream' of the motor cortex. Its ongoing activity could provide essential information used early in the planning process, and yet the first change in that activity would lag behind the motor cortex in a reaction-time task. Moreover, the motor and premotor cortex could be among the sources of central signals needed to update the area 5 kinaesthetic representation.

This view of area 5 function as a vital interface between somatosensory and motor systems is consistent with its anatomical connections. It suggests that debating whether the role of area 5 is predominantly sensory or motor is a cyclical, and ultimately sterile, exercise. Most importantly, this interpretation may point to a resolution of the apparent incompatibility between the serial organization of hierarchical models of cortical function and the massive, parallel and reciprocal connectivity of the CNS.

Acknowledgements

Martha Hyde, Dan Cohen, and Michel Prud'homme participated in the load-direction studies. Donald Crammond participated in the instructed-delay studies, and suggested many improvements to earlier drafts of this chapter. The research was supported by an establishment grant from Les Fonds de la Recherche en Santé du Québec, a Medical Research Council of Canada Scholarship, MRC grant MT-7693, and the MRC Group Grant in Neurological Sciences.

References

Alexander, G. E. (1987). Selective neuronal discharge in monkey putamen reflects intended direction of planned limb movements. *Experimental Brain Research*, **67**, 623–34.

Bioulac, B. and Lamarre, Y. (1979). Activity of postcentral cortical neurons of the monkey during conditioned movements of a deafferented limb. *Brain Research*, **172**, 427–37.

Burbaud, P., Gross, C., and Bioulac, B. (1985). Peripheral inputs and early activity in area 5 of the monkey during a trained forelimb movement. *Brain Research*, **337**, 341–6.

Bushnell, M. C., Goldberg, M. E., and Robinson, D. L. (1981). Behavioural enhancement of visual responses in monkey cerebral cortex. I. Modulation in posterior parietal cortex related to selective visual attention. *Journal of Neurophysiology*, **46**, 755–72.

Caminiti, R., Zeger, S., Johnson, P. B., Urbano, A., and Georgopoulos, A. P. (1985). Corticocortical efferent systems in the monkey: A quantitative spatial analysis of the tangential distribution of cells of origin. *Journal of Comparative Neurology*, **241**, 405–19.

Chapman, C. E., Spidalieri, G., and Lamarre, Y. (1984). Discharge properties of area 5 neurones during arm movements triggered by sensory stimuli in the monkey. *Brain Research*, **309**, 63–77.

Cheney, P. D. and Fetz, E. E. (1980). Functional classes of primate corticomoto-neuronal cells and their relation to active force. *Journal of Neurophysiology*, **44**, 773–91.

Crammond, D. J. and Kalaska, J. F. (1989a). Neuronal activity in primate parietal cortex area 5 varies with intended movement direction during an instructed-delay period. *Experimental Brain Research*, **76**, 458–62.

Crammond, D. J. and Kalaska, J. F. (1989b). Comparison of cell activity in cortical areas 6, 4 and 5 recorded in an instructed-delay task. *Neuroscience Abstracts*, **15**, 786.

Denny-Brown, D. and Chambers, R. A. (1958). The parietal lobes and be-haviour. *Research Publications of the Association for Research in Nervous and Mental Disease*, **36**, 35–117.

Duffy, G. H. and Burchfiel, J. L. (1971). Somatosensory system: organizational hierarchy from single units in monkey area 5. *Science* (Washington), **172**, 273–5.

Evarts, E. V., Fromm, C., Kröller, J., and Jennings, V. A. (1983). Motor cortex control of finely graded forces. *Journal of Neurophysiology*, **49**, 1199–215.

Georgopoulos, A. P., Kalaska, J. F., Caminiti, R., and Massey, J. T. (1982). On the relations between the direction of two-dimensional arm movements and cell discharge in primate motor cortex. *Journal of Neuroscience*, **2**, 1527–37.

Georgopoulos, A. P., Caminiti, R., and Kalaska, J. F. (1984). Static spatial effects in motor cortex and area 5: quantitative relations in a two-dimensional space. *Experimental Brain Research*, **54**, 446–54.

Hyvarinen, J. (1982). *The parietal cortex of monkey and man*, Studies of Brain Function, Vol. 8. Springer-Verlag, Berlin.

Johnson, P. B., Angelucci, A., Ziparo, R. M., Minciacchi, D., Bentivoglio, M., and Caminiti, R. (1989). Segregation and overlap of callosal and association neurons in frontal and parietal cortices of primates: A spectral and coherency analysis. *Journal of Neuroscience*, **9**, 2313–26.

Jones, E. G. and Powell, T. P. S. (1970). An anatomical study of converging sensory pathways within the cerebral cortex of the monkey. *Brain*, **93**, 793–820.

Jones, E. G., Coulter, J. D., and Hendry, S. H. C. (1978). Intracortical connect-ivity of architectonic fields in the somatic sensory, motor and parietal cortex of monkeys. *Journal of Comparative Neurology*, **181**, 291–348.

Jones, E. G., Wise, S. P., and Coulter, J. D. (1978). Differential thalamic relation-ships of sensory-motor and parietal cortical fields in monkeys. *Journal of Com-parative Neurology*, **183**, 833–82.

Kalaska, J. F. (1988). The representation of arm movements in postcentral and parietal cortex. *Canadian Journal of Physiology and Pharmacology*, **66**, 455–63.

Kalaska, J. F. (1990). What parameters of reaching are encoded by discharges of cortical cells? In *Motor control: concepts and issues* (ed. D. R. Humphrey and H.-J. Freund). Wiley, Chichester (in press).

Kalaska, J. F., and Hyde, M. L. (1985). Area 4 and area 5: Differences between the load direction-dependent discharge variability of cells during active postural fixation. *Experimental Brain Research*, **59**, 197–202.

Kalaska, J. F., Caminiti, R., and Georgopoulos, A. P. (1983). Cortical mechan-isms related to the direction of two-dimensional arm movements: relations in parietal area 5 and comparison with motor cortex. *Experimental Brain Research*, **51**, 247–60.

Kalaska, J. F., Cohen, D. A. D., Hyde, M. L., and Prud'homme, M. (1989). A comparison of movement direction-related versus load direction-related activity in primate motor cortex, using a two-dimensional reaching task. *Journal of Neuroscience*, **9**, 2080–102.

Kalaska, J. F., Cohen, D. A. D., Prud'homme, M., and Hyde, M. L. (1990). Parietal area 5 neuronal activity encodes movement kinematics, not movement dynamics. *Experimental Brain Research*, **80**, 351–64.

Künzle, H. (1978). Cortico-cortical efferents of primary motor and somatosensory regions of the cerebral cortex in *Macaca mulatta*. *Neuroscience*, **3**, 25–39.

Lamarre, Y. and Chapman, C. E. (1986). Comparative timing of neuronal discharge in cortical and cerebellar structures during a simple arm movement in the monkey. *Experimental Brain Research*, (suppl. 15), 14–27.

MacKay, W. A., Kwan, H. C., Murphy, J. T., and Wong, Y. C. (1978). Responses to active and passive wrist rotation in area 5 of awake monkeys. *Neuroscience Letters*, **10**, 235–9.

Matthews, P. B. C. (1988). Proprioceptors and their contribution to somatosensory mapping: complex messages require complex processing. *Canadian Journal of Physiology and Pharmacology*, **66**, 430–8.

Mountcastle, V. B., Lynch, J. C., Georgopoulos, A. P., Sakata, H., and Acuna, C. (1975). Posterior parietal association cortex of the monkey: command functions for operations within extrapersonal space. *Journal of Neurophysiology*, **38**, 871–908.

Pearson, R. C. A. and Powell, T. P. S. (1985). The projection of the primary somatic sensory cortex upon area 5 in the monkey. *Brain Research Reviews*, **9**, 89–107.

Pearson, C. A., Brodal, P., and Powell, T. P. S. (1978). The projection of the thalamus upon the parietal lobe in the monkey. *Brain Research*, **144**, 143–8.

Petrides, M. and Pandya, D. N. (1984). Projections to the frontal cortex from the posterior parietal region in the rhesus monkey. *Journal of Comparative Neurology*, **228**, 105–16.

Pons, T. P. and Kaas, J. H. (1985). Connections of area 2 of somatosensory cortex with the anterior pulvinar and subdivisions of the ventroposterior complex in macaque monkeys. *Journal of Comparative Neurology*, **240**, 16–36.

Pons, T. P. and Kaas, J. H. (1986). Corticocortical connections of area 2 of somatosensory cortex in macaque monkeys: A correlative anatomical and electrophysical study. *Journal of Comparative Neurology*, **248**, 313–35.

Robinson, D. L., Goldberg, M. E., and Stanton, G. B. (1978). Parietal association cortex in the primate: sensory mechanisms and behaviour modulations. *Journal of Neurophysiology*, **41**, 910–32.

Sakata, H., Takaoka, A., Kawarasaki, A., and Shibutani, H. (1973). Somatosensory properties of neurons in superior parietal cortex (area 5) of the rhesus monkey. *Brain Research*, **64**, 85–102.

Seal, J. and Commenges, D. (1985). A quantitative analysis of stimulus- and movement-related responses in the posterior parietal cortex of the monkey. *Experimental Brain Research*, **58**, 144–53.

Seal, J., Gross, C., and Bioulac, B. (1982). Activity of neurons in area 5 during a simple arm movement in monkey before and after deafferentation of the trained limb. *Brain Research*, **250**, 229–43.

Seal, J., Gross, C., Doudet, D., and Bioulac, B. (1983). Instruction-related changes in neuronal activity in area 5 during a simple forearm movement in the monkey. *Neuroscience Letters*, **36**, 145–50.

Shanks, M. F., Pearson, R. C. A., and Powell, T. P. S. (1985). The callosal connexions of the primary somatic sensory cortex in the monkey. *Brain Research Reviews*, **9**, 43–65.

Soechting, J. F. and Flanders, M. (1990). Deducing central algorithms of arm movement control from kinematics. In *Motor control: concepts and issues* (ed. D. R. Humphrey and H.-J. Freund). Wiley, Chichester (in press).

Stein, J. F. (1989). Representation of egocentric space in the posterior parietal cortex. *Quarterly Journal of Experimental Physiology*, **74**, 583–606.

Strick, P. L. and Kim, C. C. (1978). Input to primate motor cortex from posterior parietal cortex (area 5). I. Demonstration by retrograde transport. *Brain Research*, **157**, 325–30.

Tanji, J., Taniguchi, K., and Saga, T. (1980). Supplementary motor area: Neuronal response to motor instructions. *Journal of Neurophysiology*, **43**, 60–8.

Thach, W. T. (1978). Correlation of neural discharge with pattern and force of muscular activity, joint position and direction of intended next movement in motor cortex and cerebellum. *Journal of Neurophysiology*, **41**, 654–76.

Weinrich, M., Wise, S. P., and Mauritz, K.-H. (1984). A neurophysiological study of the premotor cortex in the rhesus monkey. *Brain*, **107**, 385–414.

Wiesendanger, M. (1990). The motor cortical areas and the problem of hierarchies. In *Attention and performance XII: Motor representation and control* (ed. M. Jeannerod), pp. 59–75. Erlbaum, Hillsdale, NJ.

Wiesendanger, R., Wiesendanger, M., and Rüegg, D. G. (1979). An anatomical investigation of the corticopontine projection in the primate (*Macaca fascicularis* and *Saimiri sciureus*). II. The projection from frontal and parietal association areas. *Neuroscience*, **4**, 747–65.

9

Perceptual and automatic aspects of the postural body scheme

V. S. GURFINKEL and YU. S. LEVICK

Posture and spatial orientation

Posture can be defined as a body position that an animal or human being maintains for a relatively long time. Posture is characterized by a definite set of joint angles, the maintenance of which is provided by a number of reflex mechanisms. Nevertheless, it should be stressed that, in addition to the relative position of the body parts, the definite orientation of the body with respect to external space is also important. Special systems must exist to provide the capability for orientating the body with respect to a solid supporting surface, to the flow of air or water, to the gravitational field, or to the visual environment. Such spatial orientation is necessary not only for the maintenance of basic postural attitude but also for the performance of locomotor, manipulatory, and orientational movements. Our systematic thinking about the maintenance of the relative position of body parts must be supplemented by an analysis of the physiological mechanisms required for forming the basis of spatial orientation. The notion of spatial orientation apparently includes a set of different properties, such as the ability to form the concepts of verticality and horizontality, and to determine, for example, the directions of different objects in external space, their relative positions, and the distances to them. These aspects of spatial orientation are considered in other chapters. We are going to discuss only those aspects that are connected with the maintenance of posture.

Postural regulation and the internal model of the body

At a superficial level the maintenance of the body attitude with respect to external space seems to be a rather simple task or problem that can be solved by a limited set of reflex mechanisms: for example, the labyrinthine reflexes relating head position to limbs position, the stretch reflexes in anti-gravity muscles, and the placing reactions. Nevertheless, the tasks involved in postural regulation are considerably more complex than the simple maintenance of a fixed body position in space. They include also the postural anticipation of the in-coming movement, the maintenance of equilibrium during locomotion, and the co-ordination of posture and movement. But even simple maintenance of the vertical posture in man cannot be reduced to a simple set of local stretch reflexes. Even if one assumes that this is a primary mechanism for maintaining selected joint angles, a question still remains regarding the designation of these angles, and the control of reflex characteristics during voluntary alterations of posture or during changes in external conditions. To regulate the body position with respect to the vertical, the central nervous system (CNS) must have at least an internal representation of the vertical. Such a broad spectrum of tasks in postural regulation can hardly be ensured by a simple control system based exclusively on reflex reactions. In this connection it is worth noting that in the field of artificial intelligence and robotics the interaction of an object with an environment is organized on the basis of two models: the model of the environment and the model of the object itself. Similar ideas also appeared in the early physiological record. According to this view, '. . . the organism carries in its head not only a map of external events but a small-scale model of external reality and of its own possible action' (Adrian 1947). Presumably the central organization of posture is also based on an internal model of the body, and on its internal representation in the CNS, i.e. on a system that is known in the physio-logical and clinical record as the 'body scheme'. One must stress that although the concept of the body scheme was introduced by Head and Holmes (1911–1912) at the beginning of this century and has attracted considerable attention among clinicians, physiologists, and psychologists, neither the functional role of the scheme in the system of spatial orienta-tion nor the underlying physiological mechanisms have been elucidated. However, as has been stressed by Paillard (1982), the study of the body scheme should contribute to the elaboration of an integrative approach to the solution of the main problems in the neurobiology of the behaviour. In this connection it seems to us that one needs to search for experimental approaches to the investigation of the body scheme at both the perceptual and automatic levels.

Perceptual aspects of the body scheme

Let us begin with the perceptual aspects of the body scheme. It is well known that the human hand is abundantly provided with skin receptors of pressure and touch, and with muscle, tendon, and joint receptors respond-ing to force, length, angle, velocity, etc. A superficial approach may give rise to the conclusion that such an abundance of receptors and their broad central projections allow the accurate elaboration of hand representation without addressing any additional internal model. But actually this is not so, as can be shown using the finger–nose test. One of the conditions required for successfully fulfilling this test is the availability of information about the spatial position of the finger tip. By what means can the CNS obtain such information? It is easy to see that information about this position cannot be obtained by any receptor because receptors for the 'finger tip' do not exist. Its co-ordinates can be obtained only from the values of joint angles using information about the length of kinematic links and their order. These data must be available in the CNS before the initiation of the movement. Only the internal model is capable of providing them. In this connection one is reminded of the words of Merleau-Ponty (1945), that the body scheme is not a result of association of kinaesthetic cues but rather a framework in which these cues are synthesized on the basis of some internal representation. Thus the body scheme can be thought of as a system ensuring the spatial orientation of an organism.

The conjectures about the existence of such a system arose long ago, primarily from clinical observations of 'phantom limbs' in amputees. It is interesting that a similar phenomenon can be reproduced in healthy humans (Melzack and Bromage 1973; Gross and Melzack 1978; Gurfinkel *et al.* 1986) by brachial plexus blockade or in the corresponding ischaemic blockade. In these studies it was found that with pressure-cuff ischaemia one can observe dissociation between the real and perceived positions of the limb. Sometimes this dissociation can be quite considerable. The illusory position of the hand does not remain constant. The subject frequently reports that his arm is flexing and extending, sometimes rather slowly and sometimes quite fast. It is worth noting that pressure-cuff ischaemia never leads to the sensation that a limb or a part of a limb has disappeared. This fact illustrates that some type of a list or enumeration of body parts exists in the CNS. This list has a considerable degree of resistance to changes in peripheral input. Less conservative are the representations of the length of the links: if we ask the subject to show the positions of the elbow, wrist, and finger tips (without touching them), the estimated distances between these points are usually less than the actual distances. It is thus a reasonable assumption that the positions of the body parts are perceived not on the basis of 'raw' or even substantially processed proprioceptive information but rather by means of a more complex scheme of information providing an internal representation of various compartments of the body, and having a considerable degree of autonomy. The disruption of afferent input disturbs the attachment of this model to the external space, but the model itself remains intact and serves as a basis for perception. The observations on the amputational 'phantom' show that the disappearance of internal model takes a very long time, amounting to some years.

The necessary condition for observing an experimental 'phantom' is the exclusion of vision. Opening the eyes leads to immediate merging of the 'phantom' and real limb and to the cessation of apparent movements. Presumably vision plays a leading role in the attachment of the internal model to the external space.

The consequences of dissociating the real and perceived positions are manifested strikingly in experiments in which the subject must hit a target with a finger of the ischaemic hand (Fig. 9.1). When the target (the index finger of the intact hand) was situated in a sector between the real hand and

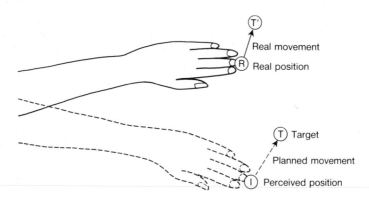

Fig. 9.1. The experimental 'phantom' produced by pressure-cuff ischaemia (for details see text).

the 'phantom' the subject, based on the wrong sensation of limb position, made a movement in the direction opposite to the one in which he should have moved to hit the target. As a result his finger did not approach the target but moved away from it. A similar effect was seen when the subjects attempted to reproduce a prescribed angle (90°) in the elbow joint. The subjects did this incorrectly, but in this case the source of the mistake was the wrong representation of the initial angle and not the inability of the subject to change the joint angle to the required value. The subject reproduced an angle differing from 90° by a difference amounting to that between the real and illusory hand positions. This experiment shows that the phenomena in question concern not only the sensory domain. The fact that the planning and execution of voluntary movements in the body-related reference system is accomplished on the basis of the illusory limb position indicates that the internal model serves not only the conscious perception of position but also the organization of motor activity.

One must stress that the functions of the body scheme are not limited to the perception of the spatial positions of body parts. In many cases the perception of external stimuli requires assessment of the position of different body parts and consequently requires the participation of the body scheme. This can be illustrated by an example dealing with the processing of tactile information.

In this respect the so-called skin writing test is most convenient. Skin writing attracted the attention of investigators because the perceived trace of the stimulus moving over the skin reflects a complex brain process, which differs substantially from a simple response to the excitation of skin receptors and depends on the integration of tactile information and information about the orientation of the receptive field. In such experiments, some stimulus, generally a digit or a letter, is traced on the subject's skin with a wooden stick (Natsoulas and Dubanoski 1964; Caffara *et al.* 1976; Gurfinkel *et al.* 1985; Parsons and Shimojo 1987). The subject must indicate which character was presented. Despite some differences in the data and their interpretation, some of the most essential results were confirmed by every investigator. First of all the interpretation of tactile stimuli by humans depends on the receptive field that is stimulated. The same character is perceived by subject as 'b' if it is traced on the front or as 'd' if it is traced on the back of the hand. This principle also extends over all the ventral and dorsal body surfaces of a standing person. In respect of position of the experimenter the characters written on the frontal surfaces (chest, abdomen) are perceived by the subjects as mirror images of the characters drawn on the dorsal surfaces (back, neck dorsum). Nevertheless the rules of perception can change as a result of a change of body position with respect to the gravitational vertical: such a change often can provoke the change of 'up' and 'down' in the perceived figures. Probably the most interesting is the outcome of skin writing on surfaces that can be turned both forward and backward. One such body surface is a palm. When the palm is turned away from the subject, the characters on it are perceived as mirror images; when the palm is facing the subject, i.e. is turned backward, the characters are perceived as 'direct'.

Based on findings in the monkey (Pons 1988), one can assume that in man also the signals from skin receptors come to the somatosensory cortex without any essential transformations. One can also assume that the trajectory of the excitation point over the projective area of cortex does not change after turning of the palm. Presumably, decoding the signals from skin receptors is done at a higher level of the CNS, where the representation of the current body position is synthesized and where the information from the receptors of different modalities converges. We can assume that this is the level of the body scheme.

The transition from drawing the characters with a stick to the use of a special vibro-tactile matrix to produce standard stimuli allowed measurement of the latent time of the response (Gurfinkel *et al.* 1990). Comparison of the response times when the palm was facing the subject and when it was turned away from him has not revealed such significant differences in latency which could be attributed to the mental rotation of the character through 180° around a vertical axis. Presumably the tactile signal comes to consciousness complete with the required 'spatial sign'. In other words, information about the position of body parts is taken into account in the still subconscious, automatic levels of processing.

The findings cited so far allow us to hypothesize that the body scheme is a supramodal organization, containing information about the kinematic structure of thc body and about the dimensions of its links and their mass–inertial characteristics, synthesizing different types of afferent signals, and presenting the results of this synthesis in the form of spatial co-ordinates and trajectories of body parts.

Analysis of the findings for skin writing shows that the widely accepted point of view, according to which the body scheme is some kind of a map (i.e. a static structure serving as a comparison with current, afferent input and usually identified with somatotopic representation), is wrong. More correct seems to be the view of Head (1920), which stressed the dynamic nature of the body scheme and assumed that body schemata are not fixed pictures or blue-prints, but flexible organizations that are responsive to changes in stimulation. For Head, schemata were processes as well as structures.

The automatic level of the postural body scheme

The above mentioned findings concern the tasks more or less directly connected with the conscious perception of body position. Nevertheless, the conscious level reflects only a small part of the CNS activity underlying the accomplishment of spatially oriented actions. It can be assumed that a considerable part of the body scheme's functions are connected not with perception but with sensorimotor processes forming the basis of postural and motor control. Such processes—for example, the transition from spatial trajectories of movements to the muscular torques that are necessary for their realization; the distribution of tonic activity between the muscle groups maintaining the selected set of joint angles; the mutual adjustment of posture and movement; the ensuring of body equilibrium in the gravitational field by control of muscular tension—are accomplished automatically, without the participation of consciousness. So it is reasonable to assume that the main part of the actions performed by the body scheme in the organization of motor acts proceeds at the subconscious level. This level, containing the internal neural model of the body and including the set of basic motor mechanisms and of algorithms for their co-ordination, represents a main, automatic part of the body scheme. We are sure that the study of this automatic part is of special value in understanding the control of posture and movement.

The primary difficulty in the study of the automatic level of the body scheme is the unsuitability of the traditional psychological and clinical approaches. We have assumed that physiological methods can bring about progress in this matter.

The problems in such studies are connected with the need to differentiate between manifestations of the functioning of the unified central organization (body scheme) and the results of interaction between a number of local postural and motor automatisms. Both centrally organized and local reactions can have similar external manifestations. Nevertheless, it can be assumed that postural reactions under the control of the body scheme must function in co-ordination with the internal representation of postural attitude. Of course, if the internal representation of the body coincides with its actual configuration, then it is very difficult to separate centrally organized reactions and reflex reactions from the more direct proprioceptive, vestibular, and visual inputs. So, to obtain the answer to the stated question it is necessary to select experimental paradigms that will allow of dissociation between the internal representation and the actual spatial configuration of the particular body. A choice of postural reactions that are sufficiently sensitive to changes of body configuration is also important.

Of the static and stato-kinetic postural reactions, thoroughly investigated by Magnus and his followers (Magnus 1924), one of the key places belongs to the so-called neck reflexes. Neck reflexes express themselves as a redistribution of the tension of the limb muscles in response to a change in the position of the head in relation to the trunk or, more precisely, to a change in the position of the trunk relative to the immobile head. The use of such reactions would be rather convenient for study of the stated problem. Unfortunately, it is difficult to observe neck reflexes in healthy adult humans. As far as they presumably still exist in humans in a latent form, it was necessary to find conditions proper for their manifestation. Convenient ways of demonstrating such influences of the neck do exist: these are methods that allow of an increase in the level of excitability of the brain stem–spinal structures mediating tonic control.

The state after the sustained voluntary activation of muscles (post-contraction effect), first described by Kohnstamm (1915), opens up such a possibility. As early as 1944, Wells (1944) attempted to use the Kohnstamm phenomenon to demonstrate the influences of the neck on the limb muscles in humans. For our observation of that phenomenon we used the following paradigm (Gurfinkel *et al.* 1989a). The subject was seated in a high armchair; his feet were not touching the floor. The subject maintained an isometric contraction of both quadriceps muscles (approximately 30 per cent of maximal voluntary contraction), pressing his calves against a stop for a period of 40 to 60 s. After a signal the subject stopped the voluntary effort and relaxed. The stop limiting the movement was removed. After 1–2 s the muscles began to contract involuntary, producing extension of the knee joints. This post-activation effect usually lasted for 30 to 60 s. If the head was in a neutral position the reactions of two legs were approximately equal. If the head was turned on the vertical axis, the extension was usually decreased on the chin-side and increased on the occipital side.

In the second type of experiment, tonic activity of the knee joint extensors was induced by bilateral vibration. In most experiments the vibrators were placed at the Achilles tendons. When there was no contact between the feet and the floor the vibration did not evoke a tonic vibration reflex (TVR; see below) in the soleus muscles, but activated the quadriceps muscles instead. The leg extension observed under these conditions also depended appreciably on the position of the head with respect to the trunk.

The performing of such experiments demands some pre-selection of subjects. They must have good reactions to muscle vibration and pronounced Kohnstamm phenomena; they must be able to relax and not resist the involuntary movements induced in the trials. We observed good neck influences on post-contractional and vibration-induced activity in nine subjects from an initial group of twenty (Gurfinkel *et al.* 1989b).

The results of a typical experiment are shown in Fig. 9.2. They were similar in both types of trial. Head rotation to the right suppressed the extension of the right knee and increased the extension of the left one; opposite reactions were observed during head rotation to the left. In the most sensitive subjects the effect was so strong that on the chin side the activity of extensors was totally inhibited, and the knee flexors were activated instead.

Nevertheless, one must stress that the pattern of neck reactions in humans is not strictly fixed; it depends on other postural factors. For example, inclination of the trunk forwards can reverse the sign of the reaction in the head rotation. In three of the subjects in standard experimental conditions these reverse reactions were observed, but inclination of the trunk backwards produced reactions in a normal form.

The general features of the reactions induced by head rotation seem to be quite similar to the known neck reflexes, as described in detail for experimental animals (Roberts 1978). Nevertheless, the results of the experiments in which dissociation between the internal representation of head position and its real position was created speak about a more complex mechanism of neck influences. We have used three different methods to obtain dissociation between the real (actual) and perceived position of the head with respect to the body. The first of these methods was based on the

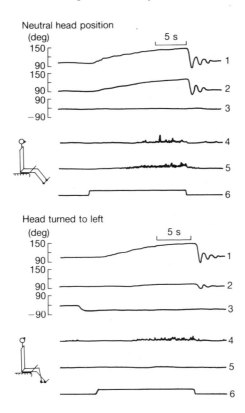

Fig. 9.2. Influence of head position on knee extension, evoked by vibration. Trace 1: knee angle of the right leg; trace 2: knee angle of the left leg; trace 3: head position (positive angles correspond to rotation to the right); trace 4: EMG of right quadriceps muscle; trace 5: EMG of left quadriceps muscle; trace 6: vibration marker.

illusions evoked by muscle vibration. It is known that vibration applied to the muscle can evoke a local TVR. The contraction of the muscle due to the TVR results in some movement. If this movement is prevented by sufficiently rigid fixation, TVR usually does not appear, and the illusory feeling of movement in the direction corresponding to the elongation of vibrated muscle appears instead. So vibration of the corresponding neck muscles can evoke head rotation, and when the head and trunk are fixed in the middle position, vibration applied to the same point evokes the illusion of head rotation in the opposite direction.

The other method of producing dissociation is based on the so-called return phenomenon. It is known that if a subject (with eyes closed) passively or actively keeps his head turned for a long time, he begins to feel that the head is slowly returning to a neutral (symmetrical) position. We used this effect in earlier studies of vestibulo-motor reactions (Gurfinkel *et al*. 1989c). In our studies of neck influences it was used to obtain dissociation between the internal representation of head position and its actual orientation. After 10 to 12 min of sitting with the head turned, the value of dissociation obtained by this method can reach 50 to 60°.

The last method of obtaining dissociation was based on the use of hypnotic suggestion. The details of experimental methods, where necessary, will be given together with the description of the results.

Let us begin with the experiments with vibration of the neck muscles. The location of the vibrator on the neck was selected in such a way as to obtain a net head rotation without any additional tilt. In the experiment illustrated in Fig. 9.3(a) the TVR in the vibrated muscle produced head rotation towards the right. After the beginning of the head turn the

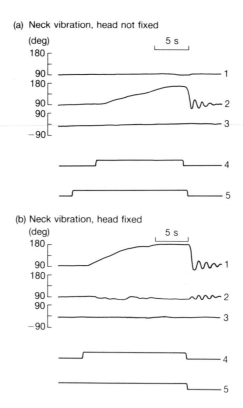

Fig. 9.3. Influence of vibration of neck muscles on knee extension evoked by vibration of Achilles tendons. (a) The head is not fixed. Vibration evokes a slight head rotation to the right. (b) The head and trunk are fixed. Neck vibration evokes an illusion of head rotation to the left. Trace 1: right knee angle; trace 2: left knee angle; trace 3: head position; trace 4: vibration marker (legs); trace 5: vibration marker (neck).

bilateral vibration of the Achilles tendons was switched on, producing extension of the left knee in accordance with the direction of head rotation. So the effect of vibration-induced head rotation did not differ from the effect of a voluntary or passive turn. An example of the vibration-induced illusion of head rotation to the left is shown in Fig. 9.3(b). The location of the vibrator was the same as in previous case [Fig. 9.3(a)], but this time the head and trunk were isometrically fixed. In the conditions of illusory head turning, extension of the right knee was observed. The asymmetry of the leg reactions during illusory rotation was even more pronounced than during the real turn. In particular, a small flexion of the left knee could be seen.

Figure 9.4 presents a sequence of trials (vibration of Achilles tendons) performed 1, 4, 6, 8, and 10 min after the subject had turned his head to the right. The subject indicated his perception of head orientation by means of a joystick. In the control test with a neutral head position the legs responded to bilateral vibration symmetrically. Immediately after the head turn the reaction in the right leg disappeared; the extension of the left knee increased. Four minutes later the effect on the left leg had diminished and a weak response had appeared in the right leg. The difference in the reactions of two sides decreased greatly in the sixth minute, when the subjective return of the head to a neutral position became obvious. The

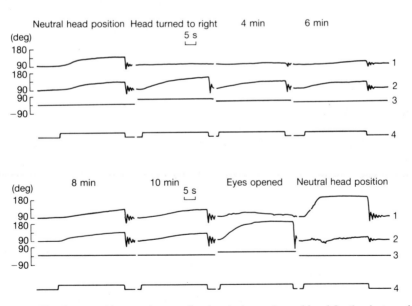

Fig. 9.4. The changes of leg reactions to vibration during prolonged head fixation in turned position (rotation to the right). Trace 1: right knee angle; trace 2: left knee angle; trace 3: perceived position of the head; trace 4: vibration marker.

asymmetry disappeared 8–10 min after the head turn, in accordance with almost total illusory return to the normal position. When the eyes were opened and the perception of the actual head position became available to the subject, the asymmetry immediately reappeared. Then the subject was ordered to close his eyes again. This time the subjective return of the head was much more rapid (3 min). Before the last test the head was passively returned to the neutral position by the experimenter. The eyes were kept closed. The subject perceived the new position of the head as slightly turned to the left. In agreement with this internal representation of the head orientation, the extension was suppressed on the left side and sharply strengthened on the right side.

The observed effect cannot be explained by adaptation of the neck receptors. The active maintenance of the head in a turned position requires the permanent activity of neck muscles, and in these conditions the responses of neck receptors do not change drastically. The reactions that appear after the re-establishment of the 'visual contact' with the real world confirm that the changes in the leg responses to vibration correspond to the perception of head orientation and are not determined by adaptation.

Hypnotic suggestion can be used as one way of producing dissociation between the real and perceived position of some body part. Furthermore, as it is known that hypnosis can induce pronounced changes in muscular tonus (catalepsy) and change the sensitivity to pain, tactile, and proprioceptive inputs, experiments under hypnosis are also of interest in the study of postural automatisms. In this connection we made a series of tests in which changes in perceived head position were suggested to subjects in a state of hypnotic sleep.

In some trials we also investigated the influences of real head rotation on the limb movements induced by hypnosis, the characteristics of such movements after asymmetrical tonic changes created by unilateral vibration or sustained voluntary contraction, and the tonic reactions under hypnotically suggested changes of sensitivity to vibration. Experiments were conducted with the participation of a specialist psychotherapist who regularly practised hypnosis. Seven subjects selected by the psychotherapist from an initial group of 15 took part in the experiments.

It is worth noting that to obtain illusions of head rotation we did not need especially deep hypnosis. Illusions were easily evoked even when the subjects had no catalepsy and the possibility of voluntary movement was not lost.

As an example let us consider the experiments on one of the subjects in more detail. Before hypnosis, a control trial was conducted, which showed the usual pattern of leg reactions. After this preliminary trial the subject was brought into hypnotic sleep. When the hypnosis was deep enough (catalepsy; accomplishment of suggested movements), it was suggested to the subject that he 'will not feel either pain or vibration'. In this situation, the activation by vibration did not evoke tonic reactions of the leg muscles. After lifting the prohibition on sensitivity to vibration the background pattern of tonic reaction fully recovered. The reactions to head rotation were also standard. Then the psychotherapist asked the subject to maintain the head in the middle position and suggested to him that, although he was looking ahead, he distinctly perceived his head as turned to the right. This illusion gave rise to a redistribution of levels of tonic activity in the leg muscles in response to vibration. The vibratory response was deeply inhibited in the right leg and increased in the left leg, as it would be during actual head rotation. The hypnotic suggestion of head rotation to the left also gave a result fully consistent with the pattern seen during an actual left turn.

These findings were reproduced in all trials on all seven subjects. It is interesting that in many cases the reaction to the suggested illusion of head rotation was stronger than with the actual turn.

In addition to trails in which a head turn was suggested, also undertook the trials in which the subject held his head turned, but it was suggested to him that he was looking directly forward. In this experimental situation the asymmetry of the leg responses disappeared or was significantly diminished.

In the course of hypnosis the subject, in response to orders such as 'your legs go up by themselves, your legs float up' often produced different movements of the upper and lower extremities. As these movements were of a slow, tonic type, we assumed that they would also be sensitive to the effects of various postural factors. So, some minutes after vibration of the right leg, the suggested knee extension turned to be asymmetrical: the motion of the right leg was significantly ahead of the left one. Only after the psychotherapist specially drew the subject's attention to his left leg did its extension become stronger.

The suggested movements were also sensitive to head rotation. In one of the trials it was suggested to the subject that his hands and legs 'are very light and are floating up'. In response to this suggestion, a slow extension of the legs at the knee joints and a gradual raising of the arms began. After the motion had begun it was further suggested to the subject that his head was turned to the left. As a result the right leg extended more than the left, and the right arm also reached a higher level than the left.

Conclusions

We have used different methods of producing dissociation between the real and perceived body position to make it possible to evaluate different aspects of the function of the body scheme. Indeed, during proprioceptive illusions induced by vibration, the internal body model obtains false information about the lengthening of corresponding muscles; in 'return phenomenon' we are probably dealing with the 'drift' of the internal model to the most habitual referent posture; and hypnotic suggestion acts on the state of internal model through the subject's consciousness.

It is evident from a number of studies (Gurfinkel *et al.* 1985; van Sonderen *et al.* 1989) that internal representation participates in the control of voluntary, goal-oriented movements.

Our experiments with the dissociation of actual and perceived head position have shown that the system of internal representation also plays a prominent role in the control of postural automatisms.

The experiments of Craske and Craske (1986), in which concentrating attention on one of the extremities gave rise to a switching of the Kohnstamm phenomenon to this extremity from the contralateral one, also suggest the essential role of internal representation in postural control.

This point of view clearly contradicts the existing concept of the system of postural regulation as a set of reflex mechanisms. One would think that within the framework of the 'Körperstellung' system there exists a set of different reflexes (proprioceptive, vestibular, optical) sufficient to assure the maintenance of posture and return to equilibrium after external disturbances. Nevertheless, one must stress that the prerequisite for study of these reflexes is strict standardization of the experimental conditions. In contrast to its activity in natural motor behaviour, each reflex depends both on the number of other reflexes and on the great variety of factors acting through the higher levels of the CNS. Such phenomena as pre-setting and anticipatory postural activity cannot be fully realized at the level of interaction of separate reflexes. We have seen that in the experiments with head return, opening the eyes, i.e. re-establishing visual contact with the environment, produces rapidly recovery of the asymmetry of the leg reactions. Thus, the postural reactions are dependent on the visual reference system of the external world. It is clear that such dependencies are impossible without some central organization responsible for the global control of posture. So, in terms of our example, it seems to be more correct to speak not about the neck reflexes but about the neck influences on the muscles of the extremities. Of course, the assumed central organization can function only using the pre-existing reflex mechanisms and connections, inhibiting or activating them according to the context. The level of internal representation of postural attitude and the levels of executive reflex mechanisms are conjugated by some intermediate system, which functions out of conscious control. We believe that this system forms an automatic, unconscious part of the body scheme. The question may arise as to whether it is justifiable to include in the body scheme an organization dealing primarily with motor control? Nevertheless, it seems to us that our findings convincingly prove the close relationship between the automatic part of the body scheme and its perceptual part. First of all, the perceptive part of the body scheme forms the internal representation of postural attitude which, according to our findings, is an essential factor, acting on the high levels of motor control. We must stress that the perceptive and automatic parts of the body scheme behave similarly with respect to their binding to the external space: visual contact evokes both the immediate merging of the experimental 'phantom' with the real limb and an equally rapid bringing of the postural reactions into balance with the actual body configuration. It is interesting also that the experimental 'phantom' reacts to the postural influences, for example on head rotation, in the same way as the actual limb does, and even a little stronger, as the 'motion' of the 'phantom' is not impeded by inertia, resistance, and other peripheral factors.

The data cited allow us to formulate some hypotheses about the organization of the internal model in the CNS. We can assume that it consists of the lower automatic level (the system of neural connections and algorithms for their use, ensuring postural control) and of a higher level—of the internal representation of body—forming the basis of conscious perception of body configuration, establishing its orientation with respect to the external world, and constructing the reference system. It is possible that on the same level of internal representation are accomplished the formulation of movement goals, and the choice of the spatial and time scales of motion. The automatic level translates these formulated tasks in terms of space-time, in the language of motor programmes. This concept can be considered as a further development of N. A. Bernstein's ideas about the hierarchical principles of multi-level movement organizations.

References

Adrian, E. D. (1947). *The physical background of perception*. Clarendon Press, Oxford.

Caffara, P., Mazzuccihi, A., and Parma, M. (1976). Osservavioni sulla percezionne cutanea degli stimoli figurati nell uomo in condizioni normali. *Bollettino della Societa Italiana di Biologia Sperimentale*, **52**, 2092–5.

Craske, B. and Craske, J. D. (1986). Oscillator mechanisms in the human motor system: investigating their properties using the aftercontraction effect. *Journal of Motor Behaviour*, **87**, 117–45.

Gross, G. and Melzack, R. (1978). Body image dissociation of real and perceived limbs by pressure-cuff ischemia. *Experimental Neurology*, **61**, (**6**), 680–8.

Gurfinkel, V. S., Debreva, E. E., and Levick, Yu. S. (1985). The dependence of the interpretation of tactile stimuli on orientation of receptive field. *Human Physiology*, **11**, 3–6. (in Russian).

Gurfinkel, V. S., Debreva, E. E., and Levick, Yu. S. (1986). The role of internal model in the perception and in the movement planning. *Human Physiology*, **12**, 769–76 (in Russian).

Gurfinkel, V. S., Levick, Yu. S., and Lebedev, M. A. (1989a). Immediate and remote postactivation effects in the human motor system. *Neurophysiology*, **21**, 343–51 (in Russian).

Gurfinkel, V. S., Levick, Yu.S., and Lebedev, M. A. (1989b). The postural automatisms revealed by the enhancement of tonic background. *Doklady USSR Academy of Science*, **305**, 1266–9 (in Russian).

Gurfinkel, V. S., Popov, K. E., Smetanin, B. N., and Shlykov, V.Yu. (1989c). Changes in the direction of the vestibulomotor during adaptation to the long-lasting static head turning in man. *Neurophysiology*, **21**, 210–17 (in Russian).

Gurfinkel, V. S., Lestienne, F., Levick, Yu. S., Popov, K. E., and LeFort, L. (1990). The egocentric references and human spatial orientation in microgravity. In *Proceedings of ESA conference on life sciences*, Trieste (in press).

Head, H. and Holmes, G. (1911–1912). Sensory disturbances from cerebral lesions. *Brain*, **34**, 102–254.

Head, H. (1920). *Studies in neurology*, Vol. 2. Oxford University Press, London.

Kohnstamm, O. (1915). Demonstration einer Katatonieartigen Erscheinung beim Gesunden (Katatonusversuch). *Neurologische Zentralblatt*, **34**, 290–1.

Magnus, R. (1924). *Körperstellung*. Springer, Berlin.

Melzack, R. and Bromage, P. R. (1973). Experimental phantom limbs. *Experimental Neurology*, **39**, 261–9.

Merleau-Ponty, M. (1945). *Phénomenologie de la perception*. Gallimard, Paris.

Natsoulas, T. and Dubanoski, R. (1964). Inferring the locus and orientation of the perceiver from responses to stimulation of the skin. *American Journal of Psychology*, **77**, 281–5.

Paillard, J. (1982). Le corps et ses langages d'espace. In *Le corps en psychiatrie* (ed. E. Jeddi), pp. 53–69. Masson, Paris.

Parsons, L. M. and Shimojo, Sh. (1987). Perceived spatial organization of cutaneous patterns on the surface of the human body in various positions. *Journal of Experimental Psychology. Human perception and performance*, **13**, 488–504.

Pons, T. P. (1988). Representation of form in the somatosensory system. *Trends in Neurosciences*, **11**, 373–5.

Roberts, T. D. M. (1978). *Neurophysiology of postural mechanisms*. Butterworths, London.

van Sonderen, J. F., Geilen, C. C. A. M., and Denier van der Gon, J. J. (1989). Motor programmes for goal directed movements are continuously adjusted according to changes in target location. *Experimental Brain Research*, **78**, 139–46.

Wells, S. W. (1944). The demonstration of tonic neck and labyrinthine reflexes and positive heliotropic responses in normal human subjects. *Science*, **99**, 36–7.

10

Motor and representational framing of space

JACQUES PAILLARD

Introduction

The intention here is to focus on some motor-oriented approaches to the spatial functions of the brain and to see how far they contribute to our understanding of the way in which the internal metric of spatial information is neurally encoded.

A motor-oriented approach assumes that the principal metric for coding spatial relationships is derived from the body's own movements in space: that is, the spatial relationship between two locations can be coded in terms of the movement required to get from one to the other. To what extent this approach can account for a plurality of sensorimotor action-spaces and also explain how a variety of spatial representations are encoded in the brain is open to question and will now be addressed.

A basic assumption of our argument is that a *sensorimotor* mode of processing spatial information coexists with a *representational* mode and that both modes are generating and storing their own mapping of space (Paillard 1987).

The *sensorimotor mode* concerns mainly that part of the physical world to which the organism is attuned by virtue of its basic sensorimotor apparatus. Local sensorimotor instruments entertain direct dialogues with that world and thus contribute to the continuous updating of a body-centred mapping of extra-corporal space where objects are located and to which actions are directed.

The *representational mode* derives from neural activities which explore and consult internal representations of the physical environment, that are embodied in memory stores. They include mental representations of local maps, spatial relationships of routes relative to landmarks, relative positions between objects, and the position of the body itself in relation to its stationary environmental frame.

The question arises as to whether the two processing modes operate in parallel, each using its own neural circuitry and generating its own mapping of space in two fundamentally different ways.

Sensorimotor dialogues and action spaces

Like a chemical molecule, the body has active sites at the cutaneous frontier that separates its internal territory from its environment. Specialized sensorimotor devices characterize these active sites: the mouth, the eyes, and the hand are prototypical examples. Each active site instantiates anatomical dispositions that are specifically tuned for a selective sensorimotor dialogue (Paillard 1971).

Each of these dialogues delimits an autonomous, regional 'sensorimotor space'. The boundaries of that space are specified by both the perimeter of its receptive field and the action radius of the motor apparatus that orients the sensory organ in its action space.

The mathematician tells us that a prerequisite for the description of a *'structure of space'* is the presence in that space of elements that are separately discernible by the observer. The discriminatory power of the sensory surface will therefore determine the basic grain of such a structure.

The mathematician also suggests that a collection of separate points is not sufficient for defining a structure of space (Arbib 1981). A rule for describing the potential relationships between the elements of the collection is mandatory. These rules, of which the choice may be arbitrary for the mathematician, defines what is called the *geometry of description* of the spatial structure. Of special interest, here, are certain metric rules which define in a structure of space what is called its *'path structure'*. These rules determine, in direction and distance, the trajectory to follow in order to move from one point to another. A 'path structure', superimposed on a collection of separate points, defines the *locality* of each of these points in a vectorial map.

A plurality of sensorimotor spaces

This kind of geometry is particularly suitable for a description of a sensorimotor space. Motor commands that displace a given sensory receptive surface from one point to another of physical space are generally prescribed in terms of direction and distance. They therefore fit the requirements for the definition of a path structure (Paillard 1987).

The visual field provides the best example of this kind of organization. The grain of the retinal receptors obviously defines the grain of the visual spatial structure. Ocular saccades are programmed in direction and distance in a retinocentric co-ordinate system. A clear mapping of these programs is known to exist in the deep layers of the superior colliculus. Saccades allow the foveal zone of the retina to be transported to visual targets located anywhere in the retinal field, by computing a 'motor error'

(Sparks 1989; and Chapter 1, this volume), i.e. the positional error of the eye, which is coded in terms of the motor command required to move it to a new position and thus cancel the error. Such motor commands could constitute the web of a path structure defining the '*visuo-ocular motor space*' within which targets are located in a retinocentric system of space co-ordinates.

Consider now what happens when the head is allowed to move. A new spatial reality emerges, delineated by the displacement of the head as carrier of the eyes. It is the head movements and their motor instruments that now impose their own path structure on visuomotor space. In this case, it is clear that visuo-ocular motor space constitutes only a sub-space of visuo-cephalo motor space. Accordingly, the same place in extra-corporal physical space can be defined by two different 'path structures': one derived from eye-movement programs and the other from the motor programs that move the head. Thus, it is imperative to establish a correspondence between these two co-ordinate systems in order to insure coherence in the visuo-ocular-cephalo mapping of the spatial surround.

This raises two problems, now well identified by experimenters in this field: the coordination of eye and head movements (Bizzi 1974; see also Chapter 3, this volume) that allows the stabilization of gaze on stable features of the environment; and the neural coding of ocular saccades in a head-centric co-ordinate system (Robinson 1975; see also Chapter 5, this volume). The analysis can, indeed, be further pursued, taking into account the orientation and displacements of the whole body as carrier of the head. A '*visuo-locomotor space structure*' then comes into play, which integrates the visuomotor sub-spaces of eye and head in order to locate objects in the stable environmental frame in which the body is moving.

Hence the concept of a *plurality* of visuomotor space structures emerges, each having its own motor descriptions of spatial relationships in the visual field. Each description conveys its own private path structure.

Conversely, the same path structures—consequently, the same motor instruments—can be associated with different sensory inputs and then mapped onto different sensorimotor space structures which may vary according to the sensory channel involved (Paillard 1982). This is obviously the case for head-orienting movements towards visual, auditory or olfactory targets, and even toward peribuccal tactile targets to be seized by the mouth. Consequently, the light, the sound, and the smell that emanate from sources located in the same direction of physical space, which then trigger the same orienting movement of the head, would therefore have a common encoding in the head-centred path structure. This encoding, however, is restricted to the common direction of the different sensory sources and ignores their distances. Distance coding depends on mechanisms different from those of direction and is generally modality-specific.

Vision, audition, and smell, for instance, have each a very specific mode for encoding the distance of sensory sources in the head-centric system of reference.

The positioning of the hand within 'reach space' is another striking example. Motor commands that actively displace the arm (as carrier of the hand) define a path structure that relates the position of the hand within the proprioceptive field of postural body space. The hand, however, can also be looked upon as a visual target and positioned in a visuo-cephalo-motor space structure. Morcover, tactile contact with physical matter in extra-corporal space, or even with the cutaneous interface of the body space, serves to calibrate autonomous tactilo-motor spaces. Here, for example, the luminous target that I touch with my finger-tip has the same encoded location in the proprioceptive path structure of my motor reach space.

Likewise, the manipulation operates in a 'hand space' which has its own private hapto-motor organization. Depending on the functional goal of the action (power grip, precision grip, or palpation), a diversity of private manual-motor spaces—proprioceptive, tactile, haptic or visuo-motor (Lederman and Klatzky 1987)—is available for selection according to the demands of the task. A recent demonstration by Strick and Preston (1982) of two separate hand maps in the motor cortex—one mainly afferented by proprioceptive, and the other by cutaneous information—points in this direction; and data from single unit recordings that dissociate power and precision grip (Gotschalk *et al.* 1981) support this approach. Rizzolatti *et al.* (1987) also describe, in the inferior premotor area, units associating peri-buccal tactile space with 'hand–mouth' path structures.

By the same token, a subdivision of the retinal field into two distinct sub-spaces has been suggested (Frost and Pöppel 1976). They can be related respectively to the motor space of a small saccade system (cortically controlled and operating in central vision) and to the motor space linked to peripheral vision involving the system of large ocular saccades (generally co-programmed with concomitant head movements).

Likewise, a similar problem emerges in the sensorimotor fields associated with depth vision, which are related to two motor systems : binocular vergence and accommodation of the crystalline lens (Poggio and Talbot 1981).

In brief, we suggest that the properties of local sensorimotor spaces provide the conditions required for the registering of proprioceptive information (or any other signals associated with motor commands) derived from orienting movements, together with co-variant information (visual, tactile, auditory and any combination thereof) about the positional changes of targets within the sensory map of the receptive surface. Thus, the location of these targets becomes encoded within a hierarchy of specific sensorimotor path structures. Accordingly, there must be as many sensorimotor mappings as there are associations between existing sensory channels and motor path structures (Paillard 1971, 1982).

So defined, a local sensorimotor space corresponds to a 'field of interaction' in the Lieblich and Arbid (1982) model, with the same mandatory requirement: the integration of multiple regional space structures into a super-ordinate system of space co-ordinates. Thus, the same locus of physical space—whatever the local sensorimotor space in which it is primarily registered and referred—has to be located at the same place in the spatial map of this super-ordinate system.

Although efferent copy signals appear to be a plausible component in the construction of visuo-ocular-motor path structures (without excluding the potential contribution of ocular proprioception), the generalization of their role to the somatic musculature seems unlikely (McCloskey 1978). In the latter case, the proprioceptive mapping of path structures is assumed to play a major role, and the problem of the integrative function of a 'body schema' emerges.

The body schema as a postural path structure

The basic assumption, here, is that every movement of articulated body segments is calibrated within the proprioceptive field of a postural space structure. Body space is envisaged as a proprioceptive-motor space where the distinct states of body postures are related by muscular activities that induce transition from one posture to another.

The existence of a repertoire of postural stereotypes, or motor synergies, (see Massion 1984), originally suggested by Ioffe (1973), has been clearly demonstrated by Nashner (1976). This repertoire of path structures may serve to specify the position of body segments within a space structure geocentrically oriented in the field of gravity (Paillard 1971). This *postural space structure* can be identified as the 'body schema' in the precise sense of Head and Holmes' (1911–1912) original definition: 'a combined standard against which all subsequent changes of posture are measured' and which intervenes in organizing spatially oriented activities 'before the change of posture enters consciousness'.

This postural space co-ordinate system is anchored to the invariant direction of gravity forces through the powerful mechanisms of maintaining an upright body posture. In agreement with Roberts (1973), who considered that the chief aim of postural regulation, in many species, is to stabilize the head in space, we have long emphasized (Paillard 1971) the pivotal role of the head segment in maintaining a 'geotropic statural referential', both in the stance of a static body and in its dynamic balance when moving (Berthoz and Pozzo 1989 and Berthoz in Chapter 6, this volume; Assaiante and Amblard 1990).

We consider this 'statural referential' to be the basic framework in which a superordinate integrated sensorimotor space could operate. It would allow the organization of the body-centred, egocentric space coordinates to which every position (or change of position) of sensory targets in physical space could be referred, whatever the sensory channel used for their detection. We are, then, in the presence of very elaborate sensorimotor machinery which can account for all the automatic posturo-kinetic adjustments that are required for the appropriate execution of spatially oriented movement.

As an illustration of these properties, we will consider two sets of experiments carried out in this laboratory: one dealing with the segregation of sensorimotor channels in the tactile modality; the other with a partition of the body-schema into a proximo-distal hierarchy of visuomotor subspaces.

Encoding the same tactile form in two different motor spaces

In an earlier study (Paillard 1971), a distinction was proposed between a 'location space' ('*un espace des lieux*') and a '*shape space*' ('*un espace des formes*'). This distinction was, of course, consonant with the then emerging dissociation of the 'two visual systems' (Ingle 1967; Schneider 1969; Trevarthen 1970; Held 1970) and with a functional segregation between 'identification' and 'location' in the processing of visual information. Emphasis was placed on the distinction between an 'object channel' and a 'space channel', the first dealing with the analysis of the various features of the object (including its shape) and the second with spatial problems (more specifically, the extra-personal space where objects are located). The distinction initially proposed between a shape space and a location space drew attention to the fact that visual identification and location processes both had to solve spatial problems, but within two different reference frames: one in an *object-centred* co-ordinate system, the other in a *body-centred* one. The former may use either the path structure of the ocular saccade motor system that palpates the object shape in central vision (see the scan-path hypothesis of Noton and Stark 1971), or an evaluation of the relative positions of the elements whose configuration composes the shape of the retinal image. The second uses the registration of gaze direction in a body-centred extra-personal space.

It follows that, depending on its size, a shape may be encoded either in the object-centred, retinal image system or in the body-centred, co-ordinate system.

An experiment carried out by Martinez (1971) addressed this type of spatial problem transposed it to tactile modality. In shape-recognition tasks, the analogy between the digital palpation of an object and its visual 'palpation' by the fovea is obvious. Likewise, the antecedent ocular saccade (often associated with a head movement) that centres the subject's gaze on the object and allows its subsequent palpation by the fovea has an obvious analogy with the transport of the hand in reaching space to a location where the object can be seized and palpated.

Palpation is clearly object-centred: once the object is grasped, exploration can proceed whatever the change of hand position in space. In contrast, the positioning of the hand to be within reach of the object is body-centred. Thus, we are, in the presence of two different sensorimotor spaces: one *hapto-digital*, which combines cutaneous and proprioceptive information with the palpating movements of the fingers in hand space; the other *visuo-brachial*, which links visual and proprioceptive information with the proximal movements that position the hand in its grasping space.

Martinez's experiment stemmed primarily from her observations of congenitally blind children learning bimanual Braille reading. They made many more mirror-image confusions when reading than sighted children of the same age. The hypothesis was therefore that tactile information collected by the tips of left and right index fingers from Braille symbols by movements of the arm, is calibrated in a body-centred frame of reference. Because of the bilateral symmetry of the motor system with respect to the mid-saggital plane, and the facility with which we can generate simultaneous, bilaterally symmetrical movements, it was envisaged that tactile forms encoded within two symmetrically arranged path structures could be perceived as identical, although mirror-framed in physical space. But then the question immediately arises: what would happen if the two tactile forms were encoded in the two hand spaces, which are independent of body space, postural constraints, and probably dependent on object space?

Between the ages of five and six years, sighted children also make frequent mirror-image confusions in matching shapes both visually and tactilely. In the experimental study, 40 children aged between five and a half and six, were given a task requiring the bimanual discrimination of symmetrical, tactile forms. The children were divided into two matched groups of two different conditions of tactile motor exploration. The first group relied entirely on digital manipulation; the wrist and the arm were immobilized. The second group explored the figures with the tip of the index finger by movements involving proximal limb joints, thus mobilizing the whole arm in its reaching space. The results, shown in Fig. 10.1, confirmed the initial hypothesis. Tactilo-motor exploration, referred to the sensorimotor space of palpation, did not produce significantly more errors than the analogous visual discrimination task. By contrast, the error rate increased very significantly when tactilo-motor exploration was referred to the sensorimotor space of hand positioning in 'reaching space' and thus related to the postural body frame. It is an open question whether a comparable interpretation is applicable to the domain of visual space.

J. Paillard

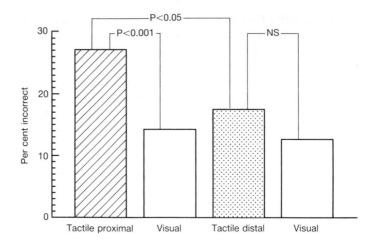

Fig. 10.1. Visual and tactile discrimination of symmetrical form (based on the data of Martinez 1971). Two matched groups of 20 children (between the ages of 5.6 and 6 years) were administered visual and tactual discrimination tests of symmetrical forms. The tests were identical for the two groups in the visual modality but differed in the tactile modality: one group used multi-digital manipulation with the arm and wrist immobilized (the tactile-distal condition: dotted column), and the other group used finger tip exploration using whole arm movements (the tactile proximal condition: hatched column). In the visual modality (white columns), both groups of children produce approximately 13 per cent mirror-image confusions when matching symmetrical visual forms. In the bimanual tactile condition, a comparable percentage of errors was found when subjects were required to identify, among three figures explored by one hand, the target form presented simultaneously for manipulation by the other hand. In this case, the exploration was multi-digital and restricted to motor hand space. In contrast, the error rate increased to 28 per cent when subjects used only the tip of their index finger and swept the figures with exploratory movements of the whole arm.

There is, however, preliminary evidence which suggests that this might be the case.

As previously mentioned Frost and Pöppel (1976) have proposed a subdivision of the retinal field into two distinct subspaces: one corresponding to the field of central vision (up to 10 per cent of eccentricity), where the small saccade system is strongly dependent on cortical control; the other related to the peripheral retina and associated with a system of large ocular saccades that are generally co-programmed with concomitant head movement. The latter movement obviously serves the need of orienting the gaze at different places in location space whereas the former operates within the object frame of shape space, where the scan-path theory of shape perception does not accommodate much of the experimental data. Consider the analogy with the tactile modality. The palpation of an object, whose size extends beyond the manipulation space of the hand, forces the displacement of the hand along the object surface and its contours. In like fashion, depending on the size of a visually-presented object, the encoding of its form could occur in either of the two systems or might even encompass both. The validation of such an hypothesis, however, would have to take into account the dominant strategy of the subject and the need to distinguish between 'eye movers' and 'head movers', a distinction recently introduced in a study of eye–head co-ordination in pointing (Bard *et al.* 1990). In the same vein, mirror-image confusions may be related to the observation that most young children are head-movers. They therefore appear to manipulate their visual space predominantly within a location space where the symmetrical organization of the postural schema presumably imposes its specific constraints.

A partition of the body schema into a hierarchy of local visuomotor spaces

The next set of experiments illustrates how the spatial problems involved in visuomotor reorganization after prismatic deviation of the visual field may shed light on the intrinsic organization of the body schema.

Subjects wearing prismatic goggles that displace their visual array, say 12° degrees to the right with regard to the saggital plane of the head, misreach visual targets located in their visual field by about the same angular error: that is, they point about 12° too far to the right of the real target. In other words, they see objects that are located straight ahead of them by looking 12° to the right in head-centric space. Their normal daily experience of visuomotor spaces, however, demonstrates that motor reaching programs are more effective when oriented in the direction of gaze. This normal calibration takes into consideration the position of the eye with respect to the head and, additionally, the position of the head with respect to the trunk. If the discrepancy introduced by the prisms between eye-position calibration with respect to the trunk is not experienced in the form of an error that can be corrected with feedback, then misreaching will persist. If, however, subjects are allowed to see their moving limb through the prisms for a short exposure period, then a readjustment occurs that results in a pointing program redirected toward the correct location of the target. It is still a matter of speculation as to where this recalibration takes place and it will not be further discussed here (but see Paillard *et al.* 1981). Suffice it to say that the remarkable capacity of the system to reorganize the structure of its visuomotor space offers an interesting opportunity for study of the properties of our putative local sensorimotor spaces.

The possibility of segregating the visuomotor sub-spaces involved in the recalibration process has been studied by Hay (1970) in conditions where the visual recalibrating exposure was restricted to a single joint movement.

Subjects were asked to point (without seeing their arms) in the direction of three visual targets distributed in the frontal plane. The directional accuracy of aiming was measured for single joint movements involving either the wrists (W), the elbow (E), or the shoulder (S). The same measurements were made in a condition where subjects wore prismatic goggles that displaced the visual field 12° to the right.

After these pre-tests, there was a period of exposure in which subjects were instructed to look at their hand moving to and fro in the visual field, for 5 min. in three different experimental conditions, using movement either of the wrist, of the elbow, or of the shoulder.

Each period of exposure was followed by a series of post-tests. Accuracy of aiming was again measured for each of the three single joint movements, vision of the limb again being occluded as in the pre-test condition. Comparison of accuracy in pre- and post-tests evaluates the amount of recalibration that follows each condition.

Without entering into the details of the experimental procedure, we may focus on the results shown in Fig. 10.2. In the condition (W), where the recalibrating experience is limited to wrist joint, there is a significant recalibration of aiming with the wrist, but accuracy of aim depending on elbow or shoulder movement does not show any significant readjustment.

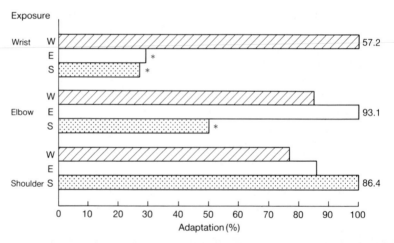

Fig. 10.2. Effects of single joint exposure on the recalibration of aiming movements after prismatic displacement of the visual field (based on the data of Hay 1970). Aiming movements were performed by movements restricted to one joint: wrist (W), elbow (E) or shoulder (S). The histograms show results obtained from 10 subjects who carried out 20 target-pointing movements for each joint. Depending on the joint whose movement was observed during the exposure period (wrist, elbow or shoulder), performance in aiming with the two other 'non exposed' joints expressed as a percentage of the amount of recalibration measured with the 'exposed' joint. The actual score (amount of readaptation) of the 'exposed' joint is given at the end of the corresponding column. The adaptation obtained from vision of shoulder movements during the exposure period generalizes significantly to elbow and wrist, whereas elbow adaptation generalizes only to the distal joint; wrist adaptation is not transferred to distal joints. Asterisks indicate significant effects.

When the period of exposure restricts vision to self-induced movements of the elbow (E), then aiming movements using the elbow joint are recalibrated, but those using the wrist joint are also significantly readjusted whereas pointing via the shoulder joint remains incorrect. Finally, the three joints are recalibrated when exposure is limited to vision only of the shoulder (S). Thus it follows that the recalibration involves the path structure of a local sensorimotor space defined by the motor field covered by the range of movement of a given joint. Moreover, a proximo-distal hierarchical subordination links these various sub-spaces. In fact, the recalibration observed with an exposed joint always transfers to the more distal joints (see Fig. 10.2). Moreover, as was often claimed in studies of prismatic adaptation, restriction of head movements is necessary to limit adaptation in the exposed limb, otherwise the recalibrating effect generalizes to all body joints. In a recent study (Paillard and Hay 1989), we were able to confirm the generalized recalibrating effect of active movement restricted to rotation of the head on the trunk, even in conditions when the eyes were stabilized by a gaze-fixation point attached to the head.

In brief, the segmentation of the body schema into sub-spaces interleaved in a proximo-distal hierarchical structure and dominated by the head segment clearly illustrates the plurality of bodily motor spaces. Thus, the body schema can be fractionated into sensorimotor sub-systems representing the motor synergies that are involved in specifying the path structures of the visuomotor sub-spaces. One additional feature of these sub-spaces is worth mentioning: visuomotor experience limited to only one direction of movement of a multi-dimensional ball joint recalibrates movements in any direction of three-dimensional space. It is also worth mentioning that this concept of a partition of motor space into a diversity of local action spaces has been recently brought forward by Rizzolatti and Gallese (1988) in a motor-oriented theory of attention.

From sensorimotor spaces to spatial representations

As already emphasized, spatial knowledge comes from a variety of sources and uses a variety of codes for its storage. The most basic knowledge is obviously that derived from Darwinian evolutionary selection. Printed in the in-built sensorimotor circuitry, it tunes neural mechanisms to the spatial constraints of both their body architecture and their environment.

Later acquisitions will enrich the basic repertoire of the sensorimotor machinery without changing radically the direct way in which sensory input is linked to motor commands. This machinery automatically surmounts the constraints of its action spaces and does not require any elaborate 'computational mapping' in order to generate 'data-driven', goal-directed behaviour (the 'taxon' systems of O'Keefe and Nadel 1978). In which case does knowledge, which is presumably embodied in some kind of internal map and which shapes anticipatory, memory-driven spatially oriented actions, depend on other sources of spatial information and require a specific encoding mode?

Internal representations are described by psychologists either as *images* embodied in an iconic code or as *mental representations* encoded in abstract or symbolic form. Neurobiologists, for their part, distinguish between *projectional maps*, which are relatively isomorphic with the peripheral arrangements of sensory receptors, and *computational maps*, which extract place codes from different input signals, without preserving any topographical arrangement of their constituent neurons. Sensory and motor maps of the neocortex are projectional whereas the place map of the hippocampus is assumed to be computational (see Chapter 16). The last term, borrowed from the field of artifical intelligence, may be misleading when applied to neural mapping, as Konishi (1986) has suggested. He proposed, instead, 'centrally synthesized maps' as a more neutral concept.

In fact, one important feature of biological systems (when compared with neuron-like networks) is their astonishing capacity to extract co-variant signals from the flow of sensoryinput that impinges on their sense organs, and to stabilize in the neural circuitry selective configurations of synapses that are co-variantly activated (Phillips *et al.* 1984).

The visible world and the body structure contain many redundancies and stable features. The static nature of the physical, visual background provides a stable environmental frame within which the moving body may orient itself and navigate.

Regularities of the physical environment are progressively encoded in the structure of central networks. Central space structures then emerge from the processing of a polymodal inflow of changing re-afferent information, generated by the displacements of the body within its environmental frame. Subsequently, this processing gives rise to a hierachy of distributed and layered populations of neurons from which some kind of 'central synthesized map' could be made.

The construction of these maps, however, might differ from that of conventional neuromimetic networks, which generally do not close the external loop between motor output and re-afferent input (see, however, Kupferstein 1988; and Chapter 22, this volume). In other words, computational networks are generally not able to entertain a sensorimotor dialogue with an extended environment that is, nevertheless, a source of parametric spatial knowledge.

It is these dialogues that allow the brain and its neural network to detect and register the spatial features of its environment that remain invariant or co-variant across the transformations generated in the sensory inflow by their own motor activity. The basic concept here is that of *re-afference*—a term coined by von Holst and Mittelstaedt (1950) to denote the consequences of self-produced movement on the sensory inflow.

Representational space maps would also differ from sensorimotor path structures in that they are predominantly tied to visual information about the environmental frame, whereas the path structures are closely linked to a proprioceptively defined, postural frame of reference. This is obviously the case for the locomotor space.

All mobile species, whatever their propulsive mechanism depending upon the supporting medium—earth, air, or water—have to structure their locomotor space. In contrast with activities that move individual body segments within the postural frame of reference, locomotor programmes involve rhythmical reproduction of an ordered sequence of limb movements, resulting in a displacement of the body as a whole. In this case, and in contrast with arm movement, the corresponding proprioceptive re-afferent information cannot provide the relevant information for encoding the parameters of locomotor trajectories and hence for the construction of a 'body-centred path structure'. That structure, however, may be defined by a system of inertial navigation using vestibular afference and computing the head position in an absolute physical space (see Potegal 1982; and Chapter 6). But there are also many co-variant changes in the retinal image of the outside world when the body moves, and these signals might also well serve to generate an internal representation of a stable environmental frame (Gibson 1950).

Thus, a motor-oriented interpretation of the construction of basic space structures may apply equally well to both the geotropic, body-centred frame of reference (to which most of our spatially directed actions are to be referred) and the central representation of space, which assumes an allocentric, stable environmental frame of reference (in which the ever-changing position of a moving body has permanently to be updated).

Representation of the environmental frame, however, does not exhaust the gamut of the various cognitive, mental representations of space studied by psychologists. Egocentric and allocentric descriptions of spatial relationships both refer to primitive adaptive processes in the affordance of an organism to its environment and, as such, lend some plausibility to the hypothesis of an inherited, allocentric frame of the kind envisaged by O'Keefe and Nadel (1978). Alternatively, more elaborate and abstract mappings of spacial relationships might evolve in man, especially in relation to the development of language with its propositional function, and also to the extension of topographical memory within the rich resources of spatial thinking.

Focusing on the two—egocentric and allocentric—reference frames, a central issue is to understand how these two co-ordinate systems may interact and co-operate together in the transactional processes that bind perception to action. Pointing tasks have provided a good experimental paradigm for exploring this question.

Egocentric versus allocentric reference frame in pointing

Inaccuracy in pointing at visual targets can usually be ascribed to imprecision in specifying information about the location of the target. Depending on the reference frame used by the organism, however, this location may be defined either egocentrically or allocentrically. When head and body position are fixed so that only the eyes are allowed to move, then the perceived oculocentric direction of the target is critical. In this condition, Conti and Beaubaton (1980) have shown that accuracy of pointing at a luminous target in complete darkness is significantly less than when pointing at a target illuminated in a structured visual field. The interpretation of this finding is that the perceived oculocentric direction of the target in both cases relies on two different modes of encoding. In darkness, the extra-retinal signal of eye position in the orbit (presumably derived from the oculomotor command signal) is the only one that can be used to calibrate the position of the target in relation to head position. The location of the target is then defined in an egocentric reference frame. In contrast, in a structural and visual array, additional visual cues are present which allow the target to be located in the environmental frame to which the position of the body has also to be referred.

The experimental dissociation of these two encoding modes for locating visual targets has been obtained in two ways: first, in dissociating the 'perceived' and the 'registered' location of the target in a motor pointing task; second, in separating the eye-position signal from the perceived oculocentric direction of the target.

Perceived and registered location

An experiment by Bridgeman *et al.* (1979) illustrates the former line of investigation. Subjects were asked to detect if a central target, flashed on during a saccadic eye movement, was moving or not moving and, if moving, whether toward the right or the left. They were also requested to point to the actual location of the target. The striking finding was that subjects consistently pointed correctly to the right or to the left, despite their failure (due to saccadic perceptual suppression) to perceive any displacement of the target. The conclusion was that the sensorimotor system had direct access to information that was not available at the perceptual level. More specifically, we may assume that egocentric information, as measured by pointing, is available to subjects even when exocentric information regarding displacement of the stimulus has been masked at the perceptual level.

A similar dissociation is observed in the 'blind sight' phenomenon: hemianopic patients who are not able to detect a target presented in their blind field can nevertheless point to it when forced to guess its location (see review in Weiskrantz 1989). A similar phenomenon has been observed in the tactile modality (Paillard *et al.* 1983). A patient with a de-afferented arm was able to locate correctly with her left hand punctate stimuli on her insensitive right arm. Her astonishment was particularly interesting: 'I don't understand why I am going there because I don't feel anything . . . Where does it come from?' Asked to describe her feelings more precisely, she tried unsuccessfully to use the vocabulary of seeing and hearing, and finally said: 'It's so tenuous, so tenuous you know . . . but I know that there is a place where you were going and I went there too.' Interestingly, she was describing this very unusual experience of space without identifiable sensory content in terms of 'knowing how to get there' (see Epilogue, this volume).

Another striking example of this dissociation is displayed by the 'Roelofs effect' exploited in an experiment by Bridgeman (1989). Stable targets, presented inside a moving frame, appear perceptually to move in a direction opposite to that of the frame. Subjects invited to state the position of the target verbally gave an incorrect location, whereas they pointed at the target in its real, physical position.

In conclusion, spatially oriented movements can be accurately directed by a sensorimotor mapping of path structures, even when the perceptual system is receiving inadequate or erroneous information, or even no information at all.

Location and dependency on eye position

The above conclusion has been further strengthened by the second line of investigation, which intervenes at the level of the extra-retinal signal. These experiments (reviewed by Jeannerod 1983 and Paillard 1987) used either reversible paralysis of the ocular muscles by D-tubocurarine (Matin *et al.* 1982) or a technique of 'eye press' (Stark and Bridgeman 1983) to suppress or reversibly modify the signal of eye–head position. The following conclusions have been drawn from these experiments. When the luminous target is inaccurately located, perceived position and manual pointing coincide, in darkness because of the incorrectly biased eye-position signal which displaces the egocentric frame of reference. When, however, the target is set within a visually textured frame, its perceived position no longer depends on the extra-retinal signal that calibrates it within the egocentric co-ordinate system. Instead, it is referred to the allocentric system of space co-ordinates in the environmental frame. Then, a correct perceptual evaluation of its real position in that frame (which coincides with the reality of the physical surrounding) is achieved. In contrast, the pointing movement continues to be driven to the wrong location corresponding to the incorrectly biased, extra-retinal signal.

Interactive contribution of egocentric and allocentric frames

Finally, we can observe the co-operative and interactive contribution of these two co-ordinate frames in experiments concerned with the recalibration of pointing programmes consequent upon prismatic displacement of the visual field. Without going into the procedural details of this experiment, (Paillard *et al.* 1981), consider here its main findings.

The two adaptation processes were dissociated, depending on the two different conditions of exposure: one condition permitted vision of hand movements against an homogeneous visual background; the other the presence of a stationary visual target or a whole structured visual field in which free hand movements were made. The former recalibration condition operates preferentially in *peripheral* vision (more than 40° eccentricity) and is suppressed by stroboscopic illumination of the visual field (at 3.5 pulses per second). Recalibration in the latter condition operates mainly in *central* vision and is not dependent upon whether the illumination is continuous or intermittent (Paillard *et al.* 1981).

The distinction made in this experiment between the recalibrational efficacy of *active* compared with *passive* movement provides an additional argument for making a clear, functional distinction between these two systems. Peripheral vision does not process visual information coming from a limb that is passively displaced during the period of exposure, whereas central vision, provided that there is a structured visual background, processes information from either the actively or the passively displaced limb to recalibrate the pointing program (see Fig. 10.3).

Our interpretation, therefore, was that adaptation provided by peripheral vision might be driven by a reshaping of path structures in the egocentric frame of reference, which needs proprioceptive, self-induced re-afferent information. In contrast, adaptation provided by central vision requires the visual localization of a moving limb within the stationary framework of a visual surround, where position and change of position of the hand are calibrated relative to the stationary cues of the visual frame. In the latter case, interestingly, the nature of the movement—active or passive—is irrelevant for the recalibration process.

We tentatively ascribed (Paillard and Amblard 1985) the central and peripheral vision system, respectively, to the X and Y visual channels described in the visual system of the cat. We now know that they may be assigned in man to the 'parvocellular' and the 'magnocellular' channels,

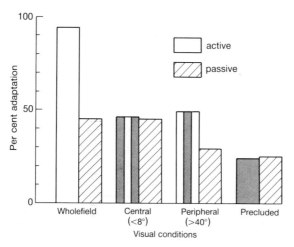

Fig. 10.3. Self-induced versus passive movements in prismatic adaptation (based on the data of Paillard *et al.* 1981). The histograms display percentage of adaptation shown after a 10 minute exposure period of the moving limb (moved actively or passively) in four different visual conditions (whole field, central, peripheral and occluded). The data were obtained from four subjects (selected as good adapters). In whole field vision, i.e. when both peripheral and central vision were involved, active movement led to near complete adaptation (94 per cent). In contrast, with vision of passive movement the amount of adaptation was significantly less, and did not exceed 48 per cent.

When restricted to central vision (<8° eccentricity) the percentage of adaptation remained virtually unchanged (46 versus 45 per cent) whether the observed movement was active or passive.

When only the peripheral field was involved (>40° eccentricity), the percentage of adaptation, which was 49 per cent with active movement, was reduced to 29 per cent with passive movement—i.e. to the basic level of adaptation that is observed when vision of the moving limb was totally precluded, and adaptation is attributed to extra-retinal factors.

respectively, according to the recently proposed division of visual pathways in primates (De Yoe and van Essen 1988). If so, the parvocellular system can be considered the main instrument for the processing of relative position both within object-centred space (where information about the shape and size of the object is mainly extracted by central vision), and world-centred space (where the relative position of objects to one another is measured within the allocentric frame of the stabilized, visual world). The magnocellular pathway, for its part, conveys information about the visual changes co-variant with self-induced, proprioceptive, re-afferent information from the moving limb. Here, there is a contribution from the peripheral retina to the elaboration of visuomotor space structures, whatever the motor instrument (eyes, head, limb, body as a whole) implicated in the specification of the path structure concerned.

This notion is obviously reminiscent of the 'exproprioceptive vision' as defined by Lee (1977) and derived from the Gibson concept of 'kinesthetic vision'. An important goal for future research, therefore, is to specify how

180   *J. Paillard*

and where proprioceptive and visual information converge in central nervous structures to align their space maps and how and where self-induced motor activities acquire their privileged role in calibrating or recalibrating our sensorimotor spaces.

References

Arbib, M. A. (1981). Perceptual structures and distributed motor control. In *Handbook of physiology*, Vol. 2, *Motor control* (ed. V. B. Brooks), pp. 1449–80. American Physiological Society, Bethesda, ML.
Assaiante, C. and Amblard, B. (1990). Head stabilization in space while walking: effect of visual deprivation in children and adults. In *Proceedings of the Xth international symposium on disorders of posture and gait* (ed. T. Brandt), pp. 262–6. Thieme Verlag, Stuttgart.
Bard, C., Fleury, M. and Paillard, J. (1990). Head orienting and aiming accuracy. In *Head–neck co-ordination* (ed. A. Berthoz, W. Graf, and J.-P. Vidal). (In press.)
Berthoz, A. and Pozzo, T. (1989). Intermittent head stabilization during postural and locomotory tasks in humans. In *Posture and gait: development, adaptation and modulation* (ed. B. Amblard, A. Berthoz, and F. Clarac), pp. 189–98. Elsevier, Amsterdam.
Bizzi, E. (1974). The coordination of eye–head movements. *Scientific American*, **231**, 100–6.
Bridgeman, B. (1989). Separate visual representations for perception and for visually guided behavior. In *Spatial instruments and spatial displays*, (ed. S. Ellis, M. Kayser, and A. Grunwald), p. 40.1–40.16, NASA, Mountain View, California.
Bridgeman, B., Lewis, S., Heit, G., and Nagle, M. (1979). Relation between cognitive and motor-oriented systems of visual position perception. *Journal of Experimental Psychology* and *Human Perception Performance*, **5**, 692–700.
Bridgeman, B., Kirch, M., and Sperling, A. (1981). Segregation of cognitive and motor aspects of visual function using induced motion. *Perception and Psychophysics*, **29**, 336–42.
Conti, P. and Beaubaton, D. (1980). Role of structural visual field and visual reafference in accuracy of pointing movements. *Perception and Motor Skills*, **50**, 239–41.
De Yoe, E. A. and Van Essen, D. C. (1988). Concurrent processing stream in monkey visual cortex. *Trends in Neuroscience*, **11**, 219–26.
Frost, D. and Pöppel, E. (1976). Different programming modes of human saccadic eye movements as a function of stimulus eccentricity: indications of a functional subdivision of the visual field. *Biological Cybernetics*, **23**, 39–48.
Gibson, J. J. (1950). *The perception of the visual world*. Houghton Mifflin, Boston.
Gotschalk, M., Lemon, R. N., Nijs, H. G. T., and Kuypers, H. G. J. M. (1981). Behaviour of neurons in monkey periarcuate and precentral cortex before and during visually guided arm and hand movements. *Experimental Brain Research*, **44**, 113–16.

Hay, L. (1970). Contribution à l'étude de l'organisation de l'espace postural chez l'Homme: étude expérimentale de l'adaptation des différents segments du corps à une déviation prismatique du champ visuel. *Cahiers de Psychologie*, **13**, 3–24.

Head, H. and Holmes, G. (1911–1912). Sensory disturbances from cerebral lesions. *Brain*, **34**, 102–245.

Held, R. (1970). Two modes of processing spatially distributed visual stimulation. In *The neurosciences second study program* (ed. F. O. Schmitt), pp. 317–24. The MIT Press. Cambridge, Massachussetts.

Ingle, D. J. (1967). Two visual mechanisms underlying the behaviour of fish. *Psychologische Forschung*, **31**, 44–51.

Ioffe, M. E. (1973). Pyramidal influences in establishment of new motor coordinations in dogs. *Physiology and Behavior*, **11**, 145–53.

Jeannerod, M. (1983). How do we direct our action in space? In *Spatially oriented behavior* (ed. A. Hein and M. Jeannerod), pp. 1–13. Springer-Verlag, Berlin.

Konishi, M. (1986). Centrally synthesized maps of sensory space. *Trends in Neuroscience*, **9**, 163–8.

Kupferstein, M. (1988). An adaptive neural model for mapping invariant target position. *Behavioral Neuroscience*, **102**, 148–62.

Lederman, S. J. and Klatsky, R. L. (1987). Hand movements: a window into haptic object recognition. *Cognitive Psychology*, **19**, 342–68.

Lee, D. N. (1977). The functions of vision. In *Modes of perceiving and processing information* (ed. H. L. Pick and E. Salbman). Erlbaum, Hillsdale, NJ.

Lieblich, J. and Arbib, M. A. (1982). Multiple representations of space underlying behavior. *Behavorial and Brain Science*, **5**, 627–59.

Martinez, F. (1971). Comparison of two types of tactile exploration in a task of a mirror-image recognition. *Psychonomic Science*, **22**, 124–5.

Massion, J. (1984). Postural changes accompanying voluntary movements. Normal and pathological aspects. *Human Neurobiology*, **2**, 261–7.

Matin, L., Picoult, E., Stevens, J., Edwards, M., and MacArthur, R. (1982). Oculoparalytic illusion: visual-field dependent mislocalization by humans partially paralysed with curare. *Science*, **216**, 198–201.

McCloskey, D. I. (1978). Corollary discharges: motor commands and perception. In *Handbook of physiology*, Vol. 2, *Motor control* (ed. V. Brooks), pp. 1415–47. American Physiological Society, Bethesda, MD.

Nasher, L. M. (1976). Adapting reflexes controlling the human posture. *Experimental Brain Research*, **26**, 59–72.

Noton, D. and Stark, L. (1971). Scan paths in saccadic eye movements while viewing and recognizing patterns. *Vision Research*, **11**, 929–42.

O'Keefe, J. and Nadel, L. (1978). *The hippocampus as a cognitive map*. Oxford University Press, Oxford.

Paillard, J. (1971). Les déterminants moteurs de l'organisation spatiale. *Cahiers de Psychologie*, **14**, 261–316.

Paillard, J. (1982). Le corps et ses languages d'espace. In *Le corps en psychiâtrie* (ed. E. Jeddi), pp. 53–69. Masson, Paris.

Paillard, J. (1987). Cognitive versus sensorimotor encoding of spatial information. In *Cognitive processing and spatial orientation in animal and man* (ed. P. Ellen and C. Blanc-Thinus), pp. 43–77. Martinus Nijhoff, Dordrecht.

182   *J. Paillard*

Paillard, J. and Amblard, B. (1985). Static versus kinetic visual cues for the processing of spatial relationships. In *Brain mechanisms and spatial vision* (ed. D. J. Ingle, M. Jeannerod, and D. N. Lee), pp. 299–330. Martinus Nijhoff, Dordrecht.

Paillard, J. and Hay, L. (1989). Head contribution to visuomotor recalibration after prismatic displacement of the visual field. Abstracts *Head–neck symposium* (ed. A. Berthoz, W. Graf, and J. P. Vidal) Fontainebleau, France.

Paillard, J., Jordan, P. L., and Brouchon, M. (1981). Visual motion cues in prismatic adaptation: evidence for two separate and additive processes. *Acta Psychologica*, **48**, 253–70.

Paillard, J., Michel, F., and Stelmach, G. (1983). Localization without content: a tactile analogue of 'blind sight'. *Archives of Neurology*, **40**, 548–51.

Phillips, C. G., Zeki, S., and Barlow, H. B., (1984). Localization and function in the cerebral cortex: past, present and future. *Brain*, **107**, 326–61.

Poggio, O. F. and Talbot, W. H. (1981). Mechanisms of static and dynamic stereopsis in foveal cortex of the rhesus monkey. *Journal of Physiology*, **315**, 469–92.

Potegal, M. (1982). Vestibular and neostriatal contributions to spatial orientatio. In *Spatial abilities: development and physiological foundations* (ed. M. Potegal), pp. 361–87. Academic Press, New York.

Rizzollati, G. and Gallese, V. (1988). Mechanisms and theories of spatial neglect. In *Handbook of neuropsychology*, Vol. 1 (ed. F. Boller and J. Grafman), pp. 223–46. Elsevier, Amsterdam.

Rizzolatti, G., Gentilucci, M., Fogassi, L. Luppino, G., Matelli, N., and Panzoni-Maggi, S. (1987). Neurons related to goal directed motor acts in inferior area 6 of the macaque monkey. *Experimental Brain Research*, **67**, 220–4.

Roberts, T. D. M. (1973). Reflex balance. *Nature*, **244**, 156–63.

Robinson, D. A. (1975). Oculomotor control signals. In *Basic mechanisms of ocular motility and their clinical implications* (ed. D. Lennerstrand and P. Bach y Rita), pp. 337–74. Pergamon, Oxford.

Schneider, G. E. (1969). Two visual systems: brain mechanisms for localization and discrimination area dissociated by tectal and cortical lesions. *Science*, **163**, 895–902.

Sparks, D. L. (1989). The neural coding of the location of targets for saccadic eye movements. *Journal of Experimental Biology*, **146**, 195–207.

Stark, L. and Bridgeman, B. (1983). Role of corollary discharge in space constancy. *Perception and Psychophysics*, **34**, 371–80.

Strick, P. L. and Preston, J. B. (1982). Two representations of the hand in area 4 of a primate. III. Somatosensory input organization. *Journal of Neurophysiology*, **48**, 150–9.

Trevarthen, C. (1970). Two mechanisms of vision in primates. *Psychologische Forschung*, **31**, 299–337.

Von Holst, E. and Mittelstaedt, H. (1950). Das Reafferenzprinzip. *Die Naturwissenschaften*, **37**, 464–76.

Weiskrantz, L. (1989). Blindsight. *Handbook of neuropsychology*, Vol. 2 (ed. F. Boller and J. Grafman), pp. 375–85. Elsevier, Amsterdam.

PART 3

The parietal cortex and spatial disorders

11

Space and the parietal association areas

J. F. STEIN

In this chapter I will attempt to evaluate the evidence that the main function of the posterior parietal association area is to begin the transformation of sensory input into signals of use for controlling movement by mediating the accurate, spatial direction of attention. To do this I will show that the association areas behind the primary somaesthetic cortical areas 1, 2, and 3, which are collectively known as the posterior parietal cortex (PPC), are not merely passive association areas in which different sensory inputs are integrated; rather, that first and foremost they are sensorimotor association areas, where sensory, motor, and motivational inputs are brought together so that they can be correctly interpreted in the light of how the animal is moving. Sensory and motor signals about the position and movements of our bodies and of surrounding objects of interest are evaluated in the PPC by neural networks that enable us to direct our attention to them and then to shift our gaze to look at or move towards them.

One important question is whether these functions are mediated by a representation of physical space. Does the PPC employ a body-centred frame of reference or a stabilized frame of the visual surrounding (Paillard 1987; Stein 1989)? In other words, is there a map of environmental, 'real' space in the PPC which is independent of body position? Normal humans cannot imagine an object that occupies no volume nor has any established position in space; likewise we cannot conceive of an object being in two places at the same time, despite what the physicists tell us about what takes place at a quantal level. So we take it as self-evident that our conception of space corresponds to physical reality, and that it exists independently of our observing it. Whether the sensations we use to define it are delivered to our consciousness by the retina, eye movements, the ear, touch, palpation, or locomotion, all seem to operate in the same real space. Despite visual impressions starting off in retinal co-ordinates, in somaesthetic signals arriving in cutaneous co-ordinates, and in movements of the limbs operating in 'joint co-ordinates', we relate all these inputs to the same conception of real space.

But the facts that we can do this, and that we believe in real space, are not sufficient grounds for supposing that a distinct map of space must exist in a particular location in our brains. We need direct evidence of its existence before we can be sure. In fact, no such evidence has emerged. Instead, recent experimental findings suggest that primary sensory representations may be transformed directly into appropriate motor vectors (Goldberg and Bruce 1990)—retinal to oculomotor, proprioceptive to limb movement, etc.—rather than an intermediate stage being interposed which converts each primary sensory representation into a common co-ordinate system representing real, physical space.

Frequently, after a stroke, particularly if it involves the posterior part of the right parietal lobe, patients find that their conception of space completely alters. The left half shrinks or disappears; the right half may dilate; and the apparent positions of objects become jumbled up, even though often each can still be recognized correctly. Such patients are very inaccurate when attempting to reach out for things. They tend to bump into them when walking around; and they lose their way, even when following formerly familiar routes.

Such distortions of perceptual space are not confined to the neurologically impaired. Deviation of the apparent position of objects follows a few minutes of looking through laterally displacing prisms; and this gives rise to a relatively long-lasting adaptation of spatial co-ordinates (Paillard *et al.* 1981), which is not unlike that caused by lesions of the PPC.

Thus, even though we think of physical space as having objective reality, our perceptual reconstruction of it can vary; and our moment-to-moment view of it depends to a large extent upon how much weight we apply to different sensory inputs and the movements they evoke.

Nevertheless, we normally do manage to relate visual, somaesthetic, proprioceptive, and motor spaces successfully to each other, even though from the point of view of the primary, sensory receiving areas, these signals arrive couched in different co-ordinate systems. Visual space is constructed from a series of retinal snapshots that have to be pieced together by incorporating information about the direction in which the eyes are pointing, to give a mind's eye view of visual space. Similarly, somaesthetic space is a reconstruction built from the somatotopic maps of the skin represented in the primary somaesthetic cortex, and from the motor and proprioceptive signals that indicate what the limbs were doing when objects were encountered.

Reconstruction of the location of sound sources by the auditory system is even more indirect. The direction of a sound is computed from monaural sources such as the frequency filtration—'coloration'—provided by the pinna; and in animals with mobile ears this depends on the orientation of the pinna. Also, differences in the amplitude and timing of sounds arriving at the two ears are interpreted in the light of movements of the head to give additional information about the location of a sound.

Yet all these different versions of external space—visual, somaesthetic, motor, and auditory—are successfully brought together in the PPC and somehow used to direct attention, eye, and limb movements accurately. It will be the task of this chapter to see what light anatomical and physiological techniques can throw on how these processes are achieved.

Historical background

The question whether things in the outside world really do exist, or are merely inventions created by the minds of their perceivers, has dominated Western philosophy. Plato introduced his famous concept of 'Ideas', now better translated as 'Universals', around 400 BC. Universals describe the physical properties of an object or the relations between objects, whereas 'Particulars' are particular examples of such Universals apprehended by an individual's senses. Thus space is a Universal, as are shape, colour, and location, but a 100 cm blue box positioned 2 m away is described by Particulars. Different observers seeing the box would each receive different sensory impressions of it, but all would agree about its fundamental properties and relations.

Many people would argue, therefore, that Plato solved the problem over 2000 years ago: Universals reflect the real world, whilst Particulars describe our sensing of it. But arguments about whether there really is a real world continue to our own day (Morgan 1977).

At the beginning of the twelfth century, Abelard established 'nominalism' by successfully undermining the concept of Universals. He argued that they could all be considered names for collections of objects with similar properties perceived by the senses. Thus Universals could not be said to have independent reality because they were merely summarizing many people's sense data. This view was developed further by Hume, Locke, Leibniz, and Berkeley, to the extreme of solipcism—the view that nothing actually exists except in the minds of some observer, including God. In contrast, Kant inverted the argument, maintaining that qualities apprehended by the senses really do reveal real physical objects; whereas relations between objects, such as my being in my study, and the impossibility of a dog also not being a dog but being a cat at the same time, were purely consequences of our mental ways of ordering things, and might be different in a race of Martians or Manvetarians.

For scientists these arguments are very perplexing. *De facto* they have to believe in the reality of objects and the space in which they are located. For it is essential to science that an object should lie in a defined space. But the physical space in which it is may not be exactly the same space that we see or feel, because none of these spaces is identical. The space that we see is not the same space as that which we touch. Probably it is only by learning in infancy how to interpret the feel of things, to correspond with how they look, that the two senses of vision and touch come to correlate with each other satisfactorily. Similarly, we learn how to relate the sound of objects in different locations to their appearance.

But scientists assume that physical space is neutral as between hearing, touch, and sight. Physical space is not itself the space of touch or the space of sight, but we believe that they must share a common co-ordinate system. The real shape of objects in real space, which is what concerns science, is not necessarily the same as anybody's personal private space, however. Real space is public; apparent space is a construction of the individual's mind, private to him or her. Hence the physical space (the perception of which I am going to argue that the PPC is responsible for), though it is connected with the perceptual spaces that we see, hear, and feel, is not identical with any of them. The manner in which they are related with each other is what we are going to be investigating when we consider the functions of the PPC.

If, as common sense would lead us to believe, there is one public, all-embracing, physical space in which objects are located, their relative positions must more or less correspond to the relative positions of the sense data supplied about our private spaces. We can know all these kinds of thing about physical space that a man who was born blind might know through other people telling him about the space of sight. But the kinds of thing that a man born blind could never appreciate about the space of sight, such as the colour red, or the three-dimensional appearance of objects, we also cannot know about physical space.

Newton held strongly to the view that the billiard-ball world of action and reaction that he described has a physical reality, independent of those observing it. As mentioned earlier, this view contrasted with that of his co-inventor of the differential calculus, Leibniz, and later with that of Locke and Bishop Berkeley, who held the 'idealistic view' that what appears as matter is really something mental, i.e. either the world collection of rudimentary minds (Leibniz) or ideas in the mind of God (Berkeley).

Idealists denied the existence of matter as something intrinsically different from mind, though they did not deny that sense data signify that something might exist independently of our private sensations. But Berkeley asserted that nothing can ever be known except what is in some mind, and that whatever is known without being in my mind must be in some other mind, i.e. God's. Thus the idealists fought vigorously against the concept that there could be any *a priori* ideas, independent of the senses. Real space could not be common to vision, hearing, and touch, because if it were, space would have to be an absolute—innate, instinctive, universal; and it was the life's work of the idealists to prove that there were no such things as Universals. They believed that even what appears as matter is really mental.

Hence Berkeley and Leibniz would be very unhappy with any notion of internal cerebral representations of physical space—cognitive maps common to all the senses. Kant, on the other hand, believed in *a priori* Universals; and, like Newton, he held that space is objectively real, not purely a construction created by the make up of our brains. Such 'realists' would therefore not be in the least surprised to encounter a part of the brain set aside to represent real space.

Arguments in favour of localization of functions in the brain, such as that of the representation of space, began with the phrenologists, Gall and Spurtzheim. These two men made important neuroanatomical discoveries, for example, about the significance of the grey matter of the cerebral cortex, the site of the decussation of the pyramidal tracts, and of the nature of the cerebral commissures, but their ill-substantiated phrenological theories attracted justified scepticism. Their stretching of phrenological theory far beyond the evidence that was then available severely hampered acceptance of the very idea that functions might be localized in different parts of the brain. Thus, although Gall described, as early as 1810, how an injury in the left frontal lobe deprived a soldier of speech, and therefore suggested that the faculty of speech resided there, it is not Gall but Broca to whom this idea is credited.

Gall attributed to the parietal lobe the faculties of 'cautiousness, conscientiousness and self esteem', with characteristic lack of any supporting evidence. It was not until Theodore Mynert traced the sensory fibres of the spinal cord through the thalamus to the post-central gyrus in the anterior part of the parietal cortex that any inkling of the true somaesthetic functions of this area emerged. Head and Holmes (1911) confirmed that the primary somaesthetic cortex is indeed situated in the anterior part of the parietal lobe.

But the true functions of the posterior part of the parietal lobe did not prove so easy to determine. Flechsig taught that it was a purely somaesthetic association area. Modern conceptions of its function started with David Ferrier's celebrated mistake (Glickstein 1985)! Shortly after confirming in monkeys Fritz and Hitsig's seminal discovery that electrically stimulating the pre-central gyrus of the dog led to movements of the contralateral limbs, Ferrier began stimulating other parts of the monkey's brain. When he stimulated the posterior part of the parietal lobe he found that the animal's eyes deviated contralaterally. When he cauterized this area the animal behaved as if it was blind; so Ferrier, not unnaturally, concluded that the PPC contained the primary visual centres of the brain. This conclusion led him to contradict the celebrated Herman Munk, Professor of Physiology in Berlin, who reported that the occipital not the parietal lobe contained the primary visual receiving areas. Munk was excessively rude about Ferrier's claim and in the process managed to destroy his own scientific reputation. Nevertheless, he was proved right and Ferrier mistaken.

Mitchell Glickstein has pointed out that Ferrier's first experiments on the parietal lobe were performed without the benefit of any aseptic techniques, and that most of his animals did not survive long enough to be studied for more than two days after ablation. In 1871, however, Ferrier moved to King's College, London, where Joseph Lister was now a professor of surgery; he introduced Ferrier to the mysteries of asepsis. Thereafter, Ferrier was able to study the monkeys for a much longer time after ablation. He rapidly revised his opinion and came to the conclusion that Munk was right after all. Parietal lesions led to apparent loss of vision only very temporarily. But even after a long period of time they continued to cause misreaching and poor visual guidance of eye and arm movements.

At about the same time, Hughlings-Jackson (1870) was developing his theories of the hierarchical organization of the central nervous system. From observing the pattern of the dissolution of control in focal or generalized neurological disease, he had reached the conclusion that the nervous system can be conceived of as having three levels. The lowest comprised the spinal and brain-stem, motor and sensory systems; the middle level encompassed the primary, motor and sensory, cortical receiving areas; whilst the highest level was represented by the cortical association areas. Among these the PPC held pride of place in Hughlings-Jackson's scheme, as it is situated behind the primary somaesthetic cortex, in front of the primary visual cortex, and medial to the primary auditory cortex. So, despite prevailing views, and even though Hughlings-Jackson himself had predicted the existence of the primary motor cortex, he did not accord to the motor strip the seat of the Will. Instead he saw clearly that areas feeding into the motor cortex probably had greater significance for the planning of voluntary actions. Accordingly, he believed that the PPC played a most important role in initiating movement and behaviour.

Moreover, he was prescient about the possibility of separate specialized roles for the right, as compared with the left, parietal regions. He attributed, to the left, contributions to speech, language, comprehension, reading, and writing—as did Dax, Broca, and Dejerine; but he emphasized the importance of the complementary specialization of the right parietal cortex for cross-modal and visuo-spatial perception.

The next figure we must deal with is Reszo Balint. Although the syndrome that bears his name rest on his description of only one case (J.K.), his methodical approach and meticulous observation, coupled with his having provided detailed *post mortem* findings, make it still one of the most useful accounts of impaired visuomotor control in the literature (Husain and Stein 1988). J.K. suffered from three main symptoms: (a) impaired visual guidance of movement, which Balint named optic ataxia—this was analogous to the sensory ataxia found in tabes; (b) psychic paralysis of gaze—this was an inability to attend to more than one object at a time; (c) deviation of the field of attention to the right-hand side.

These symptoms were not due to any sensory or oculomotor impairment, as Balint found that the patient's visual fields and his eye movements were all normal. Instead J.K. appeared to suffer from interruption of the information-processing stages that lie between sensation and movement. He was not able to make proper use of visual information to direct either his attention, his eyes, or his limbs accurately. In short, he exhibited failure of 'active sight'. Subsequently, J.K. came to post-mortem; and he was found to have lesions in the posterior part of the parietal lobe on both sides.

In 1918, Gordon Holmes published an account of six soldiers with disturbances of visual and spatial orientation following gunshot wounds that involved the PPC on both sides (Holmes 1918). The patients were severely disorientated, being unable to find their way around or to judge where they were in relation to surrounding objects. They were inaccurate when determining direction and distance; and they missed visual targets when reaching out for them. These are further symptoms of failure of 'active sight'. Nevertheless, following the warnings of Hughlings-Jackson, Holmes was well aware that finding a lesion which causes spatial disorientation does not necessarily localize a centre for spatial orientation. He cautiously concluded, therefore, that damage to the angular and supramarginal gyri in the PPC interrupted a central association pathway connecting occipital visual areas with the rest of the brain.

Up to this time, most neurologists had concentrated on potential visual functions for the PPC, ignoring any possible significance that might be attributed to its site just posterior to the primary somaesthetic cortex. However, in 1924, Gerstmann published details of a patient with finger agnosia, right/left disorientation, dysgraphia, and discalculia, all caused by a localized lesion in the left angular gyrus (Gerstmann 1924). Nowadays, whether Gerstmann's syndrome is a distinct entity is much debated (Gerstmann 1957) and doubted; but the first two symptoms he described, faulty finger localization and left right confusion, which particularly affected spatial identification of the parts of the patient's own body, emphasize that the functions of the PPC include not only representation of external space but also that of personal space, i.e. the disposition of a subject's own limbs and body, and the mediation of 'active touch'. Gerstmann's syndrome suggests that the PPC may hold not only the neural apparatus responsible for directing movement in relation to external space but also that in relation to a subject's own body image. Head had earlier recognized the necessity for such an internal model of a subject's own body, which he called the body 'schema', as early as 1911 (Head and Holmes 1911).

The evolution of these clues to parietal lobe function in the hands of more recent neurologists and neuropsychologists will be taken up in later chapters; but the question raised by Hughlings-Jackson about the special-ization of the right and left parietal regions for different functions may be briefly considered here. Following Gall, Dax, Broca, Wernicke, and Dejerine, the fashion in the late nineteenth and early twentieth centuries was to consider the left hemisphere dominant for speech and language comprehension, whereas the right hemisphere was thought to be completely subservient, and to have no special functions itself. Indeed, as recently as 1950, J. Z. Young wondered why nature bothered to furnish us with a right hemisphere at all! Despite Hughlings-Jackson's championship of the per-ceptual powers of the right hemisphere, what evidence there then was pointed either to bilateral involvement in visuo-spatial functions (Balint, Holmes) or to the pre-eminence of the left parietal cortex (Gerstmann). It was not until the 1940s and another World War to provide the clinical material, that Brain (1941) and Zangwill (McFie *et al.* 1950) were able to demonstrate that the right hemisphere does indeed play its own special part in visuo-spatial function.

By the middle of the twentieth century, therefore, clinical neurology had provided us with a complex set of systems to explain following post-parietal damage. These comprise visual inattention, poor visual guidance of move-ment, spatial disorientation, and disturbances of the body image—together with dyslexia, dysgraphia, and dyscalculia following left hemisphere lesions; and more pronounced visuo-spatial disorders following right hemisphere lesions. In the remainder of this chapter, I shall review the evidence, mainly from animal work, that indicates how these results of PPC lesions may be explained by postulating that the PPC contains a neural representation of the rules whereby sensory input data are used to control shifts of a subject's attention, hence to help guide movements of body, limbs, and eyes.

Anatomy

Macdonald Critchley (1953) termed the PPC the 'parieto–temporo–occipital crossroads', but even this description of its cross-modal connec-tions does not do adequate justice to their complexity. Over 70 inputs and outputs of areas 5 and 7 have been identified in the monkey. I will not attempt to review the whole of this massive record here; this has been done recently much better than I could by Hyvarinen (1982), Andersen (1987), and Husain (1991). I merely emphasize that the PPC is concerned with bringing together visual, somaesthetic, proprioceptive, auditory, vestibular, oculomotor, limb motor, and motivational signals to create a network for transforming sensory input into signals suitable for motor control.

The PPC in humans is the area lying between the post-central sulcus anteriorly, the sub-parietal sulcus on the medial aspect of the hemisphere, the parieto-occipital sulcus posteriorly, and laterally the postero-medial part of the superior temporal sulcus. Figure 11.1 illustrates its location. The area consists of the superior parietal lobule, which in monkeys consists

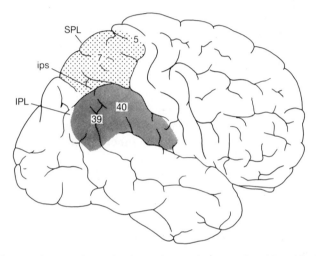

Fig. 11.1. In man the posterior parietal cortex comprises areas 5 and 7 and in the superior parietal lobule (SPL), and areas 39 and 40 in the inferior parietal lobule (IPL)—ips, intra-parietal sulcus.

of Brodman's area 5, but in humans contains both areas 5 and 7 (Bonin and Bailey 1947), and the inferior lobule; in monkeys, this contains areas 7a and 7b, whereas in man it comprises the supra-marginal gyrus, Brodman's area 39, and the angular gyrus, Brodman's area 40. These regions are also known in the terminology of von Economo as areas PE, PG, and PF (von Economo 1929). It has been suggested that areas 39 and 40 in the human correspond to areas 7a and 7b in the inferior parietal lobule of the monkey; whereas areas 5 and 7 in the human are equivalent to the superior parietal lobule of the monkey (areas 5a and 5b). But this view is controversial (Bonin and Bailey 1947; Mesulam 1985). In addition to these areas, the motion-sensitive areas of the superior temporal sulcus, middle temporal (MT) or V5, and MST, are functionally related to the posterior parietal lobe, although they are not classically designated part of the PPC.

It will be apparent that the evolution of the human brain has been associated with massive enlargement of the PPC, particularly of the inferior parietal lobule, areas 39 and 40. The general principle of the connections of the PPC is that it receives and returns reciprocally projections from and to all second-order sensory cortices, together with motor and motivational structures.

Area 5

The main cortical inputs to area 5, the superior parietal lobule, in the monkey come from somaesthetic areas S1 and S2—Brodman's areas 1, 2, and 3 in front, and from area 7 posteriorly (Jones and Powell 1969; Pandya and Kuypers 1969). Also, the ipsilateral motor and pre-motor cortex areas 4 and 6 project to it, as do contralateral areas 5 and 7 connecting via the corpus callosum. The vestibular cortex (lateral area 2) also feeds into area 5 (Divac *et al.* 1977; Grusser *et al.* 1982; Pandya and Seltzer 1982). In addition, the cingulate gyrus sends a dense projection.

The main sub-cortical input is from the pulvinar and the posterior group of thalamic nuclei, which receive many other inputs from the oculomotor- and neck movement-related areas of the superior colliculus (SC) (Pearson *et al.* 1978; Powell *et al.* 1989).

The main efferent projections from area 5 within the cerebral cortex are to the pre-motor and supplementary motor areas (lateral and medial area 6, respectively) and into the lateral intra-parietal area (LIP) posteriorly (Andersen and Gnadt 1989). Its connections with the cingulate gyrus mentioned earlier are reciprocal. Contralaterally it projects reciprocally via the corpus callosum to the opposite areas 5 and 7 (Pandya and Kuypers 1969). Sub-cortically, it projects to the thalamus, caudate nucleus, and putamen (Petras 1971), to the tectum, and to the pontine nuclei (Brodal 1978), thence to the cerebellar hemispheres.

Area 7

The main cortical inputs to area 7 in the monkey come from the somaesthetic, auditory, and visual systems. It receives from ipsilateral somaesthetic cortex (S1 and S2) (Pandya and Seltzer 1982) and from area 5 in front (Caminiti and Sbriccoli 1985), and from areas 18 and 19 behind (Pandya and Kuypers 1969; Rockland and Pandya 1979). Laterally, auditory areas 22 and the planum temporale project into it (Divac *et al.* 1977). Although the somaesthetic projection may be crudely somatotopic, and possibly there is a residual, retinotopic order in the visual projection, there is no evidence of tonotopicity in the auditory projection.

With regard to visual inputs, area 7a (PG) in the monkey is the best understood. It is the site of convergence of two broad streams of visual information. First, it receives such information from the primary visual, striate cortex by way of extra-striate cortical areas (Rockland and Pandya 1979; Ungerleider and Desimone 1986). Second, it receives visual and oculomotor information from the SC by way of the pulvinar (Asanuma *et al.* 1985).

The major input from the striate cortex travels by two routes (Andersen 1987): the first is via V3a, the dorsal pre-lunate region, and area MST (Ungerleider and Desimone 1986a). The second projection is directed by way of MT mainly towards the intra-parietal sulcus (Ungerleider and Desimone 1986b; Maunsell and Van Essen 1983a). Areas V3a, MT, and MST in turn each receive inputs from the striate cortex and/or other visual areas. These pathways are outlined in Fig. 11.2. They constitute part of the dorsal visual pathway, which is thought to be important in localizing, rather than identifying visual targets—the 'where' pathway of Ungerleider and Mishkin (1982) (see also Mishkin *et al.* 1983; Ungerleider and Desimone 1986a, b).

The important sub-cortical projections to area 7 and the intra-parietal sulcus are as follows: those layers of the SC that receive from the retina project to the intra-parietal sulcus in area LIP, whereas area 7a receives from the deep, non-retinotopic, oculomotor, layers of the SC (Andersen 1987). The retino–collicular–intra-parietal pathway is a fast system, which is involved in orienting the eyes to novel objects in the visual surround. The projection from the deep layers of the SC to area 7a is, on the other hand, probably more important for spatial perception, updating the cortex about eye movements that have been executed.

Visual information is directed anteriorly and dorsally towards area 7a; but somatosensory information, touch, position, and vibration sense, is relayed posteriorly from the post-central gyrus, which contains the primary somatosensory cortical areas 1, 2, and 3, not only to area 5 but also to area 7b (Pandya and Seltzer 1982). Area 7b also receives visual inputs from area 7a (Divac *et al.* 1977; Seltzer and Pandya 1980). Again, the principle is that both the visual route through area 7a and the somatosensory route through areas 5 and 7b converge on the intra-parietal sulcus. Also, auditory and vestibular inputs are relayed, respectively, through area TPT (tempo-parietal area—a higher-order auditory area) and the vestibular cortex, which is situated postero-laterally to the somasthetic cortex (Schwartz and Frederickson 1971).

Thus many modalities of sensory information converge in the PPC. Associations may be made within modalities: visual, somatosensory, auditory, and vestibular. The highest level of this convergence seems to be located in the intra-parietal sulcus.

One particular area within the intra-parietal sulcus is especially involved with saccadic eye movements; this is LIP, which sends dense projections to

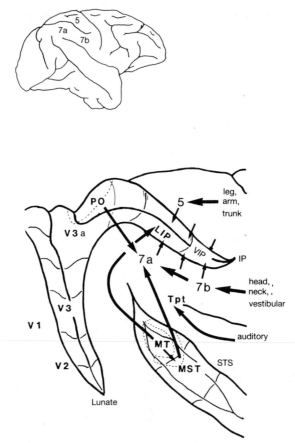

Fig. 11.2. *Top:* posterior parietal cortex in monkey (areas numbered). *Bottom:* Lunate, superior temporal (STS) and intra-parietal (IP) sulci spread out. Areas 5 and 7 converge on the lateral (LIP) and ventral intra-parietal (VIP) areas. Tpt: temporo-parietal area; PO: Bonin and Bailey notation middle temporal area (MT); MST: middle superior temporal area.

the frontal eye fields and to the SC (Andersen and Gnadt 1989), and may therefore be considered an output station for the networks within the PPC that control eye movements.

Area 7 also receives from the frontal eye field (area 8) as well as prefrontal area 46 (Andersen *et al.* 1985). In addition it is connected via the corpus callosum with contralateral areas 5 and 7 (Pandya and Kuypers 1969). Finally, and most importantly, it is reciprocally connected with the limbic system via the cingulate gyrus (Mesulam *et al.* 1977; Stanton *et al.* 1977).

The main sub-cortical inputs to area 7 come from the oculomotor (deep) layers of the SC via the pulvinar, as we have seen, and from the cerebellum and basal ganglia via the VA nucleus of the thalamus (Hyvarinen 1982). The main sub-cortical outputs are to the pulvinar, basal ganglia, SC, and the massive projection to the cerebellar hemispheres via the pontine nucleus (Glickstein *et al.* 1980).

In summary, area 5 connects somaesthetic with limbic and motor structures, and area 7 connects visual and auditory areas with limbic and motor structures. Thus area 7 exhibits the connections summarized earlier; marrying retinal, somaesthetic, proprioceptive, vestibular, and auditory sensory signals, together with information about movements of the eyes, neck, body, and limbs. In addition, it receives motivational signals from the limbic system. In return it projects back to the limbic, sensory, and motor areas feeding it. It provides large outputs back to the motivational centres in the cingulate gyrus and to motor centres in basal ganglia, frontal eye fields, pre-motor cortex SC, and cerebellum. Therefore, on anatomical grounds, we can consider the PPC a 'multimodal, sensorimotor association' area for the direction of attention, and eye and limb movements.

Single unit responses

Physiological recording of the responses of single neurons in the PPC tells us much more about how these connections may mediate sensorimotor transformations. These recordings must be made in awake animals trained to perform tasks designed to reveal the functions of the PPC. Such work has made one thing very clear. Neuronal responses there are exceedingly complex. As expected, their activity is related to many influences—sensory inputs, motor outputs, states of intention and attention.

Area 5

In area 5 the sensory properties of neurons are an order of magnitude more complex than those recorded in S1. Eighty per cent are related to joint position; but they are activated best when the joints are moved in a natural sequence, and when appropriate areas of skin are stimulated in the same way as they would be during a normal movement (Sakata *et al.* 1973). Bilateral interactions are common: for instance, flexion of one hip can inhibit the normal excitatory responses to flexion of the other (Sakata 1985). Sakata termed many of these area 5 neurons 'matching' because they are maximally stimulated by bringing two appropriate body parts together, e.g. rubbing the palms together with the shoulders adducted, or brushing the fur on the left forearm with the right hand.

An important observation, first made by Mountcastle and his colleagues (Mountcastle *et al.* 1975), and confirmed by all subsequent workers, is that even if PPC neurons can be activated by passive sensory stimulation, their discharge is markedly enhanced if the stimulation is caused by the animal's own movement. Some movement-related neurons in area 5 fail to respond at all to passive cutaneous stimulation; but they discharge briskly when the animal actively reaches out for an object. Kalaska (see Chapter 8) has shown that their discharge is relatively unaltered by loading the arm, but continues to reflect the direction of the arm movement unambiguously even when loaded. These cells do not respond to visual stimuli or to any associated eye movements. Mountcastle called them arm projection units. Others—hand manipulation units—respond only during active palpation of food, etc.

Area 7

The study of responses in area 7 has been dominated by a controversy about whether their activity is best described as sensory, sensorimotor, motor, or attentional. The characteristics of 7a neurons have therefore been intensively studied in order to try to settle the matter.

The great majority of neurons in this area are visually driven (Motter and Mountcastle 1981). Such 'light-sensitive' neurons have very large receptive fields and they will often respond to flashed, stationary stimuli even if they are of no particular significance to the animal. Their receptive fields often cover the entire contralateral hemi-field, and they usually expand over the midline, well into the ipsilateral field. Often they have a region of insensitivity around the fovea itself (foveal sparing). They therefore seem ideally suited to detecting novel stimuli in the visual periphery.

These neurons have another interesting property. Although they do not encode stimulus speed, they are sensitive to movement either way (centrifugal) or towards (centripetal) the fovea. This is referred to as 'radial opponent vector' organization. The combined output of a population of such neurons can readily encode, to within 9°, the true direction of a stimulus. It has therefore been suggested (Paillard 1982) that these neurons play an important role in tracking the movement of a limb in the visual periphery as it is directed towards a target upon which the eyes have alighted. They may also play a role in detecting 'optic flow', the pattern of motion of elements in the visual scene experienced by an observer moving through the environment (Lee 1980). They are probably stimulated best by textured, moving stimuli, like those in areas MT and MST; but they do not display selectivity for orientation, colour, or shape.

A most important characteristic of many light-sensitive neurons in area 7a is their additional responsiveness to the position of the eye in the orbit (Andersen *et al.* 1988). Their discharge rate modulates even when the animal moves its eyes around in a totally dark room. Also, when these neurons are stimulated at the optimum site in their receptive field, their discharge rate is only maximal when the eyes are in a particular position. It falls off for other eye positions, even when the stimulus is kept at the same retinal locus, i.e. when the visual stimulus is moved by the same amount and in the same direction as the eyes when they move, in order to keep it in the same position on the retina despite such movements (Andersen *et al.* 1985). In general, the best combination of retinal and eye position is that which places the 'hot spot' in the visual cell's receptive field on a saggital plane through the animal's 'egocentre' (see below).

Whether the eye-position signal carried by these cells comes from stretch receptors in the ocular muscles, or from corollary discharges arising in oculomotor centres, or both, is not yet definitely known. But many of these light-sensitive neurons also respond to saccadic eye movements (Motter and Mountcastle 1981; Steinmetz *et al.* 1987). Because the visual response to the appearance of a target interacts with the animal's saccadic eye movement, delineation of what is a visual and what is a motor component of the response has been somewhat difficult. For instance, it has been suggested that the apparent saccade response could, in fact, be merely an artefact, simply representing the visual stimulation of the cell by the appearance of the target. Or it could be a consequence of the target moving across the retinal receptive field during a saccade. However, these suggestions cannot explain the response of neurons to saccades that are made totally in the dark. Hence it is generally agreed that most visually responsive neurons also respond independently to saccadic eye movements.

The saccade neurons are active when the monkey makes a saccade to a new visual target of interest. But they are not active when the eye movement is made spontaneously, and not in response to a distinct visual target, whether currently displayed or memorized (Gnadt and Andersen 1988). They are selective for the direction of the saccade, but not for its amplitude. In many, their discharge only follows saccades made in the dark, or to the remembered position of a target. So these cells cannot be said to be controlling the eye movement. They merely reflect ongoing saccades. One must remember that there is a complete sub-cortical system in the SC for controlling reflex saccades. Post-saccadic parietal cells may therefore merely be monitoring the activity of cells in the SC, or the frontal eye fields.

However, in the LIP there are many neurons, comprising nearly 20 per cent of those found in the area, that discharge during the period over which a monkey has been trained to wait to make an eye movement to a remembered position (Gnadt and Andersen 1988); i.e. they fire well before the saccade, and they seem to code for the intended direction of movement. Clearly these may control such saccades. The responses of light-sensitive cells to visual stimuli are often enhanced if the stimulus is behaviourly relevant. Indeed, Mountcastle (Mountcastle *et al.* 1975) at first thought that they were light-sensitive only if the animal subsequently made an actual saccade to the target. But it was later shown by Robinson *et al.* (1978) that many neurons show small responses even to passive visual stimulation, and even in the absence of any movement. Active oculomotor reaction of the animal most definitely enhances these responses, however.

In most oculomotor regions, such enhancement only occurs if overt eye movements are actually made; but in the PPC it is sufficient for the animal merely to direct its attention to the stimulus. Mountcastle tested the light-sensitivity of these neurons under three different attentional conditions (Mountcastle *et al.* 1981). In the first, the animal was alert, watching a fixation light but not required to do anything. In the second, it was awaiting the signal for a trial to begin. In the third, it had to detect dimming of the fixation light in order to earn a reward. In none of these trials did the animal actually move its eyes. Yet in the third condition, when the monkey's attention was explicitly directed at the dimming light, the light-sensitivity of the neuron was greatly enhanced.

Bushnell *et al.* (1981) examined the role of directed attention in these neurons in greater detail, by training monkeys to fixate a central light whilst attending to the dimming of a peripheral one; but they were trained not to turn their eyes to look at it. They found that if the peripheral light was in the large, visual receptive field of a PPC neuron its discharge was increased when the monkey attended to the target, even though the monkey made no eye movement towards it. Often this enhancement was larger than the firing that preceded an actual saccade because making a saccade often inhibits the discharge. This effect contrasts with neurons in the SC and frontal eye fields, where enhancement only occurs if the animal actually shifts its gaze to look at the target.

Another group of cells that have been identified in area 7a are 'fixation' cells (Mountcastle *et al.* 1984). These discharge most vigorously when an animal fixates an object of interest. But their activity falls off when the animal makes a saccade to fixate another stimulus. Like the light-sensitive neutones, these cells also carry an eye-position signal, which can be demonstrated by having the animal fixate different remembered positions in the dark (Gnadt and Andersen 1988). The modulation of their discharge by eye position may also be affected by the degree of convergence of the two eyes.

The light-sensitive and fixation cells are the two most important classes of neurons in area 7a. Functionally they may be considered to serve two different but complementary roles. The light-sensitive ones are activated by new events occurring in the periphery. In contrast, fixation neurons respond best when the animal is fixating a visual target of interest. The common features of these two classes are their modualtion by the direction of attention, and also by the eye position of the animal.

Although there may be neurons in area 7a that discharge specifically in relation to smooth, pursuit-tracking eye movements, the majority of these neurons are now thought to lie in area MST rather than area 7a proper.

Area 7b

As mentioned earlier, area 7b receives both visual and somaesthetic inputs. Hence most of the neurons here respond to somatosensory stimulation and a substantial proportion (10–20 per cent), particularly on the borders of 7a and 7b in area VIP, respond to both visual and somatosensory stimulation (Hyvarinen 1981; see also Chapter 12). The somatosensory and visual fields match in the sense that those with upper visual receptive fields have cutaneous fields on the forehead whilst those in the lower visual field have forelimb cutaneous fields; also they have the same directional selectivity in their visual and cutaneous fields.

Area LIP

As mentioned earlier, many neurons here discharge in advance of saccades. Many units within area LIP encode 'motor error': this defines the direction and size of the saccade required to bring a new visual target onto the fovea—the 'saccade vector' (Barash *et al.* 1989). Like the area 7a neurons which feed them, the activity of LIP neurons is also modulated by eye position (Andersen and Gnadt 1989). The LIP sends strong projections both to the SC and to the frontal eye fields. Hence one can probably consider these neurons as providing the control signal for the visual direction of contralateral, saccadic eye movements.

As Ferrier first suggested, stimulation of PPC elicits contralaterally directed saccades. But the current intensities required to elicit saccades from the PPC are considerably greater than those required from the SC or the frontal eye fields.

Neurons in the LIP may start their response over a second before the onset of a natural saccade. This property has been demonstrated by training monkeys to make saccades to the remembered position of targets (Gnadt and Andersen 1988). They are required to withhold their saccade for a few seconds after the peripheral light had been flashed on and off again. This activity preceding a saccade, but lasting long after the peripheral stimulus had disappeared, may therefore be considered the neural representation of the motor error that drives the movement. Under the conditions of these experiments, this error signal had to be held in memory until the saccade was allowed to take place.

Area MST and MT (V5)

The middle superior and middle temporal areas (MST and MT) are particularly concerned with moving rather than stationary stimuli. The properties of MT (V5) neurons have been most studied. Their firing is sensitive to the direction and speed of movement, but not to colour or form (Dubner and Zeki 1971). They are organized in columns (Albright 1984; Albright *et al.* 1984); but it is speed rather than direction that is represented in different columns. The preferred direction of movement gradually shifts with depth. The discharge of the majority of MT neurons encodes stimulus velocity (Maunsell and Van Essen 1983b), and cells recorded in the same vertical penetration have similar speed sensitivities. In addition to direction and speed, many MT neurons are highly sensitive to monocular disparity (Maunsell and Van Essen 1983c). Thus MT is probably important for motion perception in three dimensions.

When two stimuli composed of gratings moving in different directions are superimposed, the observer usually sees coherent motion of a 'plaid' moving in one direction, rather than two gratings moving over one another. A quarter of neurons in the MT respond to this global motion, rather than to the direction of motion of either of the gratings alone (Movshon *et al.* 1985). In contrast, neurons in the primary visual cortex only respond to the direction of motion of the individual gratings.

In a similar way the properties of MT neurons correlate well with the spatial and temporal characteristics of 'apparent motion'. This is the situation when motion is perceived without there being any real movement of anything. An example is when two lights at different locations are flashed sequentially. The spatial and temporal limits of the responses of MT neurons to apparent motion have been found to correspond well with those obtained from psychophysical investigations (Mikami et al. 1986), whereas those of striate and pre-striate cortical neurons are very different.

Newsome *et al.* (1989) have shown that the responses of MT neurons correspond to monkeys' psychophysical performance, even on a trial-to-trial basis in a motion detection task. The monkeys were trained to detect the direction of motion in a random-dot kinematograph, in which only a proportion of the dots moved in the same direction and the rest moved randomly. The firing of the MT cells corresponded to the monkeys' reported perception of the dots moving, rather than to the actual motion of the spots on the retina.

In about a third of MT neurons, even though they are selective for orientation, their best orientation is roughly parallel to their preferred orientation (Albright 1984; Albright *et al.* 1984). This contrasts with those in V1 or V2, whose best motion direction is always at right angles to their preferred orientation.

Pursuit-tracking cells

Most pursuit-tracking neurons in the MT give the same responses whether the animal tracks the target with its eyes alone and the head is fixed, or the head is allowed to move and the eyes remain fixed in the orbit (Komatsu and Wurtz 1988b). Thus it seems that they carry a signal which corresponds to the change in the line of sight—the gaze—rather than to movements of the eyes *per se*. The signal of gaze motion is obtained by adding signals for head and eye movement together after suitable scaling. As the modulation of pursuit-tracking cells precedes eye movements, and lesions in this area disrupt smooth pursuit, it is again reasonable to suggest that these neurons are not only correlated with pursuit eye movements, but, in fact, are used to control them.

Many pursuit cells also exhibit visual-motion sensitivity (Komatsu and Wurtz, 1988a). The favoured direction may be the same or opposite to that of the eye movement. Those sensitive to the 'anti' direction may contribute to the perception of movements of objects with respect to the environmental background, because they are stimulated by the apparent motion of the background during the tracking. This is known to be an important extra cue to the accurate estimation of the speed of a target being tracked (Tanaka *et al.* 1986).

Neurons within MT that represent movements around the fovea (so-called MTF cells) are also active during smooth pursuit. They respond best to small, moving spots of light, and they are directionally selective. Their rate of discharge falls off when the visual target is transiently blanked, even if the eyes remain moving, or when the target is stabilized on the retina (Newsome *et al.* 1988). Thus some of their response depends upon image motion over the retina, i.e. retinal 'slip'. These neurons have minimal sensitivity to background motion and their preferred direction of visual motion is the same as the direction of their preference for smooth-pursuit eye movements. Thus these MTF neurons probably encode both retinal slip—the difference between target and retinal velocity—and the eye velocity itself.

As the gaze usually lags the target during smooth pursuit, the direction of image motion on the retina as the observer tracks is usually in the direction of the pursuit. Thus MT neurons may encode the direction of motion irrespective of whether it is signalled by image movements across the retina or by successful pursuit eye movements.

It seems that inputs from the striate cortex are not necessary for these responses. Up to two thirds of neurons in MT still show motion selectivity, even after ablation of the striate cortex (Rodman and Albright 1989). Hence the SC probably provides important inputs for these responses.

Summary

These recording experiments have added greatly to our understanding of the PPC. Area 5 neurons are related to somaesthesia, proprioception and active limb movements helping to mediate 'active touch'; whereas area 7 cells are concerned with auditory, visual, and eye movements, and the visual guidance of movement ('active sight'). All PPC neurons seem to share four important characteristics: (a) they receive combinations of sensory, motivational, and related motor inputs; (b) their discharge is much enhanced when the animal is interested in a target; (c) when it attends to it; and (d) when the animal makes a movement in relation to it. Thus they are well suited to play the role suggested earlier, namely to participate in the transformation of sensory input into signals suitable for guiding motor output.

Event-related potentials in the posterior parietal cortex

Event-related, potential correlates of the activity of neurons in the PPC have now been reported in humans. A negative wave occurs 100 to 200 ms after a visual event. Its amplitude is largest, not at the occipital pole, but over the parietal cortex (Hillyard *et al.* 1985). It is usually bigger on the contralateral side; and it has been shown to be greatly enhanced when a subject attends to a particular location within that field, rather than when the attention is directed elsewhere (Neville and Lawson 1987).

A positive wave often follows the negative one at a latency of 300 to 500 ms. It appears to belong to the family of responses that relates to decision-making and stimulus selection.

Whilst the early *n* wave probably correlates with the discharge of light-sensitive neurons in the parietal cortex, the later wave may correspond to the discharge of fixation neurons. The amplitude of the later wave is particularly attenuated in patients with visual neglect (Lhermitte *et al.* 1985).

Not only are the visual-evoked potentials maximal over the PPC, but also the pre-motor positivity (PMP), which precedes saccadic eye movements by 100 to 200 ms, is largest over the parietal cortex (Thickbroom and Mastaglia 1985). It occurs 80 to 100 ms earlier if the target of a saccade is predictable compared to when it is unpredictable (Husain and Stein, unpublished observations). This result is in keeping with the idea that the PMP in the parietal cortex is the physiological correlate of the formulation of the required oculomotor plan.

Regional cerebral blood flow

Investigations of changes in regional cerebral blood flow during tasks that require subjects to direct their attention to particular targets also reveal specific responses in the human PPC (Roland 1982). There is preferential activation of the right PPC, a finding that accords with the evidence from lesion studies that both attentional and visual-direction deficits are much more serious following lesions to the right rather than the left hemisphere (Reivich *et al.* 1983).

Parietal lobe function in non-human primates

Recording the activity of neurons can only tell us what signal transformations the cells might be performing, however; they tell us that they are sufficient for the task, not whether they are necessary. Therefore single-unit findings must be supplemented by careful analysis of the outcome of lesions, in order to confirm that what we believe the cells might be doing is eliminated when they are destroyed. In this section, therefore, I shall interpret some of the results of lesion experiments in animals and of neurological damage in humans in the light of the hypothesis that the PPC is responsible for the first stage of sensorimotor transformation—the direction of attention.

Cross-modal matching

The question of whether apes and monkeys are capable of successful cross-modal matching has attracted a great deal of interest, not only because it is important for skilled motor control but also because it is considered a prerequisite to language (Luria 1958; Geschwind 1965). However, both apes and monkeys have been shown to be fully able to make successful cross-modal matches (Davenport *et al.* 1973). PPC lesions affect this ability, particularly on the left side, because primates are superior at cross-modal matching with their left hemisphere. Yet still they do not speak. Hence poor cross-modal matching cannot be an explanation for the fact that the language skills of non-human primates are at best only modest.

Superior parietal lobule

Lesions confined to the superior parietal lobule (area 5) have been shown to cause astereognosis, impaired weight discrimination, and unco-ordinated manipulatory and palpatory movements of contralateral arm

(Stein 1978). These symptoms confirm that the superior parietal lobule (area 5 in the monkey) is more concerned with representing the position of the limbs and body, and with active touch, than with visual space.

Spatial ability

Monkeys with parietal lesions have impaired ability to locate objects (Stein 1978). They have problems with finding routes, oculomotor disorders (Lynch 1980), and aiming deficiencies. The latter are said to be confined to the contralateral arm; but if care is taken to inactivate only area 7, the inferior parietal lobule, it can be shown that the deficit is of visual guidance of the movements of both arms in contralateral hemi-space (Stein 1978). They mis-aim with both arms in contralateral space, independently of where their eyes are pointing.

Visual symptoms

Visual hemi-neglect after posterior parietal lesions is said to be less prominent in animals than in humans. However, if it is searched for it is often found. Hemi-inattention may be less conspicuous in animals only because they cannot report their perceptions. Also their brains are less lateralized. Inaccurate aiming at visual targets is particularly associated with lesions of the inferior parietal lobule (Stein 1978), but most experimenters have removed both superior and inferior parietal lobules.

Thus both monkeys and men display much the same kinds of symptom, though of different magnitude, after posterior parietal lesions. These may be summarized as disturbances of the direction of attention and of the guidance of eye, limb, and body movements.

Parietal lobe lesions in man

The neuropsychological effects of parietal lobe lesions are considered in Chapter 13 in this volume, so this is not the place to go into them in great detail. However, it is worth giving an outline of the different kinds of symptom following PPC lesions in order to show that this multiplicity can be reduced to a relatively simple statement—namely that PPC lesions lead to a failure of directed attention, which disrupts the transformations of sensory into motor co-ordinate systems that are essential for the accurate guidance of attention and movement. This impairment applies not only to attending and pointing to objects in the outside world but also the patient's own body. Hemispheric specialization in humans has led to these spatial functions being located mainly in the right hemisphere. Specifically human attributes requiring both spatial and linguistic skills, such as reading, writing, and calculation, are damaged by lesions in both PPCs.

Superior parietal lobule

Tactile perception

It was not until well after the Second World War that it became clear that the only cortical lesions which could render the skin permanently anaesthetic were those affecting the anterior parietal cortex (post-central gyrus). But as Ferrier learnt (see above), it is often not easy to distinguish between primary loss of a sensory area and manifestations that are secondary to a patient's inability to direct attention to sensory inputs. Thus Penfield and his colleagues thought that devastating effects on tactile perception resulted from lesions far back in the right supra-marginal gyrus of the PPC (Evans 1935). But it later became clear that the threshold of these patients' detection of passive touch, texture, or roughness, to which their attention had been forcibly drawn, was unaffected by posterior parietal lesions (88b). But their skin is rendered totally anaesthetic by anterior parietal lesions.

Thus it is mainly the more complex somaesthetic judgements that are affected by posterior parietal lesions. By complex in this context I mean perceptual processes in which not only external stimulation of cutaneous receptors must be taken into account, but also the subjects' own movements, which caused the receptors to be stimulated in the first place (sensory re-afference). This is 'active touch' (Gibson 1950).

Amorphosynthesis

The best known example of disordered active touch is astereognosis, otherwise known as tactile agnosia. This is the inability of patients to recognize the shape of objects by touch alone. This is difficult to separate from the more generalized deficit which Denny-Brown termed amorphosynthesis (Denny-Brown and Chambers 1958). This is the inability to achieve a correct summation of the spatial impressions of the positions of the patient's limbs and body, in order to build up a satisfactory body image (morphosynthesis). Adequate representation of the body image clearly requires precise association of motor signals about the movements of the limbs and body, with re-afferent proprioceptive and cutaneous feedback about what stimulation of these receptors was the result of the movements themselves. This particular set of associations probably takes place in the superior parietal lobule in humans, as in monkeys. It will be recalled that this is the region which is in close anatomical connection with the primary somaesthetic and motor cortical areas.

Asomatognosia, the denial of the existence of a part of the body, is clearly related to amorphosynthesis, though more dramatic. It is one of the most extraordinary symptoms seen in any patient with brain damage. The denial is so complete that the patient may not dress the left side of his body (dressing apraxia); and he may even deny that his left limbs belong to him. One of Oliver Sach's most memorable patients was one who kept falling out of bed (Sachs 1985). It turned out that the poor man, who had suffered a right posterior parietal stroke, was trying to get away from the dead limb that he kept finding in bed with him. Of course, it was in reality his own left leg. On occasions, patients' denial of an affected limb is so extreme that they may attribute pain in it, which presumably they feel but cannot localize, to someone else; for example, the patient in the next bed (Critchley 1953).

Cross-modal matching

As in primates, one class of symptom that we might expect quite commonly in patients with PPC lesions is impairment of cross-modal matching, as this part of the brain is a visual/auditory/somaesthetic crossroads. Yet there is curiously little published information on this topic. Both left- and right-sided parietal lesions can give rise to problems of cross-modal matching (Mishkin 1980) but it is not at all clear that the deficit is specifically cross-modal. The difficulty is to distinguish cross-modal impairments from disturbances of sensory motor control that may give rise to inability to recognize the required tactile or visual shapes even before the patients start to attempt to compare them. Nevertheless, probably cross-modal matching (Butters *et al.* 1970) is specifically impaired after PPC lesions. But this rarely occurs in isolation from impairment of sensorimotor integration.

Inferior parietal lobule

Visual inattention and neglect

As we have seen, Reszo Balint (*vide* Husain and Stein 1988) was the first to describe a disorder of visual attention following damage to the posterior parietal lobe. Balint observed that his patient had difficulty in looking at objects other than the one he was fixating on; so much so that on cursory examination he was considered to have paralysis of gaze. More careful investigation revealed that the patient's eye movements were intact and his apparent paralysis was due to an inability spontaneously to notice visual objects other than the one he was fixating. Thus, once his attention was engaged, this patient was simply unable to direct his attention voluntarily to other objects in the visual surround. Interestingly, even when prompted he always directed his attention to objects on the right.

Balint's patient was found to have bilateral damage to the PPC but, since this original description, numerous reports of visual inattention following unilateral damage to the PPC have been published. Following the resurgence of interest in the right hemisphere since the Second World War, the special association between disorders of visual attention and the right hemisphere has been clearly recognized (see Bisiach, Chapter 14; Heilman 1979; Jeannerod 1988). Left hemi-neglect is very common clinically. Patients omit one side when asked to draw or copy a picture. When asked to cross out elements in an array they miss those on the left. When asked to bisect a line they veer towards the right. In less formal testing it is obvious that the tend to ignore the food on the left side of their plate and people on their left side.

This neglect extends also into the sphere of visual imagery. Bisiach and Luzzatti (1978) asked Milanese patients with left neglect to recall the features of Piazza la Scala in Milan, first from the perspective of standing at one end of the square, then from the other end. They found that, in both cases, patients omitted to describe features on the left. Thus the building that they had not been able to describe from one end of the square, they were able to describe when imagining themselves at the other end of the square and vice versa. Hence, features on both sides of the square must have been stored in memory but the patients with left neglect could consciously recall only those on their right from any imaginary position in the square. It is almost as if the patients were unable to inspect the left side of their 'visual mind's eye', just as they are unable to inspect the left side of the current visual world surrounding them.

Usually left visual neglect results from damage to the inferior, rather than to the superior, parietal lobule (Vallar and Perani 1987). This conclusion is supported by both pathological and blood-flow studies, and confirms the view propounded earlier that the inferior parietal lobe is most important for visuomotor transformations whereas the superior parietal lobe is more important for somatomotor control.

Visual extinction (Chapter 14) is failure to detect a stimulus on one side when the corresponding point on the other side is stimulated simultaneously. This symptom is also associated with lesions of the PPC; but unlike neglect it has been claimed that it occurs equally after lesions in either hemisphere in humans (De Renzi 1982). Thus it may be considered a milder disorder of visual attention following damage to the parietal lobes.

Cognitive spaces and their co-ordinate systems

The nature of the 'space' that is neglected following lesions of the parietal cortex is of great interest. As we have seen, the problem of the congruence of sensory co-ordinate systems has troubled thinkers from the time of Plato onwards. The primary input from the eye is retinotopically organized, that from the skin somatotopically organized, whilst the spatial origin of sounds is computed in craniotopic co-ordinates. Moreover, the position of the limbs is expressed in terms of the angles of joints and the lengths of muscles. Are all these different spatial metrics reduced to a common co-ordinate system, centred on a point midway between the eyes, and often known as the egocentre; or is there no necessity for them to be converted into a common co-ordinate system defining 'real space', as maintained by Locke and Bishop Berkeley? Common sense suggests that there must be correspondence between somaesthetic, visual, motor, and other spaces. Otherwise it would be impossible for us to operate as accurately within them as most of us effortlessly manage. But Berkeley confidently denied the existence of real space, common to all the senses, as it would have to be a Universal, independent of the senses observing it.

In fact, the requirement of the brain to convert from sensory into motor co-ordinates does not necessarily mean that there must be an explicit topographical map of real space somewhere in the brain. Berkeley and Locke may have been right about this point after all. There is no evidence of any topographical correspondence between points in the parietal cortex and points in real space. The information required to convert retinotopic into oculomotor control signals, for example, may be stored as a distributed 'look-up table' in a way analogous to a computer memory. So $3°$ up and to the right may be stored next door to $15°$ down to the left at one moment, then $20°$ up, $10°$ down to the right at the next, when the contents of that memory location are changed.

Thus the rules for transformations of sensorimotor co-ordinates are probably distributed across the whole PPC. Except possibly in the hippo-campus (O'Keefe and Nadel 1978), no individual cells have been found in any region of the brain that code for absolute position in space. They tend to carry the combination of signals that is necessary for sensorimotor transformation, e.g. retinotopic plus eye-position signals.

Maybe there is no neural representation of physical space as such. Rather, the 'real' space that common sense persuades us to believe in operationally may be an emergent property of networks of neurons, which are particularly concentrated in the parietal cortex. Each cell carries a small proportion of the instructions necessary to convert, for example, retinotopic into oculomotor control signals, rather like the elements of a hologram. Thus the activity of the whole PPC is required for accurate direction of attention, eye, or limb movements. Hence also, loss of a small part of the PPC does not create a 'hole' in contralateral space, but it causes partial degradation of the accurate direction of attention, etc. After damage the system 'degrades gracefully'. This is one of the most advantageous properties of all distributed processing systems (Rumelhardt and McClelland 1987).

Nevertheless, the ways in which sensory input is transformed into motor control, output signals give rise to a number of 'psychological' spaces with which we think and work. 'Personal' space is that occupied by our own body; its co-ordinates are defined by the body's orientation with respect to gravity, and the position of our head and limbs. It provides the datum point for 'egocentric' localization. As we have seen, it is probably modelled and serviced by the superior parietal lobule.

'Peripersonal' space is the space immediately surrounding us within which we can reach out and touch objects. Localization is most accurate in this region. It requires the association of retinal foveal vision, and oculomotor and limb-movement signals; and it is probably serviced by area 7b in the monkey, and perhaps area 39 in the human.

'Extra-personal' space is the space beyond which we have only teleceptive information about the location of objects. Auditory, peripheral retinal, oculomotor, and whole-body signals are required for this. It is probably represented in area 7a in the monkey (area 40 in the human).

We tend to think of personal, peri-personal, and extra-personal space as all being defined in relation to our egocentre. As we have seen this belief is probably an emergent mental construct, which results from the nature of the rules our brains use to transform, for example, retinal, oculomotor, limb, and motor signals into each other. These rules are part of the 'hardware' of the system.

The results of these computations probably do not get stored in long-term memory. This would be pointless because the location of targets with respect to the eyes, head, or body remains relevant only so long as these stay in roughly the same place. For example, the direction of the door of a room with respect to our nose is no longer particularly important when we move into the next room. So for longer-term storage, only the location of objects with respect to each other is retained. This is known as 'allocentric' reference; and the 'place' cells in the hippocampus may be the ones that store spatial information in this way. North and south are allocentric relations that are specified by the positions of the earth's poles. Similarly, upstairs and downstairs are defined by the stairs, not the person climbing them. On the other hand, left and right are egocentric because their direction depends upon which way you, the observer, happen to be facing.

'Parietal space'

Bisiach and his colleagues performed another of their ingenious experiments to investigate the reference point of the co-ordinate system defining the space that is neglected by patients with visual neglect (Bisiach *et al.*

1985). They asked them to explore a tactile array and noted which parts of the array were omitted when the patients held their heads at different positions with respect to the body. They asked themselves whether the boundary of the neglect moved with the retinal visual fields or whether it was anchored to another co-ordinate system in the brain. They concluded that there were probably two frames of reference, one related to the body axis, the other tied to the line of sight; the latter would be either head-centric or retinotopic.

Bisiach *et al.* (1981) showed that the representation was not retinotopic, however, by having neglect patients view, through a narrow slit, pictures that were passed behind it. So they had to build up their image of the scene from the sequence of views passing behind the slit, using only foveal vision and without making any eye movements. When asked to reproduce the picture, they consistently missed out the left side, confirming that their ability to form the left side of mental images was disturbed, even though neither the left nor right hemi-retina had been stimulated, and no eye movements had taken place. Gazzaniga and Ladavas (1987) have now confirmed that parietal neglect is indeed independent of which retinal location is stimulated.

Thus the nature of the space that is neglected in patients with PPC lesions can now be defined a little more clearly. It does not move each time the eyes move; rather it is centred on a point passing through the centre of the body and head—the 'egocentre'. It is tempting, therefore, to assume that there is a representation of egocentric space in the parietal cortex into which all other co-ordinate systems are converted.

However, I believe this is going to turn out to be a misleading interpretation. There is no evidence of a topographical map of egocentric space in the PPC. What appeared to be a representation of the position of objects in the outside world is now turning out to be a table of signal-processing rules, setting out the way in which sensory reference frames must be transformed into appropriate attentional co-ordinates in order to produce the correct vectors necessary to shift attention towards them (Goldberg and Segraves 1987). This information can then be passed on to motor centres for the guidance of eye or limb movements.

Thus it is the location of whole objects with respect to the observer, rather than their absolute position in real space, which appears to be defined; how to reach objects rather than how different parts of space are filled.

Zipser and Andersen (1988) trained a computer simulation of a three-layered neural network to transform retinotopic and gaze-angle input into a signal indicating the direction of a stimulus with respect to the observer. The 'hidden' middle-layer units in their simulation developed properties very similar to those of the PPC neurons that Andersen and colleagues have recorded from the PPC of trained monkeys.

Even though this simulation is compatible with many theories of PPC function, it has clearly shown that this new approach to elucidating the processing operations of whole networks of neurons in different cortical areas offers enormous promise for the future. The simulation did not generate a 'map' of real space but rather a set of rules for working out the direction of objects; and this set was distributed over the whole network. This, of course, is highly reminiscent of the 'holographic', gracefully degrading, properties of the PPC mentioned earlier.

Visuomotor control

As we have seen, the projections leading forward from the primary visual cortex and the occipital lobe have been simplified into two broad streams termed by Ungerleider and Mishkin the 'what' and the 'where' pathways. The former passes laterally and ventrally into the infero-temporal cortex and it carries information about the colour and shape of objects. Here this information is used to identify what the object is by matching it with visual templates stored there.

The 'where' pathway carries information about the position and movement of visual targets; and, as we have seen, it passes dorsally and anteriorly, ending in the PPC, where it mingles with projections from the SC relaying in the pulvinar. Thus it provides some of the most important information required to determine where targets of interest in the outside world are located with respect to the observer.

What transformations are necessary to localize visual targets in space? First we require some incentive, or intention, to localize them in the first place. This motivational input is probably supplied by the cingulate gyrus to the PPC, according to its distillation of limbic opinion about whether any action, mental or physical, is required at all in relation to the object. This drive results from the identification of the object, which is taking place at the same time in the inferior temporal cortex. The latter area also projects to the cingulate gyrus.

Supposing this decision to be affirmative, the next stage in localization is the swinging of the mental 'searchlight' of attention on to the target (Crick 1984). This is the first stage of active sight. It is the operation that is central to understanding how objects are localized in the world, at least in so far as conscious localization is concerned. One cannot conceive of consciously localizing the position of an object without first attending to it.

Accurately pin-pointing the location of a target requires more information than the retina alone can provide. We actively explore our environment by ceaselessly realigning our eyes, head, or body to inspect it. But each time we shift our gaze, images stream across the retina. As a result the retinal positions of these images do not reliably indicate where objects in

J. F. Stein

the real world are. In order to specify the position of targets independently of where the retina is pointing, we therefore need also to know the direction of our gaze at the time each was inspected. This information is then linked in some way with what the object was identifed to be.

Thus retinotopic co-ordinates may be transformed into oculomotor co-ordinates by associating retinal signals with those provided by the oculomotor system, and the head and body movement systems. These indicate the direction of gaze at the time.

It is probably this act of directing attention towards targets of interest that is, in itself, the operation which makes the necessary associations between retinal images and relevant motor signals, in order to localize objects. An accurate sense of visual direction therefore depends upon the accurate direction of attention; and it is the latter which accomplishes efficient transformation of retinotopic into motor co-ordinates.

Exactly analogous transformations are also required in the somatic sphere, for active touch. In order to aim my hand towards a glass I have to be aware not only of the location of the glass but also where my hand now is, before starting the movement. To know where it is consciously I have to direct attention to that part of my body image, and thus localize it in my personal space, my body image.

Only when these preliminary operations of localization have been completed by attentional mechanisms has the perceptual system generated enough information for accurate motor control. Then these signals may be passed on to the frontal lobes, superior colliculus, basal ganglia, or cerebellum to help guide head, eye, body, or limb movements. Thus the PPC appears to be the site where the sensory/motor co-ordinate transformations underlying the direction of attention, and which underpin 'active sight' and 'active touch', take place. They are needed to localize targets in the outside world and to keep in accurate track of the position of the body and limbs.

Control of saccadic eye movements

The example of saccadic eye movement will serve as a specific example of the probable function of the PPC in visuomotor control. In Robinson's model of how saccades are generated an essential feature of the control system is the stage of transforming the retinal co-ordinates of the image of a target into an explicit signal coding the position of the target with respect to the head, i.e. a measure of the position of the target in real space (Robinson 1973). Then a motor-error signal is derived by subtracting current eye position from this measure of target position in real space. This error is what is used to drive the saccadic pulse generator. However, as we have seen, no such signal representing the absolute location

of visual targets in real space with respect to the head has yet been discovered.

An alternative model (Goldberg and Bruce 1990) of how saccades may
be generated, which does not rely upon computing a signal of target
position in real space, is to cause the control system to calculate from
retinal cues that amplitude and direction of the saccade that would be
required to bring the fovea on to the target. The current motor error could
then be calculated by subtracting from the desired, retinotopically defined,
saccade amplitude a signal equivalent to how far the current saccade had
progressed. Thus the control signal to move the eyes would be obtained by
subtracting from the retinotopic vector linking the fovea to the target of
interest, a vector signalling the amount by which the eye had moved so far.
Thus saccades need never be encoded in 'real space' co-ordinates, with the
necessity for transformation into and out of this system. Instead they could
be directly transferred from retinal into motor-output vectors. Spatial
accuracy would be achieved by the accuracy of the transformation of the
co-ordinates of the retinal map into the required saccade vector. Thus, in
the saccadic system, it would probably be possible to transform the retinal
vector of the target position directly into the motor-output vector, without
the necessity for an intermediate step of transforming the position of the
target into real space co-ordinates.

This possibility casts doubt on whether there is any necessity for the sort
of 'super map' of real space into which all sensory maps must be converted.
Locke and Bishop Berkeley may well have been right after all. Real space
may be an artificial construction of our minds rather than an explicit map in
the brain. Further advances in the computer simulation of neural networks
(Crick 1989) will help to clarify the information-processing operations that
have to take place in order to perform these vector transformations.

The functions of the posterior parietal cortex

We are now in a position to attempt a summary of the probable functions
of the PPC. The main features that have to be explained are the failure of
active sight and active touch in humans and other primates after PPC
lesions, and the role of PPC neurons in the direction of attention and the
guidance of movement in monkeys. I have attempted in this chapter to
show that all these findings can be explained by a 'simple' hypothesis,
namely that the PPC is the part of the brain devoted to the direction of
attention in space. The possible role of the left PPC in humans for directing
attention in time could not be addressed here, but it is a fruitful topic for
future research.

The key idea is that the act of shifting attention in order to concentrate on an object, rather than any eye or limb movements that might follow, is the crucial information-processing operation for which the PPC is responsible. This is the step that transforms retinotopic or limb-position co-ordinates into those centred on the egocentre, which enable the accurate guidance of movements. The evidence in favour of this idea is that PPC lesions interfere with patients' ability to direct their attention to the contra-lateral side, and that this leads to mislocalization of their own limbs and of objects in the outside world, even though they can see them perfectly well. Moreover, in monkeys, PPC neurons discharge as readily before shifts of attention as before movements. These findings suggest that the prime function of the PPC is the accurate direction of attention, and that it is this operation that mediates the sensorimotor associations that are required for the successful direction of movements.

We have seen that this direction of attention does not necessarily lead to an explicit representation of 'real space' in the PPC. There is no point-to-point correspondence between points in the PPC and points in real space. Thus, direction of attention is not an anatomically topographical process analogous to the projection of the retina or skin onto the primary visual or somaesthetic cortical areas. Rather, the PPC portrayal of the world seems to be an emergent property of the way in which neurons there are linked together in a network to encode the rules by which different primary sensory representations may be converted into guidance of movement in relation to them. No one cell carries complete information about a locus in space. Instead the strength of linkages between neurons represents the rules for guiding attention, and hence movement.

It must be admitted, however, that at the present time there is only circumstantial evidence for these conjectures. We do not yet have a clear idea how one would recognize the signs of such a distributed system in action. What would it look like recorded at the end of an electrode, or imaged by position-emission tomography? Nevertheless, much evidence suggests that it is in the PPC that the first stage takes place. Here multi-modal sensory, motivational, and motor inputs are put together to direct attention to different locations in space, so that movements may be sub-sequently directed towards them. Thus the PPC probably does not contain a representation of space, but rather a representation of the rules that must be followed in order to direct attention, and hence eye, limb, or body movements, towards objects in space.

References

Albright, T. D. (1984). Direction and orientation selectivity of neurons in visual area MT of the macaque. *Journal of Neurophysiology* **51**, 1106–30.

Albright, T. D., Desimone, R., and Gross, C. G. (1984). Columnar organization of directionally selective cells in visual area MT of the macaque. *Journal of Neurophysiology*, **51**, 16–31.

Andersen, R. A. (1987). Inferior parietal lobule function in spatial perception and visuomotor integration. In *Handbook of physiology* (ed. F. Plum and V. B. Mountcastle, pp. 483–518. American Physiological Society, Rockville, MD.

Andersen, R. A. and Gnadt, J. W. (1989). Posterior parietal cortex. In *The neurobiology of saccadic eye movements, reviews in ocularmotor research*, Vol. 3 (ed. R. Wurtz and M. Goldberg), pp. 315–55. Elsevier, Amsterdam.

Andersen, R. A., Asanuma, C., and Cowan, W. M. (1985). Callosal and prefrontal associational projecting cell populations in area 7a of the macaque monkey: a study using retrogradely transported fluorescent dyes. *Journal of Comparative Neurology*, **232**, 443–55.

Andersen, R. A., Essick, G. K., and Siegel, R. M. (1985). Encoding of spatial location by posterior parietal neurons. *Science*, **230**, 456–8.

Andersen, R. A., Essick, G. K., and Siegel, R. M. (1988). Neurons of area 7 activated by both visual stimuli and oculomotor behavior. *Experimental Brain Research*, **67**, 316–22.

Asanuma, C., Andersen, R. A., and Cowan, W. M. (1985). The thalamic relations of the caudal inferior parietal lobule and the lateral prefrontal cortex in monkeys: divergent cortical projections from cell clusters in the medial pulvinar nucleus. *Journal of Comparative Neurology*, **241**, 357–81.

Barash, S., Bracewell, R. M., Gnadt, J. W., Fogassi, L., and Andersen, R. A. (1989). Quantitative analysis of sacade-related activities in areas LIP and 7a of macaque. *Society For Neurosciences Abstracts*, **15**, 1203.

Bisiach, E. and Luzzatti, C. (1978). Unilateral neglect of representational space. *Cortex*, **14**, 129–33.

Bisiach, E., Capitani, E., and Porta, E. (1985). Two basic properties of space representation in the brain. *Journal of Neurology and Neurosurgical Psychiatry*, **48**, 141–4.

Bisiach, E., Capitani, E., Luzzatti, C., and Perani, D. (1981). Brain and conscious representation of outside reality. *Neuropsychologia*, **19**, 543–51.

Bonin, G. von and Bailey, P. (1947). *The neocortex of Macaca mulatta*. University of Illinois Press, Urbana.

Brain, R. (1941). Visual disorientation with special reference to lesions of the right hemisphere. *Brain*, **64**, 244–72.

Brodal, P. (1978). Principles of organisation of the monkey corticopontine projection. *Brain*, **148**, 214–28.

Bushnell, M. C., Goldberg, M. E., and Robinson, D. L. (1981). Behavioral enhancement of visual responses in monkey cerebral cortex. I. Modulation in posterior parietal cortex related to selective visual attention. *Journal of Neurophysiology*, **46**, 755–72.

Butters, N., Barton, M., and Brody, B. A. (1970). Role of the right parietal lobe in the mediation of cross-modal associations and reversible operations in space. *Cortex*, **6**, 174–90.

Caminiti, R. and Sbriccoli, A. (1985). The callosal system of the superior parietal lobule in the monkey. *Journal of Comparative Neurology*, **237**, 85–99.

Chavis, D. A. and Pandya, D. N. (1976). Corticofrontal connections in rhesus monkey. *Brain Research*, **117**, 369–86.

Crick, F. (1984). Function of the thalamic reticular complex: the searchlight hypothesis. *Proceedings of the National Academy of Sciences USA*, **81**, 4586–90.

Crick, F. (1989). The recent excitement about neural networks. *Nature*, **337**, 129–33.

Critchley, M. (1953). *The parietal lobes*. Hafner, New York.

Davenport, R. K., Rogers, C. M., and Russell, I. S. (1973). Cross-modal perception in apes. *Neuropsychologia*, **11**, 21–8.

Denny-Brown, D. and Chambers, R. A. (1958). The parietal lobes and behavior. *Research Publications of the Association for Research in Mental Disease*, **36**, 35–117.

De Renzi, E. (1982). *Disorders of space exploration and cognition*. Wiley, Chichester.

Divac, I., Lavail, J. H., Racic, P., and Winston, K. R. (1977). Hetereogeneous afferents to the inferior parietal lobule of the rhesus monkey revealed by the retrograde transport method. *Brain Research*, **123**, 197–207.

Dubner, R. and Zeki, S. M. (1971). Response properties and receptive fields of cells in an anatomically defined region of the superior temporal sulcus in the monkey. *Brain Research*, **35**, 528–32.

Evans, J. P. (1935). A study of the sensory defects resulting from excision of the cerebral substance in humans. *Research Publications of the Association for Research in Mental Disease*, **15**, 331–70.

Gazzaniga, M. S. and Ladavas, E. (1987). Disturbances in spatial attention following lesion or disconnection of the right parietal lobe. In *Neurophysiological and neuropsychological aspects of spatial neglect* (ed. M. Jeannerod) pp. 203–13. Elsevier, Amsterdam.

Gerstmann, J. (1924). Fingeragnosie: Ein unschriebene Storung der Orientierung am eigenen Korper. *Wiener Klinische Wochenschift*, **37**, 1010–12.

Gerstmann, J. (1957). Some notes on the Gerstmann syndrome. *Neurology*, **7**, 866–9.

Geschwind, N. (1965). Disconnection syndromes in animals and man. *Brain*, **88**, 237–94.

Gibson, J. J. (1950). *The perception of the visual world*. Houghton Mifflin, Boston.

Glickstein, M. (1985). Ferrier's mistake. *Trends in Neuroscience*, **8**, 341–4.

Glickstein, Cohen, J. L., Dixon, B., Gibson, A., Hollins, M., Labossière, E., and Robinson, F. (1980). Corticopontine visual projections in macaque monkeys. *Journal of Comparative Neurology*, **90**, 209–29.

Gnadt, J. W. and Andersen, R. A. (1988). Memory related motor planning activity in posterior parietal cortex of macaque. *Experimental Brain Research*, **70**, 216–20.

Goldberg, M. J. and Bruce, C. J. (1990). Primate frontal eye fields: Maintenance of a spatially accurate signal. *Journal of Neurophysiology* (in press).

Goldberg, M. E. and Segraves, M. A. (1987). Visuospatial and motor attention in the monkey. *Neuropsychologia*, **25**, 107–18.

Grusser, O. J., Panse, M., and Schreiber, V. (1982). Neuronal responses in the parieto-insular vestibular cortex of alert Java monkeys (*Macaca fascicularis*). In *Physiological and pathological aspects of eye movements* (ed. A. Roncoux and M. Crommelink), pp. 251–70. Junk, The Hague.

Head, H. and Holmes, G. (1911). Sensory disturbances from cerebral lesions. *Brain*, **34**, 102–24.

Hecaen, H., Penfield, W., Bertrand, C., and Malmo, R. (1956). The syndrome of apractognosia due to lesions of the minor cerebral hemisphere. *Archives of Neurology and Psychiatry*, **75**, 400–34.

Heilman, K. M. (1979). Neglect and related disorders. In *Clinical neuropsychology* (ed. K. M. Heilman and E. Valenstein), pp. 268–307. Oxford University Press.

Heilman, K. M. and Valenstein, E. (1985). *Clinical neuropsychology*. Oxford University Press.

Hillyard, S. A., Munte, T. F., and Neville, H. J. (1985). Visuospatial attention, orienting and brain physiology. In *Attention and performance* (ed. M. I. Posner and O. S. Martin), pp. 63–84. Erlbaum, Hillsdale, NJ.

Holmes, G. (1918). Disturbances of visual orientation. *British Journal of Ophthalmology*, **2**, 449–80.

Hughlings-Jackson, J. (1870). *Selected writings* (ed. J. Taylor). Hodder and Stoughton, London.

Husain, M. (1991). Visuospatial and visuomotor functions of the posterior parietal lobe. In *Vision and visual dyslexia* (ed. J. Stein), Chapter 13. Macmillan, London. (In press.)

Husain, M. and Stein, J. F. (1988). Rezso Balint and his most celebrated case. *Archives of Neurology*, **45**, 89–93.

Hyvarinen, J. (1981). Regional distribution of functions within in parietal association area 7 of the monkey. *Brain Research*, **206**, 287–303.

Hyvarinen, J. (1982). *The parietal cortex of monkey and man*. Springer-Verlag, Berlin.

Jeannerod, M. (1988). *The neural and behavioural organization of goal directed movements*. Oxford Psychology Series 15. Oxford University Press, Oxford.

Jones, E. G. and Powell, T. P. S. (1969). Connections of the somatic sensory cortex of the rhesus monkey. I. Ipsilateral cortical connections. *Brain*, **92**, 477–502.

Komatsu, H. and Wurtz, R. H. (1988a). Relation of cortical areas MT and MST to pursuit eye movements. I) localization and visual properties of neurons. *Journal of Neurophysiology*, **60**, 580–603.

Komatsu, H. and Wurtz, R. H. (1988b). Relation of cortical areas MT and MST to pursuit eye movements. II. Interaction with full-field visual stimulation. *Journal of Neurophysiology*, **60**, 621–44.

Lee, D. N. (1980). The optic flow field. *Philosophical Transactions of the Royal Society*, (B) **290**, 167–79.

Lhermitte, F., Turell, E., LeBrigand, D., and Chain, F. (1985). Unilateral visual neglect and wave P300. A study of nine cases with unilateral lesions of the parietal lobes. *Archives of Neurology*, **42**, 567–73.

Luria, A. R. (1958). Brain disorders and language analysis. *Language and Speech*, **1**,

Lynch, J. C. (1980). The functional organization of posterior parietal association cortex. *Behavioral and Brain Science*, **3**, 485–534.

Maunsell, J. H. R. and Van Essen, C. (1983a). The connections of the middle temporal visual area (MT) and their relationship to a cortical hierarchy in the macaque monkey. *Journal of Neuroscience*, **3**, 2563–86.

Maunsell, J. H. R. and Van Essen, C. (1983b). Functional properties of neurons in Middle Temporal visual area of the macaque monkey. I. Selectivity for stimulus direction, speed, and orientation. *Journal Neurophysiology*, **49**, 1127–47.

Maunsell, J. H. R. and Van Essen, C. (1983c). Functional properties of neurons in Middle Temporal visual area of the macaque monkey. II. Binocular interactions and sensitivity to binocular disparity. *Journal of Neurophysiology*, **49**, 1148–67.

McFie, J., Piercy, M. F., and Zangwill, O. L. (1950). Visual spatial agnosia associated with lesions of the right cerebral hemisphere. *Brain*, **73**, 167–70.

Mesulam, M.-M. (1985). Attention, confusional states and neglect. In *Principles of behavioral neurology* (ed. M.-M. Mesulam), pp. 125–68. Davis, Philadelphia.

Mesulam, M.-M., Van Hoesen, G. W., Pandya, D. N., and Geschwind, N. (1977). Limbic and sensory connections of the inferior parietal lobule (area PG) in the rhesus monkey: a study with a new method for horseradish peroxidase histochemistry. *Brain Research*, **136**, 393–414.

Mikami, A., Newsome, W. T., and Wurtz, R. H. (1986). Motion selectivity in macaque visual cortex. II. Spatiotemporal range of directional interactions in MT and V1. *Journal of Neurophysiology*, **55**, 1328–39.

Mishkin, M., Ungerleider, L. G., and Macko, K. A. (1983). Object vision and spatial vision: two cortical pathways. *Trends in Neuroscience*, **6**, 414–17.

Morgan, M. J. (1977). *Molyneux's question*. Cambridge University Press.

Motter, B. C. and Mountcastle, V. B. (1981). The functional properties of the light sensitive neurons of the posterior parietal cortex studied in waking monkeys: foveal sparing and opponent vector organization. *Journal of Neuroscience*, **1**, 3–26.

Mountcastle, V. B., Lynch, J. C., Georgopoulis, A., Sakata, H., and Acuna, C. (1975). Posterior parietal association cortex of the monkey: command function for operations within extrapersonal space. *Journal of Neurophysiology*, **38**, 871–908.

Mountcastle, V. B., Andersen, R. A., and Motter, B. C. (1981). The influence of attentive fixation upon the excitability of the light-sensitive neurons of the posterior parietal cortex. *Journal of Neuroscience*, **1**, 1218–35.

Mountcastle, V. B., Motter, B. C., Steinmetz, M. A., and Duffy, C. J. (1984). Looking and seeing: the visual functions of the parietal lobe. In *Dynamic aspects of neocortical function* (ed. G. M. Edelman, W. E. Gall, and W. M. Cowan), pp. 159–64. John Wiley, New York.

Movshon, J. A., Adelson, E. H., Gizzi, M. S., and Newsome, W. T. (1985). The analysis of moving patterns in pattern recognition. *Experimental Brain Research* (suppl. 11), 117–51.

Neville, H. J. and Lawson, D. (1987). Attention to central and peripheral visual space in a movement detection task: an event-related potential and behavioral study. I. Normal hearing adults. *Brain Research*, **405**, 253–67.

Newsome, W. T., Wurtz, R. H., and Komatsu, H. (1988). Relation of cortical areas MT and MST to pursuit eye movements. II. Differentiation of retinal from extraretinal inputs. *Journal of Neurophysiology*, **60**, 604–20.

Newsome, W. T., Britten, K. H., and Movshon, J. A. (1989). Neuronal correlates of a perceptual decision. *Nature*, **341**, 52–4.

O'Keefe, J. and Nadel, L. (1978). *The hippocampus as a cognitive map*. Oxford University Press.

Paillard, J., Jordan, P. L., and Brouchon, M. (1981). Visual motion cues in prismatic adaptation. *Acta Psychologica*, **48**, 253–70.

Paillard, J. (1982). The contribution of peripheral and central vision to visually guided reading. In *Analysis of visual behavior* (ed. D. J. Ingle, M. A. Goodale, and R. J. W. Mansfield), pp. 367–88. MIT Press, Cambridge, Mass.

Paillard, J. (1987). Cognitive v. sensorimotor encoding of spatial information. In *Cognitive processes and spatial orientation* (ed. P. Ellon and C. Thinns-Blanc). Martinus Nijhoff, Dordrecht.

Pandya, D. N. and Kuypers, H. G. J. M. (1969). Cortico-cortical connections in the rhesus monkey. *Brain Research*, **13**, 13–36.

Pandya, D. N. and Seltzer, B. (1982). Intrinsic connections and architectonics of posterior parietal cortex in the rhesus monkey. *Journal of Comparative Neurology*, **204**, 196–210.

Pearson, A., Brodal, P., and Powell, T. P. S. (1978). The projection of the thalamus upon the parietal lobe in the monkey. *Brain Research*, **144**, 143–8.

Petras, J. M. (1971). Connections of the parietal lobe. *Journal of Psychiatric Research*, **8**, 189–201.

Petrides, M. and Iverson, S. D. (1979). Restricted posterior parietal lesions in the rhesus monkey and performance on visuospatial tasks. *Brain Research*, **161**, 63–77.

Reivich, M., Gur, R., and Alavi, A. (1983). Positron emission tomographic studies of sensory stimuli, cognitive processes and anxiety. *Human Neurobiology*, **2**, 25–33.

Robinson, D. A. (1973). Models of the Saccadic eye movement system. *Kybernetik*, **14**, 77–83.

Robinson, D. L., Goldberg, M. E., and Stanton, G. B. (1978). Parietal association cortex in the primate: sensory mechanisms and behavioral modulation. *Journal of Neurophysiology*, **41**, 910–32.

Rockland, K. S. and Pandya, D. N. (1979). Laminar origins and terminations of cortical connections of the occipital lobe in the rhesus monkey. *Brain Research*, **179**, 3–20.

Rodman, H. R. and Albright, T. D. (1989). Single unit analysis of pattern–motion selective properties in the middle temporal visual area (MT). *Experimental Brain Research*, **75**, 53–64.

Roland, P. E. (1982). Cortical regulation of selective attention in man. A regional cerebral blood flow study. *Journal of Neurophysiology*, **48**, 1059–78.

Rumelhardt, D. E. and McClelland, J. L. (1987). *Parallel distributed processing*. MIT Press, Cambridge, Mass.

Sachs, O. (1985). *The man who mistook his wife for a hat*. Duckworth, London.

Sakata, H. (1985). The parietal association cortex: Neurophysiology. In *Scientific basis of clinical neurology* (ed. M. Swash and C. Kennard), pp. 226–36. Churchill Livingstone, Edinburgh.

Sakata, H., Takoaka, A., Kawarasaki, A., and Shibutani, H. (1973). Somatosensory properties of neurons in superior parietal cortex (area 5) of the rhesus monkey. *Brain Research*, **64**, 85–102.

Schwartz, D. W. F. and Frederickson, J. M. (1971). Rhesus monkey vestibular cortex, a bimodal projection field. *Science*, **172**, 280–1.

Seltzer, B. and Pandya, D. N. (1984). Further observations on parieto-temporal connections in the rhesus monkey. *Experimental Brain Research*, **55**, 301–12.

Stanton, G. B., Cruce, W. L. R., Goldberg, M. E., and Robinson, D. L. (1977). Some ipsilateral projections to areas PF and PG of the inferior parietal lobule in monkeys. *Neuroscience Letters*, **6**, 243–50.

Stein, J. F. (1978). Effects of parietal lobe cooling on manipulation in the monkey. In *Active touch* (ed. G. Gordon), pp. 79–90. Pergamon, Oxford.

Stein, J. F. (1989). Representation of egocentric space in the posterior parietal cortex. *Quarterly Journal of Experimental Physiology*, **74**, 583–606.

Steinmetz, M. A., Motter, B. C., Duffy, C. J., and Mountcastle, V. B. (1987). Functional properties of parietal visual neurons: radial organization of directionalities within the visual field. *Journal of Neuroscience*, **7**, 177–91.

Tanaka, K., Hikosaka, K., Saito, H.-A., Yukie, M., Fukuda, Y., and Iwai, E. (1986). Analysis of local and wide-field movements in the superior temporal visual areas of the macaque monkey. *Journal of Neurosciences*, **6**, 134–44.

Thickbroom, G. W. and Mastaglia, F. J. (1985). Cerebral events preceding saccades. *EEG and Clinical Neurophysiology*, **62**, 277–89.

Ungerleider, L. G. and Desimone, R. (1986a). Projections to the superior temporal sulcus from the central and peripheral field representations of V1 and V2. *Journal of Comparative Neurology*, **248**, 147–63.

Ungerleider, L. G. and Desimone, R. (1986b). Cortical connections of visual area MT in the macaque. *Journal of Comparative Neurology*, **248**, 190–222.

Ungerleider, L. G. and Mishkin, M. (1982). Two cortical visual systems. In *The analysis of visual behavior* (ed. D. J. Ingle, M. A. Goodale, R. J. W. Mansfield), pp. 549–86. MIT Press, Cambridge, Mass.

Vallar, G. and Perani, D. (1987). The anatomy of spatial neglect in humans. In *Neurophysiological and neuropsychological aspects of spatial neglect* (ed. K. Jeannerod), pp. 235–58. North-Holland, Amsterdam.

von Economo, (1929). *The cytoarchitectonics of the human cerebral cortex*. Oxford University Press.

Zipser, D. and Andersen, R. A. (1988). Back propagation learning simulates response properties of a subset of posterior parietal neurons. *Nature*, **331**, 679–84.

12

Congruent representations of visual and somatosensory space in single neurons of monkey ventral intra-parietal cortex (area VIP)

JEAN-RENÉ DUHAMEL, CAROL L. COLBY, and
MICHAEL E. GOLDBERG

Introduction

We perceive the space in which we live by the use of all of our senses. Vision is the pre-eminent sense in primates, but we can also use audition, somatic sensation, and even olfaction. Our perception of space is calibrated by the accuracy of our movements through it. This calibration requires an intermodality equivalence, such that stimuli of disparate modalities ultimately evoke equivalent responses at some place in the nervous system. Clinical and experimental evidence has long implicated the posterior parietal cortex in the process by which the brain constructs an image of space (Critchley 1953). The posterior parietal cortex lies at the junction of visual and somatosensory cortices, and although historically it was thought to be a somatosensory association cortex, recent work has emphasized its visual nature (Hyvarinen and Poranen 1974; Lynch *et al.* 1977; Robinson *et al.* 1978). Such studies also demonstrated some convergence between vision and somatic sensation in the posterior parietal cortex of the monkey (Robinson *et al.* 1978; Leinonen *et al.* 1979).

Recent work on the primate extra-striate cortex has brought to light the existence of numerous, independent representations of the visual field (Van Essen & Maunsell 1983), and connectional studies in the macaque indicate that there are a number of separate areas within the posterior parietal cortex. Within the intra-parietal sulcus alone there are at least four distinct areas as defined on the basis of their connections to other cortical and sub-cortical regions: the medial intra-parietal area (MIP), connected to area PO (Colby *et al.* 1988a); the posterior intra-parietal area (PIP), connected to V3, V4, and PO (Felleman and Van Essen 1983; Colby *et al.* 1988a); the lateral intra-parietal area (LIP), connected to the frontal cortex (Andersen *et al.* 1985) and superior colliculus (Lynch *et al.* 1985); and the ventral intra-parietal area (VIP), connected to areas MT and MST, the motion-sensitive regions in the superior temporal sulcus (STS) (Maunsell and Van Essen 1983b; Ungerleider and Desimone 1986). We have mapped out these areas physiologically by recording the activity of single neurons in the intra-parietal sulcus in alert, active monkeys, trained in a wide variety of tasks, using a recording grid for reliable placement of electrodes (Crist et al. 1988).

We describe here the responses of cells in a single physiologically defined zone, area VIP, which our histological reconstruction shows to be located in the fundus of the intra-parietal sulcus. Cells in this region have visual motion-detection properties similar to those in MT and MST, from which they presumably receive their visual input, but motion-sensitive cells in VIP have three additional properties not described in cells in the superior temporal sulcus: (a) behavioural modulation of visual responsiveness similar to that observed in other parietal areas (Bushnell et al. 1981); (b) depth selectivity independent of retinal disparity; and (c) somatosensory responses that correspond to the visual responses. These data suggest a role for VIP neurons in the generation of a supra-modal representation of space (Colby et al. 1988b, 1989; Duhamel et al. 1989).

Methods

Two rhesus monkeys (*Macaca mulatta*) were trained in a series of visual and oculomotor tasks, and surgically prepared under general anaesthesia for chronic neurophysiological recording by the implantation of ocular search coils, head-holding devices, and recording chambers through which electrodes could subsequently be introduced into the cerebral cortex. Behavioural monitoring, eye position, and unit sampling, as well as on-line data analysis, were done with a PDP-11/73 computer (Goldberg 1983).

Recordings were made with flexible tungsten electrodes introduced through stainless-steel guide tubes implanted nearly but not quite through the dura, which in turn were stabilized by a nylon grid held rigidly in the recording cylinder (Crist et al. 1988). The grid served as a guide to produce parallel penetrations with a resolution of 0.5 mm. The rigidity of the system and the atraumatic quality of the electrodes allowed us to make a large number of penetrations at multiple recording sites within the intra-parietal sulcus. We found that electrode penetrations made several months apart at the same grid locations yielded neurons with similar response types at similar depths. In one monkey, after having mapped the intra-parietal sulcus in both hemispheres, we recorded again at each site and placed a pattern of lesions designed to identify each electrode track and the depth at which specific types of activity were found. By sectioning the brain in the plane of the grid, we were able to reconstruct this large number of lesions

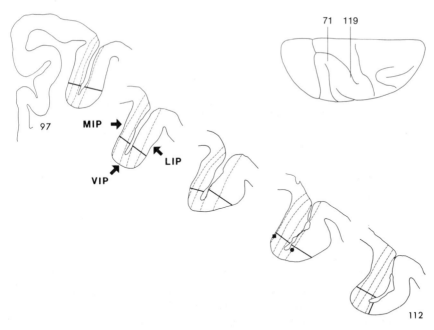

Fig. 12.1. Drawings made from a numbered series of thionine-stained sections showing the physiological borders of VIP and the electrode tracks (dashed lines) that passed through this area. The square and circle show the location of two VIP neurons as determined by marking lesions—MIP, medial intra-parietal area and LIP, lateral intra-parietal area.

reliably. In the work reported here, one hemisphere has been reconstructed completely (Fig. 12.1), and the location of the physiologically defined VIP has been confirmed in a second hemisphere.

Results

We report here on 136 neurons in area VIP. The borders of this physiologically defined area are shown in Fig. 12.1: VIP is restricted to the fundus of the intra-parietal sulcus. All of these neurons had visual receptive fields. We will describe the visual, behavioural, and somatosensory properties of these neurons.

Characteristics of the visual receptive field

Area VIP stood out from the surrounding, visually responsive cortex by the relative ease with which its cells could be driven. These neurons were strongly responsive to a wide range of visual stimuli and were particularly sensitive to stimulus motion. Their response properties were similar in several respects to those of cells in MT and MST. First, almost 70 per cent of the cells in VIP were direction-selective. For example, the neuron shown in Fig. 12.2A responded strongly to a small spot moving through its receptive field in the on direction and was completely unresponsive to the same stimulus moving in the null direction. The location at which this cell was recorded is marked by the circle in Fig. 12.1. Second, VIP neurons showed strong responsiveness to whole-field motion and were direction-selective when tested with a random-dot pattern. Third, VIP neurons, like cells in areas MT and MST, could be selective for the speed at which a stimulus moves through the receptive field. Fourth, some VIP cells exhibited crisp, transient, on/off responses to stationary stimuli flashed within the field. Finally, a small sample of direction-selective VIP neurons studied in a smooth-pursuit task showed strong responsiveness in relation to pursuit eye movements, similar to that of cells in the STS. This activity appeared to depend on visual input because the response was strongly reduced if the pursuit target was briefly blanked off and the monkey continued to move its eyes in a predictive manner. In their directional selectivity, speed tuning, and responsiveness to small, moving targets and large, field movements, VIP neurons resembled those in the MT and MST. The next three sections present data on how VIP appears to differ from these other motion areas.

Behavioural modulation of visual activity

The activity of cells in the posterior parietal cortex can be modulated by the behaviour required of the animal. When a stimulus becomes behaviourally significant, the visual response of a cell can be enhanced (Robinson et al. 1978; Bushnell et al. 1981; Yin and Mountcastle, 1977). We found enhanced visual responses in cells in the VIP. An example of such an enhanced visual response is shown in Fig. 12.2B, which compares the activity of a directionally selective neuron in a fixation task to that in a saccade task. The cell did not respond to the stimulus in the fixation task, but responded briskly to the same stimulus in the saccade task. A visual memory-guided, saccade task is shown, in which the stimulus appeared and disappeared while the monkey looked at the fixation point. When the fixation point disappeared, the monkey made a saccade to the location where the stimulus had been. This task allowed us to distinguish between activity related to the stimulus and that related to the movement itself. The neuron shown responded to the stimulus, but did not discharge before the saccade. Such enhanced activity to behaviourally significant stimuli is a common characteristic of neurons in the parietal cortex (Robinson et al. 1978; Bushnell et al. 1981; Yin and Mountcastle 1977), and our findings

(A) Response to moving stimuli

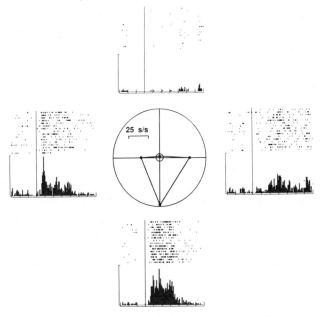

(B) Response to stationary stimuli

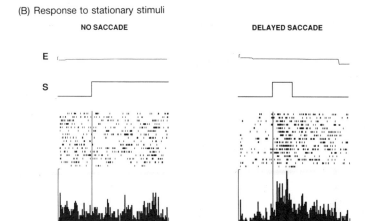

Fig. 12.2. Activity of a VIP visual neuron (62.366). (A) Direction tuning is represented by a polar plot (centre) showing the average firing rate of the cell to a small stimulus moving at 10°/s in four different directions across the receptive field. (B) Activity of the same neuron showing no response to the presentation of a stationary stimulus in the receptive field while the monkey maintains central fixation (left), and an enhanced response to the presentation of the same stimulus in a delayed saccade task (right). All displays and histograms aligned on stimulus onset (E, eye; S, stimulus—calibration bar on histograms set at 100 Hz). Histogram bin width, 16 ms; tic marks on horizontal axis occur every 200 ms.

indicate that this phenomenon extends to the depths of the intra-parietal sulcus. They contrast with previous findings in the STS, where Newsome *et al.* (1988) reported that MST neurons showed enhanced visual responses to moving but not to stationary stimuli.

Depth selectivity

Twenty per cent of the neurons in the VIP are tuned for stimulus location in depth. Half of these depth-selective neurons responded best to near stimuli, located 10 to 20 cm from the animal, while the other half responded best to 'ultra-near' stimuli presented within 5 cm of the monkey's face. These responses were characterized not by an absolute preference, but by a gradient of firing that varied as function of viewing distance. The activity of an ultra-near cell is illustrated in Fig. 12.3. This cell responded best to stimuli located on a tangential screen 5 cm from the monkey, less well to a stimulus at 10 cm, and least well to a stimulus at 57 cm. The monkey fixated a spot on a tangential screen at 57 cm during presentation

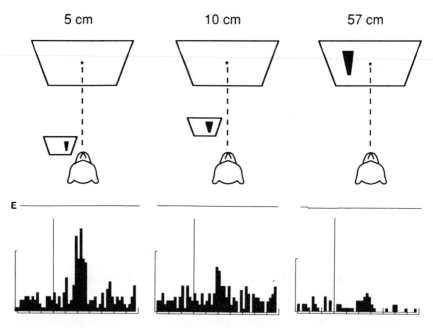

Fig. 12.3. Activity of an ultra-near VIP neuron (62.311). Top cartoons show the locations of the screens used to project the stimulus, an elongated vertical bar, at 5, 10 and 57 cm from the animal's eye (E) (drawings not to scale). The fixation point was always presented on the farthest screen. The neuron's response shown below is strongest to the ultra-near stimulus and weakest to the far stimulus. Histogram bin width, 40 ms; tic marks on horizontal axis occur every 200 ms.

of all stimuli, so the cell did not require changes in accommodation or vergence as a cue for depth. The cell also did not require retinal disparity as a cue for depth because it responded equally well to monocular and binocular stimuli, and it also discharged when the animal looked at a near object. Thus this cell appeared to respond to a near stimulus regardless of the cues used in establishing that nearness. We do not know if these neurons also respond to pure binocular disparity, in which case they would be sensitive to the depth of the object no matter what cues were used to make an estimation of depth. Depth-sensitive, STS neurons respond to disparity cues but it is not known whether they respond to depth cues other than disparity (Maunsell and Van Essen 1983a; Komatsu *et al.* 1988). Ultra-near responses similar to those observed in the VIP have also been reported in the pre-motor cortex (Rizzolatti *et al.* 1987) in an area generally assumed to be important in the generation of mouth movements, movements which can be guided only by ultra-near visual stimuli.

Somatosensory activity

Perhaps the most unexpected feature of neuronal activity in the VIP was the presence of strong and robust somatosensory responses in neurons with motion- and depth-sensitive visual properties. Careful testing of well-isolated VIP neurons with visual and somatosensory stimuli showed that 70 per cent of such neurons were truly bimodal. Both the locations and the motion requirements of the visual and somatosensory receptive fields are closely matched.

Somatosensory responses were evoked using air puffs, light pressure applied with the tip of a stationary or moving cotton applicator, and by rotating individual joints. Testing was always done with the monkey unable to see the process of somatosensory stimulation. Whenever the somatosensory receptive field could not be seen by the monkey, we tested the cell while the monkey was performing a fixation task in order to control for eye position. We found that all cells that had a somatosensory receptive field responded well to passive stimulation. Most of these receptive field were cutaneous, and over 80 per cent were located on the head and face. We found a few cells that responded to joint rotation. Area VIP contains a complete representation of the head and face region. The majority of the receptive fields were contralateral, with 24 per cent having bilateral fields and 16 per cent ipsilateral receptive fields. Most VIP cells (68 per cent) had receptive fields on the front of the face or body, but some receptive fields included the side (21 per cent) or back (11 per cent) of the head or body. Finally, for those cells in which we tested specifically for direction selectivity to somatosensory stimulation, about two-thirds showed clear selectivity.

Congruent visual and somatosensory response properties

There is a striking correspondence between the location and response
properties of visual receptive fields and those of somatosensory receptive
fields. The location, size, and motion selectivity of the receptive fields are
complementary in both the visual and somatosensory domains, as illustrated in Fig. 12.4. This neuron responds to visual stimuli presented in the
upper periphery of the ipsilateral visual field. The same cell also has an
ipsilateral, somatosensory receptive field covering the upper part of the
face and above the ear. The location and depth of this cell in the intra-
parietal sulcus was identified by a marking lesion represented by the square
symbol in Fig. 12.1, in the same section as the direction-selective neuron

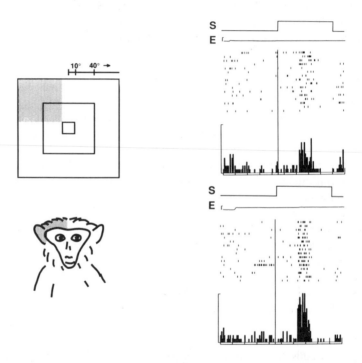

Fig. 12.4. Activity of a bimodal VIP neuron (62.340). Top diagram represents the visual field
of the monkey divided into three zones: the central 10° on either side of both visual meridians
inside the small inner square; the periphery of the visual field, up to 40°, inside the middle
square; the far periphery within the outer square. The visual receptive field corresponds to the
shaded area, and the top right displays show the cell's response to a stimulus presented within
it. The shaded area of the bottom left diagram shows the location of the somatosensory
receptive field, and the displays on the right show the cell's response to light touch of this
area. For simplicity left and right sides of the visual field and of the monkey are aligned. This
cell has ipsilateral receptive fields in both sensory modalities. S, stimulus; E, eye—histogram
bin width, 16 ms; tic marks on horizontal axis occur every 200 ms.

(A)	Somatosensory				(B)	Somatosensory		
	contra	bi	ipsi			upper	hm	lower
contra	14	3	—		upper	9	2	—
bi	—	2	—		hm	—	2	—
ipsi	—	—	4		lower	—	1	3

(Visual labels on left axis for both A and B)

Fig. 12.5. Visuo-somatosensory correspondence along the (A) vertical and (B) horizontal meridian (hm)—contralateral (contra), bilateral (bi), and ipsilateral (ipsi).

described above, but in a more medial track that reached the VIP through the medial bank of the sulcus.

The correspondence between the locations of the visual and somato-sensory receptive fields for the population of bimodal VIP neurons can be summarized as follows: (a) the vertical meridian of the visual field matches the body midline (Fig. 12.5A); (b) the visual fields above and below the horizontal meridian match, respectively, the upper and lower part of the face (Fig. 12.5B); and (c) the degree of eccentricity of the visual receptive field is related to the position of the somatosensory receptive field with respect to the mid-sagittal plane, such that cells with frontal somatosensory receptive fields have more central visual receptive fields than cells with somatosensory receptive fields on the side, top, or back of the head.

Visual and somatosensory receptive fields also corresponded in size (Fig. 12.6). Cells with fairly discrete, central, visual receptive fields had somatosensory receptive fields that were small and located on the muzzle area, while cells with larger and more peripheral visual receptive fields had somatosensory activity to stimulation of larger cutaneous zones extending to the sides of the face, head, or body.

In addition to matching in location and size, VIP receptive fields had matching direction selectivities in each modality. When direction select-ivity was present in both sensory modalities, the preferred visual direction was associated with an identical preferred direction for the somatosensory stimulus. This was true both for cutaneous responses to a moving stimulus across the surface of the receptive field and for responses to passive, joint rotation of the limbs.

Discussion

In these studies we have demonstrated that area VIP of the rhesus monkey contains a large number of neurons with directionally selective visual

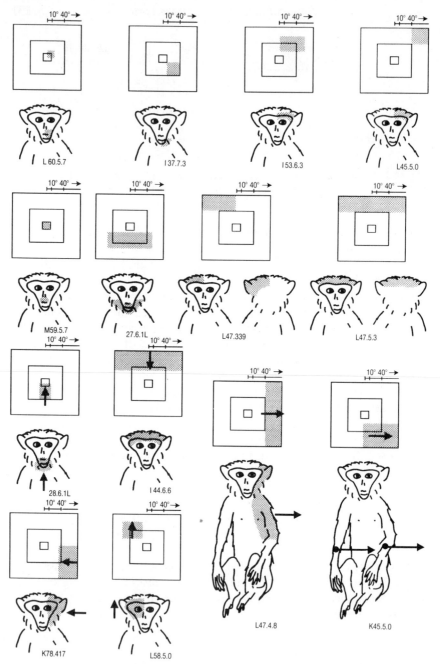

Fig. 12.6. Examples of congruent, visual and somatosensory, receptive-field properties of isolated VIP neurons. Conventions as in Fig. 12.4. Arrows within the visual receptive fields and next to the somatosensory ones represent the preferred direction for cells responsive to moving stimuli. Numbers correspond to individual neurons.

receptive fields, a finding which was to be expected on the basis of this area's strong projection from the motion-sensitive areas in the STS. We made the unexpected finding that a majority of these movement-selective, visual neurons also have somatosensory receptive fields whose tactile properties are congruent with their visual properties: their visual and somatosensory receptive fields are matched in location and size, and demonstrate identical movement selectivities. A second surprising finding was the selectivity of many of these neurons for stimulus distance. This depth selectivity was not dependent upon any single cue, such as disparity or accommodation-vergence. Rather, these neurons clearly had access to all lines of evidence that the nervous system uses to decide about the depth of the stimulus.

The function of such bimodal activity is far from clear, although there are several possibilities as to its meaning. The interpretation of a unimodal neuron is relatively simple. Activity of a neuron in the lateral geniculate nucleus implies the presence of a visual stimulus with certain properties. Activity of multimodal neurons in the motor system is also clear: these neurons do not speak to the sensory modality that evokes their discharge, but to a motor command. Thus it is likely that the auditory–visual neurons in the frontal eye field of the monkey do not so much carry a sensory message as drive a saccade of a certain amplitude and direction. The nature of the stimulus that evoked that saccade is irrelevant (Bruce and Goldberg 1985). A similar hypothesis may be made for neurons in the pre-motor mouth area that discharge before visual stimuli, regardless of retinal location, as long as they are in range of a monkey's bite (Rizzolatti *et al.* 1987). However, unlike the frontal cortex, parietal neurons do not issue unequivocal motor commands. Our neurons have the property, described by Bushnell *et al.* (1981), of giving the same enhanced response in saccade tasks and in saccade-free, peripheral attention tasks. Neurons give equivalent discharges to pursuit stimuli and to pursuit. Thus the simple, motor explanation for the meaning of these bimodal neurons is unlikely to be accurate.

A more plausible hypothesis is one of a supra-modal analysis of the environment. One example of this would be to establish a correspondence between a body-centred somatosensory representation and a retinotopic visual representation. Another would be to provide evidence of self-movement through the environment, either by optic flow or by tactile flow. The same movement through the environment that creates an optic flow should also create a tactile flow of air on the skin. Directionally sensitive neurons responsive to hair movement should be optimal for detecting tactile flow. As both somatosensory and visual flow should result in the message of self-movement, the interpretation of the neuronal discharge is again unambiguous.

Somatosensory–visual, bimodal neurons could also be involved in the

234   *J.-R. Duhamel, C. L. Colby, and M. E. Goldberg*

analysis of immediate extra-personal space. An object represented by a
tactile receptive field on the face and by a visual receptive field in nearby
space could excite a neuron representing that part of space, and could also
serve as a sensory input to the motor system concerned with movements
toward objects in space.

Finally, there is always the possibility that such bimodal activity attests
to simultaneous participation of a neuron in networks concerned with
different analyses. Richmond *et al.* (1989) have emphasized that neurons in
the visual-pattern recognition system can carry several different signals
multiplexed in the temporal modulation of their spike discharge. We,
however, do not see marked differences in the temporal wave-forms of the
somatosensory and visual responses, so this form of independent signal
transfer is unlikely to obtain here. We are left with the basic conundrum
presented by multi-modal discharges: an unambiguous signal somewhere
is necessary to decode the ambiguity of a multi-modal signal. If the unambiguous signal has equal access to any level of the nervous system, then
why does the brain generate the ambiguous signal? Understanding the
answer to this question will certainly increase our understanding of how the
brain processes space.

References

Andersen, R. A., Asanuma, C., and Cowan, M. (1985). Callosal and prefrontal
associational projecting cell populations in area 7a of the macaque monkey: a
study using retrogradely transported fluorescent dyes. *Journal of Comparative
Neurology*, **232**, 443–55.
Bruce, C. J. and Goldberg, M. E. (1985). Primate frontal eye fields: I. Single
neurons discharging before saccades. *Journal of Neurophysiology*, **53**, 603–35.
Bushnell, M. C., Goldberg, M. E., and Robinson, D. L. (1981). Behavioral enhancement of visual responses in monkey cerebral cortex: I. Modulation in
posterior parietal cortex related to selective visual attention. *Journal of
Neurophysiology*, **46**, 755–72.
Colby, C. L., Gattass, R., Olson, C. R., and Gross, C. G. (1988a). Topographic
organization of cortical afferents to extrastriate visual area PO in the macaque: a
dual tracer study. *Journal of Comparative Neurology*, **238**, 1257–99.
Colby, C. L., Duhamel, J.-R., and Goldberg, M. E. (1988b). Response properties
of neurons in macaque intraparietal sulcus. *Society for Neuroscience Abstracts*,
14, 11.
Colby, C. L., Duhamel, J.-R., and Goldberg, M. E. (1989). Visual response
properties and attentional modulation of neurons in the ventral intraparietal
area (VIP) in the alert monkey. *Society for Neuroscience Abstracts*, **15**,
162.
Crist, C. F., Yamasaki, D. S. G., Komatsu, H., and Wurtz, R. H. (1988). A grid

system and a microsyringe for single cell recording. *Journal of Neuroscience Methods*, **26**, 117–22.

Critchley, M. (1953). *The parietal lobes*. Arnold, London.

Duhamel, J.-R., Colby, C. L., and Goldberg, M. E. (1989). Congruent visual and somatosensory response properties of neurons in the ventral intraparietal area (VIP) in the alert monkey. *Society for Neuroscience Abstracts*, **15**, 162.

Felleman, D. J. and Van Essen, D. C. (1983). The connections of area V4 of macaque monkey extrastriate cortex. *Society for Neuroscience Abstracts*, **9**, 153.

Goldberg, M. E. (1983). Studying the neurophysiology of behavior: Methods for recording single neurons in awake behaving monkeys. In *Methods in cellular neurobiology, Vol. 3* (ed. J. L. Barker and J. F. McKelvy), pp. 225–48. Wiley, New York.

Hyvarinen, J. and Poranen, A. (1974). Function of the parietal associative area 7 as revealed from cellular discharges in alert monkeys. *Brain*, **97**, 673–92.

Komatsu, H., Roy, J. P., and Wurtz, R. H. (1988). Binocular disparity sensitivity of cells in area MST of the monkey. *Society for Neurosciences Abstracts*, **14**, 202.

Leinonen, L., Hyvarinen, J., Nyman, G., and Linnankoski, I. (1979). Functional properties of neurons in lateral part of associative area 7 in awake monkeys. *Experimental Brain Research*, **34**, 299–320.

Lynch, J. C., Mountcastle, V. B., Talbot, W. H., and Yin, T. C. T. (1977). Parietal lobe mechanisms for directed visual attention. *Journal of Neurophysiology*, **40**, 362–89.

Lynch, J. C., Graybiel, A. M., and Lobeck, L. J. (1985). The differential projection of two cytoarchitectonic subregions of the inferior parietal lobule of macaque upon the deep layers of the superior colliculus. *Journal of Comparative Neurology*, **235**, 241–54.

Maunsell, J. H. R. and Van Essen, D. C. (1983a). Functional properties of neurons in middle temporal visual area of the macaque monkey. II. Binocular interactions and sensitivity to binocular disparity. *Journal of Neurophysiology*, **49**, 1148–67.

Maunsell, J. H. R. and Van Essen, D. C. (1983b). The connections of the middle temporal visual area (MT) and their relationship to a cortical hierarchy in the macaque monkey. *Journal of Neuroscience*, **3**, 2563–86.

Newsome, W. T., Wurtz, R. H., and Komatsu, H. (1988). Relation of cortical areas MT and MST to pursuit eye movements. II. Differentiation of retinal from extraretinal inputs. *Journal of Neurophysiology*, **60**, 604–20.

Richmond, B. J., Optican, L. M., and Gawne, T. J. (1989). Neurons use multiple messages encoded in temporally modulated spike trains to represent pictures. In *Seeing contour and colour* (ed. J. J. Kulikowski and C. M. Dickinson), pp. 701–10. Pergamon, Oxford.

Rizzolatti, G., Gentilucci, M., Luppino, L., Matelli, M., and Ponzoni-Maggi, S. (1987). Neurons related to goal-directed motor acts in inferior area 6 of the macaque monkey. *Experimental Brain Research*, **67**, 220–4.

Robinson, D. L., Goldberg, M. E., and Stanton, G. B. (1978). Parietal association cortex in the primate: Sensory mechanisms and behavioral modulations. *Journal of Neurophysiology*, **41**, 910–32.

Ungerleider, L. G. and Desimone, R. (1986). Cortical connections of visual area MT in the macaque. *Journal of Comparative Neurology*, **248**, 190–222.

Van Essen, D. C. and Maunsell, J. H. R. (1983). Hierarchical organization and functional streams in the visual cortex. *Trends in Neuroscience*, **6**, 370–5.

Yin, T. C. T. and Mountcastle, V. B. (1977). Visual input to the visuomotor mechanisms of the monkey's parietal lobe. *Science*, **197**, 1381–3.

13

Brain and space: some deductions from the clinical evidence

GRAHAM RATCLIFF

Those neuropsychologists who, like myself, work directly with patients with cerebral lesions are uniquely placed to benefit from the kinds of data and theory discussed in this volume. Potentially, we are also in a unique position to serve as an interface between the two main sources of this information—the concrete world of neuroanatomy and neurophysiology on the one hand and the more abstract realm of cognitive theory and computational modelling on the other.

The raw material of clinical neuropsychology is the disordered behaviour of individuals with damaged or dysfunctional nervous systems, and the neuropsychologist's aim is typically to detect, describe, measure, classify, and above all understand the disorders he or she encounters in the clinic. In the case of visuo-spatial disorders, the clinical picture is so complex that we need all the help we can get in order to see it clearly. Thus, any information about the possible neural basis of spatial vision can have great heuristic value, even if it derives from experiments with non-human species or is suggested by attempts to test possible solutions to the computational problems involved in spatial orientation in artificially intelligent, computational devices. Similarly, the spatial disorders associated with cerebral damage should be of interest to cognitive neuroscientists working at both ends of that discipline; if the neural mechanisms subserving spatial orientation in the human brain are similar to those studied in the neurophysiological laboratory or have been accurately modelled, then the spatial disorders seen in the clinic should at least be consistent with data and theory from these other fields and perhaps even predicted by them.

There have been many comprehensive reviews of disorders of spatial orientation (Benton 1969, 1985; De Renzi 1982, 1985; Ratcliff 1982a; Newcombe and Ratcliff 1989) and this chapter will not attempt to describe them again. Rather, I shall attempt to identify some points of contact between the neurophysiological, clinical, and cognitive levels of explanation, where these disciplines seem to have implications for each other. The attempt will be frankly subjective, making points that seem potentially significant to me at this time. We will look first at some instances in which the physiological, clinical, and cognitive data appear to be consistent, reinforcing each other or, at most, suggesting refinements or extensions to existing theories. Then we will look at some apparent inconsistencies where the clinical data fit less comfortably and have more substantial implications for work in other areas.

Disorders of sensory analysis

My first attempts to understand spatial disorders were stimulated by the work of Alan Cowey in Oxford (Cowey 1979), which clearly outlined the behavioural implications of the evidence emerging at that time for anatomically and physiologically distinguishable visual areas in the pre-striate cortex. Although the situation is probably much more complex than we thought at that time (Ratcliff and Cowey 1979), the existence of functionally distinct sub-units within the visual system still constitutes a plausible explanation for the unusual but well-documented cases in which cerebral damage affects the processing of information about one property of the stimulus to a much greater extent than others. Thus we can see selective effects on colour vision (Damasio 1981), movement (Zihl *et al*. 1983), probably depth perception (Danta *et al*. 1978), and visual localization (Ratcliff and Davies-Jones 1972). Further, there is little evidence for hemispheric asymmetry with respect to these disorders, which typically appear in their full form only after bilateral lesions, although minor variants affecting the contralateral side sometimes appear after unilateral damage to either hemisphere. This contrasts with the general tenor of neuropsychological thinking, which emphasizes the role of the right hemisphere in visuo-spatial tasks. However, it is just what one would expect if these disorders were attributable to damage to information-processing units with contralateral reference operating 'bottom-up' on sensory information, relatively free from 'top-down' influence by higher level, lateralized processors. Such units would be analogous to those found in non-human primates with functionally symmetrical brains.

In the spatial domain, the relevant disorder in this category is the Balint–Holmes syndrome and its variants (see Newcombe and Ratcliff 1989 for a recent review). The true syndrome consists of a triad of symptoms—inability to reach accurately for visually presented stimuli, inability to shift the gaze so as to bring peripherally exposed stimuli into view, and a restriction of attention to a small part of the visual field—although incomplete versions can occur in which one component is much more prominent than the others or only one side is affected. Although the pattern of associated deficits varies between cases, it is quite clear that the difficulty these patients experience in noticing and locating visual stimuli is not necessarily the consequence of paralysis of limbs or eye muscles, or of actual cuts in the visual field. In the extreme form, the patients appear to be incapable of visually guided behaviour and feel their way around as though blind, attempting to locate by touch a stimulus of whose presence they may be aware but whose location seems not to be apparent to them. They may also have difficulty in perceiving more than one stimulus at a time and difficulty in disengaging their attention from the stimulus on which it is focused, with a consequent difficulty in appreciating the spatial context in which it appears. Yet those objects that are perceived may be recognized and named normally, and orientation may be restored when space is explored tactually.

The older published record suggested that the responsible lesion in the Balint–Holmes syndrome was in the supra-maginal and angular gyri but, more recently, cases have been described that implicate more dorsal, parietal damage in the region of Brodmann's areas 5 and 7 (Ratcliff and Davies-Jones 1972; Kase *et al.* 1977; Damasio and Benton 1979). Two pieces of circumstantial evidence support the view that damage to these areas is crucial. First, they are close to the watershed region in the border zone between the territories of the middle and posterior cerebral arteries, which is vulnerable to sudden severe hypotension, a common cause of Balint's syndrome (Damasio 1985). Second, the neurophysiological evidence suggests that neurons in these areas have the properties that would be required to subserve the function that appears to be disturbed in the Balint–Holmes syndrome.

Interestingly, this remains true for several different accounts of the clinical syndrome and several different views about area 7 neurons. Some have emphasized the misreaching component, attributing it to inadequate specification of the position of the visual stimulus caused by damage to a mechanism that provides target information to the motor system (e.g. Ratcliff and Davies-Jones 1972; Newcombe and Ratcliff 1989); and Andersen (1987) sees the posterior parietal cortex as an interface between sensory and motor systems that accomplish motor movement under sensory guidance. Others (e.g. Damasio 1985; Farah 1990) emphasize the attentional disturbance, seeing the difficulty in shifting gaze or reaching for a target as secondary to a failure to 'notice' it or, at least, to direct adequate attention to it, and Robinson *et al.* (1978) pointed out the enhancement of the firing rate shown by parietal neurons when monkeys could be assumed to be attending to a stimulus in the neuron's receptive field.

Some further support for the attentional hypotheses comes from the syndrome of unilateral spatial neglect, which may be a severe unilateral manifestation of the same kind of attentional impairment seen bilaterally in the Balint–Holmes syndrome. Morrow and Ratcliff (1988) showed that clinical neglect in patients with right hemisphere lesions was closely related to impairment of the ability to disengage attention from its current focus before shifting it to the contralateral side, an impairment which Posner *et al.* (1984) had shown was characteristic of patients with parietal lesions.

Whether the neurons of the posterior parietal cortex help to provide visual-target information to the motor system or direct attention to relevant locations in space, or both, the question arises as to the form in which they represent the space on which they are operating. As Stein (1989) points out, the input to parietal cortex ultimately is topographically organized—retinotopically in the case of vision and somatotopically in the case of sensation. However, there is neither physiological evidence of a topographical map in the posterior parietal cortex nor clear reports of 'space scotomata' after parietal lesions, such that reaching is only affected for targets in a small part of space, as would be expected if the part of the topographically organized representation corresponding to that part of space were damaged (Stein 1989). It does seem that space is represented contralaterally at this level as, with few exceptions (Perenin and Vighetto 1988), disorders of visually guided reaching after unilateral lesions predominantly affect the contralateral half of space, irrespective of the arm used in reaching, with minimal effect on ipsilateral space. Similarly, the unilateral lesions causing neglect affect one half of space. Even in the monkey, where unilateral lesions were initially thought to affect reaching with the contralateral limb (rather than in contralateral hemi-space), Stein (1978) has shown that both arms misreach in contralateral space when area 7 alone is inactivated.

Apart from this hemi-space effect, posterior parietal lesions seem to produce general impairment of reaching for all targets rather than simply those in a specific location. This argues against a topographical map of space in this part of the brain, and Stein (1989) interprets this property of parietal lesions as support for the idea that the spatial map of the posterior parietal cortex is an emergent property of a neural network functioning as a parallel distributed processing system that 'degrades gracefully' (Rumelhardt and McClelland 1987) when damaged. It differs in this respect from the strictly retinotopically organized striate cortex, where small lesions produce scotomata with minimal effects on the remainder of the visual field. It seems then that the spatial map represented in the posterior parietal cortex and putatively disrupted in the Balint–Holmes syndrome should be described as egocentric but not retinotopic or somatotopic. It seems to be involved in the direction of attention to relevant points in space and the acquisition of stimuli in the immediate environment, either by manual reaching or redirection of gaze. So far, the physiological and clinical evidence converges on very similar conclusions and can be regarded as mutually supportive.

The physiological evidence also suggests that posterior parietal cortex is the most likely candidate for updating the relationships between the moving animal and external stimuli (Leinonen *et al.* 1979) and allowing for the effects that alterations in eye and head position will have on the movement required to locate the target in a given retinal position. This would be necessary to produce a genuinely egocentric reference frame that would not allow eye and head movements to mislead reaching, but the clinical evidence really does not speak to this issue, although it is certainly not in any way inconsistent with the hypothesis. Professor Paillard, whose contributions to the field we honour in this volume, has consistently emphasized the importance of integrating sensorimotor and visual information, courteously but firmly bringing my own neglect of this issue to my attention some years ago when he kindly sent me a diagrammatic representation of his views on the neural basis of spatial information processing which made explicit the relationship between these modalities. This diagram has subsequently been published (Paillard 1990 and Epilogue, this volume) and is also remarkable for the degree to which it incorporates anatomical and computational components into the same schema.

Thus we have in posterior parietal cortex a neural system in which the properties of the 'hardware' have been thoroughly established by physiological means, but in which the mode of operation is understood in terms of computational modelling and the deductions about its function, as derived from these two descriptions, have, in a sense, been tested by observation of its dysfunction in cases of Balint–Holmes syndrome. The next step is to determine how this egocentric module located in the posterior parietal cortex fits into the broader, neural context of spatial information processing as a whole. Two properties of the human spatial information-processing system that were originally suggested by the clinical evidence have subsequently been confirmed by work in other areas.

Dorsal and ventral, cortical visual pathways

Newcombe and Russell (1969) originally demonstrated a double dissociation between the effects of right, superior parietal lesions and more inferiorly placed, temporo-parieto-occipital lesions on performance of visual tasks. Patients with superior parietal lesions were impaired in a stylus maze-learning task but not in a visual closure task in which the subject must perceive a face in an incomplete representation camouflaged by shadow. The patients with the more ventral lesions had the reverse pattern of impairment. These findings were interpreted as evidence for visuospatial deficit after parietal lesions and a different perceptual deficit, involving impaired visual recognition, after temporo-parieto-occipital lesions. This interpretation has subsequently been elaborated and refined

(Newcombe *et al.* 1987) in the light of anatomical evidence for two visual pathways in the primate brain (Ungerleider and Mishkin 1982; Ungerleider 1985).

The suggestion that spatial disorders can be distinguished from impairments of visual recognition has been supported by several other studies and, where the data allow anatomical conclusions, the clinical evidence also supports the suggestion of a parietal basis for complex, spatial information processing. Thus, Martin (1985) reported the case of a patient with callosal agenesis who performed normally on tasks requiring the identification of stimuli exposed to either half-field, but had impaired performance when asked to judge the location of stimuli initially presented to the left hemisphere via the right half-field. Given the hypothesis of right hemisphere dominance for more complex spatial functions in man, this suggests that spatial information could not be transferred from left to right hemisphere in this patient. The preservation of recognition performance, particularly the patient's ability to verbalize material perceived through the left visual field, suggests that transfer of some visual information was possible, and this is assumed to have been mediated by the anterior commissure. As information destined for transfer by this route must pass through the temporal lobe, these findings suggest that the ventral, temporal system is capable of carrying information needed to subserve recognition but not location.

The contrasting effects of damage to the visual recognition and spatial encoding systems are illustrated in particularly dramatic form by two other cases, reported separately by Ratcliff and Newcombe (1982) and by Martin (1987). Ratcliff and Newcombe's patient, M.S., was rendered agnosic after what was assumed to have been viral encephalitis. He had a marked and persistent inability to recognize objects by sight and even more severe difficulty in recognizing drawings of objects, achieving scores varying from 6 to 9 out of 36 on the Wingfield Object Naming Test in sessions separated by several years. It is quite clear that his difficulty is one of object recognition and not simply of naming, and his errors tend to suggest a visually based disorder.

Several aspects of his condition are relevant here. M.S. was able to draw very accurate, detailed copies of line drawings of objects that he could not recognize, and he was able to copy meaningless geometric drawings, such as the Rey figure, with reasonable accuracy. However, he accomplished these copies by a slavish, line-by-line strategy in which he seemed to be identifying a constituent line, reproducing it, noting the spatial relationship obtaining between the line he had drawn and another element of the stimulus, reproducing the second element in appropriate spatial relationship to the first, and so forth. In contrast, when asked to produce line drawings of similar objects with no model present, his productions were crude and frequently unrecognizable. M.S. was also able to reproduce drawings of 'impossible' figures such as the 'devil's tuning fork' (Masterson and Kennedy 1975) and their 'possible' equivalents, such that his drawings retained the geometric properties indicating the 'possibility' or 'impossibility' of the originals. Yet when asked to judge whether these stimuli could be made out of solid pieces of wood (i.e. to draw a conclusion about the 'object' represented) in an experiment modelled on that reported by Young and Deregowski (1981), he was unable to recognize the 'possibility' or 'impossibility' of what he had drawn (Ratcliff 1982b).

In contrast, Martin's (1987) patient C, with a diagnosis of Alzheimer's disease, was able to identify and name objects normally at his first evaluation, and these abilities were still relatively preserved 20 months later when other aspects of his condition had deteriorated substantially. He also had considerable artistic skill and spontaneously drew scenes and portraits while in hospital. When asked to copy realistic pictures from get-well cards and newspapers, patient C drew exceptionally good reproductions. However, unlike the copies made by M.S., they were not exact duplicates of the originals but 'captured the essential features of the model without reproducing each element in exact detail or position' and included embellishments that were perfectly appropriate to the context of the drawing but had not been present in the stimulus. In spite of his drawing skill, patient C's attempts to copy complex, meaningless material such as the Rey figure, adequately accomplished by M.S., were hesitant, frustrating, incomplete, and distorted. At follow-up, when he had deteriorated to the point at which his drawing of the Rey figure consisted of only four lines, C was still able to produce a recognizable copy of a meaningful drawing (the canoe from the Boston Naming Test), although it did not approach the quality of his earlier drawings of real objects. Interestingly, and in contrast to the performances of M.S., C's drawing of the canoe clearly indicates the intent to reproduce a meaningful sub-unit (a seat), which is marred by a failure to get the spatial relationships between the constituent lines precisely correct.

Both Ratcliff and Newcombe (1982) and Martin (1987) interpret the dissociation shown by their subjects as evidence for two routes to drawing. One, used by M.S. and described as 'data driven' by Martin (1987), seems to involve a system that allows faithful analysis of the spatial relationships obtaining between stimuli or elements of stimuli. Although one might argue that an object can be described in terms of the spatial relationships between the various parts, edges, and contours that make up its shape, the visual agnosia displayed by M.S. indicates that the spatial analysing system is not capable of subserving object recognition. The other system, used by patient C and described by Martin (1987) as 'conceptually driven', appears to involve object recognition; C's performances suggest that the spatial analysis system is not only insufficient for object recognition but is not even necessary for this ability.

The differences between these patients throw the distinction between

disturbances of spatial analysis and visual recognition into sharp relief. The
anatomical implications of these findings are less clear but computerized
tomographic scans do suggest more ventral involvement in M.S. and more
dorsal involvement in C. They also illustrate how useful it is to have some
kind of anatomical or cognitive model to guide the interpretation of clinical
data. The vastly different performances shown by each of these patients for
superficially similar visual tasks is still dramatic and intuitively surprising
even though, intellectually, we can explain it. How much more puzzling
would it be if we did not have the evidence from non-human primates showing the anatomical separation of two cortical visual systems (Ungerleider
and Mishkin 1982; Ungerleider 1985), or cognitive models of object recognition (e.g. Marr and Nishihara 1978) on which to draw in attempting to
understand them?

Disturbed appreciation of spatial relationships

Patient C, who was discussed in the preceding section, is unusual in that his
difficulty in some constructional tasks coexisted with a preserved ability to
draw realistic representations of real objects, but difficulty in copying
meaningless geometric drawings is not in itself unusual. Indeed, constructional tasks like copying the Rey figure or assembling block designs are
common clinical techniques for eliciting the higher-level spatial deficit
typically seen after damage to the posterior part of the right hemisphere.
The hallmark of this disorder is the inability to appreciate the relative
position of stimuli or their elements with respect to each other rather than
with respect to the observer, and Benton (1969) characterized the deficit as
impaired 'relative' localization as distinct from the impairment of 'absolute' localization seen in the Balint–Holmes syndrome. These disorders
can occur in the absence of symptoms of misreaching and restricted attention, suggesting that they are not attributable to damage to the egocentric
locational system discussed earlier, and that the egocentric module putatively located in posterior parietal cortex is not enough to encode the
relative positions of elements in a complex scene. Although one might
have thought it would be logically possible to deduce the relative positions
of external stimuli by calculating differences in their bearing from the
egocentre, it appears that the human nervous system does not take this
approach, preferring to use a separate module that presumably maps
relative position in an allocentric encoding system.

   Most models of spatial vision also recognize the utility of multiple forms
or levels of representation, although their number and precise nature vary.
Thus Hinton (1981) favours a three-frame model, whereas Feldman (1985)
employs four frames. Information flow in both these models proceeds from

stages at which position is referenced to the retina or egocentre towards stages at which more relational encoding takes place. Hinton (1981) uses the term 'scene frame' to describe the last stage of his model, in which the position of objects is represented in relation to the remainder of the scene. This seems to be just the kind of module that would be required to subserve the function disturbed in patients with the kind of spatial disorder typically seen after right parietal damage. The clinical record also supports the suggestion of a sequence of processing units in which egocentric encoding is a necessary precursor of allocentric encoding. With occasional exceptions, which can probably be explained in terms of disconnections, patients with symptoms of Balint–Holmes syndrome also have difficulty in drawing, route finding, and other complex spatial tasks, but the reverse is not the case. Thus, in terms of the interpretation discussed here, disturbed egocentric encoding implies disturbed allocentric mapping but not vice versa. This, in turn, suggests that the egocentric module feeds into the allocentric system.

Some potential inconsistencies

While the preceding section has suggested that current thinking about space in clinical neuropsychology, neurophysiology, and cognitive science is generally mutually complementary, there are some points on which the disciplines seem to differ.

One of these is the emphasis placed in the clinical and physiological record on the two cortical visual systems respectively specialized for handling spatial information and subserving object recognition. This does not appear to be perceived as a major constraint on cognitive modelling, although Farah (1990) does suggest an architecture that takes account of this aspect of the clinical and anatomical data. Farah's solution also accounts for a related paradox, which has been glossed over in the clinical literature. Although the spatial and object recognition systems are supposedly independent and parallel, we refer to the former system's ability to locate 'objects' as though information from the recognition system defining object boundaries were already available to it. We also refer to neglect of 'the left' without specifying how this is defined, and there is clinical evidence to suggest that patients may neglect the left half of an object even though they notice other objects further to their left (Gainotti *et al.* 1972). This suggests that 'the left' may, in this context, be defined partially with respect to an external object and Farah *et al.* (1989) have also shown experimentally that the orientation and extent of a shape (a pseudo-object) exposed to patients with unilateral neglect can influence the distribution of attention across space. This and complementary evidence of ways in which the spatial system appears to influence the object recognition system led Farah (1990) to propose separate representations for spatial attention and the representation of objects which could nevertheless influence each other by 'top-down' effects on an earlier stage of processing from which each received input.

Neglect of the left after right hemisphere lesions is more common than neglect of the right after left hemisphere lesions. This asymmetry is difficult to reconcile with the suggestion made earlier that unilateral neglect is a unilateral form of the bilateral, spatial restriction of attention seen in Balint–Holmes syndrome and that this results from damage to a system that is not asymmetrically represented in the brain. After all, unilateral misreaching is no less common in right hemi-space after left hemisphere lesions than in left hemi-space after right hemisphere damage. If misreaching and inattention result from damage to the same mechanism, one would expect a similar symmetry in the prevalence of neglect. A possible explanation lies in the fact that the allocentric representation of external space does seem to be mediated predominantly by the right hemisphere. Thus, even though damage to the left hemisphere may disturb a low-level mechanism for directing attention to contralateral hemi-space, it will leave a higher-level representation of the environment predominantly intact, thereby allowing some degree of awareness of both sides of space. A problem with this explanation, however, is that the work of Bisiach and Luzzatti (1978; see also Chapter 14) suggests that lesions which disturb attention to the left also impair the ability to attend to an internal representation of the left side of space.

There is also some difficulty in specifying exactly which spatial behaviours are supposed to be mediated by which representation and where in the brain it is to be found, particularly for more complex behaviours and more abstract representations. Some (e.g. Stein 1989) distinguish psychological spaces in terms of their physical properties or distances from the subject, while others (e.g. Hinton 1981) define frames of reference in terms of the purpose or property of the encoding they subserve. Stein distinguishes three spaces—personal, peri-personal, and extra-personal—all of which are referenced to the egocentre, and a spatial memory in which the location of external objects is allocentrically encoded in order to subserve route finding and topographical orientation. The clinical record does provide some support for the idea that topographical disorientation is an entity that can be separated from other forms of spatial disorder (Habib and Sirigu 1987) and which therefore reflects disturbance of a different or additional level of representation. On the other hand, it does seem unlikely that extra-personal space (that which is outside reaching distance) is necessarily referenced to the egocentre if the task that is being performed in it is, for example, reading a map, evaluating a position on a chessboard or deciding whether a soccer player received a pass in an offside position. It seems even less likely that the form of representation would necessarily change in the case of the map or the chessboard simply because one had moved close enough to touch them, thereby bringing them into peri-personal space in Stein's terms. To be sure, if one wished to pick up a pawn it would be an advantage, perhaps a necessity, to be able to reference its location ego-centrically but its position in relation to the other pieces would be much more important when planning the move. It seems reasonable to assume, then, that the form in which spatial information is represented is determined as much by the task to be performed as by the scale or distance involved.

The anatomical basis for the later stages of spatial information processing is less clear and the outcome of animal experimentation is less helpful than at early stages. The functional asymmetry of the human brain, which generally becomes more apparent the further one gets from basic sensory processes, complicates the interpretation of the findings in animals and, even within a given hemisphere, it is not entirely clear which structures in the human cortex are analogous to those studied in non-human primates. Certainly, the hippocampus seems to justify rather less emphasis in man, except in relation to spatial memory (Smith and Milner 1981), than it has received in animals (O'Keefe and Nadel 1978).

These potential inconsistencies should be regarded as challenges to further work rather than as problems. The interchange of ideas across disciplines cannot only help us to a better understanding of phenomena that we have found puzzling but may also cause us to rethink old familiar ideas with which we were satisfied. Professor Paillard has facilitated inter-disciplinary discussions about the neural basis of spatial orientation on a number of occasions and it is to be hoped that this volume will be another significant contribution in this regard.

References

Andersen, R. A. (1987). Inferior parietal lobe function in spatial perception and visuomotor integration. In *Handbook of physiology* (ed. V. B. Mountcastle, F. Plum, and S. R. Geiger), pp. 483–518. American Physiological Society, Bethesda, MD.

Benton, A. L. (1969). Disorders of spatial orientation in man. In *Handbook of clinical neurology* (ed. P. J. Vinken and A. W. Bruyn), pp. 212–28. Elsevier, Amsterdam.

Benton, A. L. (1985). Visuoperceptive, visuospatial, and visuoconstructive disorders. In *Clinical neuropsychology* (ed. K. M. Heilman and E. Valenstein) pp. 151–85, Oxford University Press.

Bisiach, E and Luzzatti, C. (1978). Unilateral neglect of representational space. *Cortex*, **14**, 129–33.

Cowey, A. (1979). Cortical maps and visual perception. *Quarterly Journal of Experimental Psychology*, **31**, 1–18.

Damasio, A. R. (1981). Central achromatopsia, *Neurology*, **31**, 910–21.

Damasio, A. R. (1985). Disorders of complex visual processing: agnosias, achromotopsia, Balint's syndrome, and related difficulties of orientation and construction. In *Principles of behavioral neurology* (ed. M. M. Mesulam), pp. 259–88. Davis, Philadelphia.

Damasio, A. R. and Benton, A. L. (1979). Impairment of hand movements under visual guidance. *Neurology*, **29**, 170–4.

Danta, A., Hilton, R. C., and O'Boyle, D. J. (1978). Hemisphere function and binocular depth perception. *Brain*, **101**, 569–89.

DeRenzi, E. (1982). *Disorders of space exploration and cognition*. Wiley, Chichester.

DeRenzi, E. (1985). Disorders of spatial orientation. In *Handbook of clinical neurology*, Vol. 1 (45), *Clinical neuropsychology* (ed. J. A. M. Frederiks), pp. 405–22. Elsevier, Amsterdam.

Farah, M. J. (1990). *Visual agnosia*. MIT Press, Cambridge, Mass.

Farah, M. J., Wallace, Brunn, J. L., and Madigan, N. (1989). Structure of objects in central vision affects the distribution of visual attention in neglect. *Society for Neurosciences Abstracts*, **15**, 481.

Feldman, J. A. (1985). Four frames suffice: a provisional model of vision and space. *Behavioral and Brain Science*, **8**, 265–89.

Gainotti, A., Messerli, P., and Tissot, R. (1972). Qualitative analysis of unilateral spatial neglect in relation to laterality of cerebral lesions. *Journal of Neurology, Neurosurgery and Psychiatry*, **35**, 545–50.

Habib, M. and Sirigu, A. (1987). Pure topographical disorientation: a definition and anatomical basis. *Cortex*, **31**, 73–86.

Hinton, G. E. (1981). A parallel computation that assigns canonical object-based frames of references. In *Proceedings of the Seventh International Joint Conference on Artificial Intelligence*, Vol. 2, pp. 683–5. University of British Columbia, Vancouver.

Kase, C. S., Troncosco, J. F., Court, J. E., Tapia, J. F., and Mohr, J. P. (1977). Global spatial disorientation. *Journal of the Neurological Sciences*, **34**, 267–78.

Leinonen, L., Hyvarinen, J., Nyman, G., and Linnanonski, J. (1979). Functional properties of neurons in lateral part of associative area 7 in awake monkeys. *Experimental Brain Research*, **34**, 299–320.

Marr, D. and Nishihara, H. K. (1978). Representation and recognition of the spatial organisation of three dimensional shapes. *Proceedings of the Royal Society of London*, **B200**, 269–94.

Martin, A. (1985). A qualitative limitation on visual transfer via the anterior commissure: evidence from a case of callosal agenesis. *Brain*, **108**, 43–63.

Martin, A. (1987). Representation of semantic and spatial knowledge in Alzheimer's patients: implications for models of preserved learning in amnesia. *Journal of Clinical and Experimental Neuropsychology*, **9**, 191–224.

Masterson, B., and Kennedy, J. M. (1975). Building the devil's tuning fork. *Perception*, **4**, 107–9.

Morrow, L. and Ratcliff, G. (1988). The disengagement of covert attention and the neglect syndrome. *Psychobiology*, **16**, 261–9.

Newcombe, F. and Ratcliff, G. (1989). Disorders of visuospatial analysis. In *Handbook of neuropsychology*, Vol. 2 (ed. F. Boller and J. Grafman), pp. 333–56. Elsevier, Amsterdam.

Newcombe, F. and Russell, W. R. (1969). Dissociated visual perceptual and spatial deficits in focal lesions of the right hemisphere. *Journal of Neurology, Neurosurgery and Psychiatry*, **32**, 73–81.

Newcombe, F., Ratcliff, G., and Damasio, H. (1987). Dissociable visual and spatial impairments following right posterior cerebral lesions: clinical, neuropsychological and anatomical evidence. *Neuropsychologia*, **25**, 140–61.

O'Keefe, J. and Nadel, L. (1978). *The hippocampus as a cognitive map*. Oxford University Press.

Paillard, J. (1990). Basic neurophysiological structures of eye–hand co-ordination. In *Development of eye–hand co-ordination across the lifespan* (ed. C. Bard, M. Fleury, and L. Hay), pp. 26–74. University of South Carolina Press.

Perenin, M.-T. and Vighetto, A. (1988). Optic ataxia: a specific disruption in visuomotor mechanisms. I. Different aspects of the deficit in reaching for objects. *Brain*, **111**, 643–74.

Posner, M. I., Walker, J. A., Frederick, F. J., and Rafal, R. D. (1984). Effects of parietal injury on covert orienting of attention. *Journal of Neuroscience*, **4**, 1863–74.

Ratcliff, G. (1982a). Disturbances of spatial orientation associated with cerebral lesions. In *Spatial abilities: development and physiological foundations* (ed. M. Potegal), pp. 301–31. Academic Press, New York.

Ratcliff, G. (1982b). An apperceptive deficit in associative visual agnosia. Paper presented at the annual meeting of the International Neuropsychological Society. Pittsburgh, February, 1982.

Ratcliff, G. and Cowey, A. (1979). Disturbances of visual perception following cerebral lesions. In *Research in psychology and medicine*, Vol. 1 (ed. D. J. Oborne, M. M. Gruneberg, and J. R. Eiser), pp. 307–14. Academic Press, London.

Ratcliff, G. and Davies-Jones, G. A. B. (1972). Defective visual localisation in focal brain wounds. *Brain*, **95**, 49–60.

Ratcliff, G., and Newcombe, F. (1982). Object recognition: some deductions from the clinical evidence. In *Normality and pathology in cognitive function* (ed. A. W. Ellis), pp. 147–71. Academic Press, London.

Robinson, D. L., Goldberg, M. E., and Stanton, G. B. (1978). Parietal association cortex in the primate: sensory mechanisms and behavioral modulations. *Journal of Neurophysiology*, **41**, 910–32.

Rumelhardt, D. E. and McClelland, J. L. (1987) *Parallel distributed processing*. MIT Press, Cambridge, Mass.

Smith, M. L. and Milner, B. (1981). The role of the right hippocampus in the recall of spatial location. *Neuropsychologia*, **19**, 781–93.

Stein, J. F. (1978). Effect of cooling parietal lobe areas 5 and 7 on visual and tactile performance of trained monkeys. In *Active touch* (ed. G. Gordon), pp. 79–90. Pergamon, Oxford.

Stein, J. F. (1989). Representation of egocentric space in the posterior parietal cortex. *Quarterly Journal of Experimental Psychology*, **74**, 583–606.

Ungerleider, L. G. (1985). The corticocortical pathways for object recognition and spatial perception. In *Pattern recognition mechanisms* (ed. C. Chagas, R. Gattas, and C. Gross), pp. 21–33. Pontifical Academy of Sciences, Vatican City.

Ungerleider, L. G. and Mishkin, M. (1982). Two cortical visual systems. In *The analysis of visual behavior* (ed. D. J. Ingle, R. J. W. Mansfield, and M. S. Goodale), pp. 549–86. MIT Press, Cambridge, Mass.

Young, A. W. and Deregowski, J. B. (1981). Learning to see the impossible. *Perception*, **10**, 91–105.

Zihl, J., VonCramon, D., and Mai, N. (1983). Selective disturbance of movement vision after bilateral brain damage. *Brain*, **106**, 313–40.

14

Extinction and neglect: same or different?

EDOARDO BISIACH

I will start with two concise, albeit imperfect, definitions for the benefit of those who are not familiar with neurological jargon. The term 'extinction' refers to a phenomenon discovered by Loeb in 1884 (see Loeb 1885): a stimulus addressed to an area which projects to a disordered component of the central nervous system may, in some instances, be adequately perceived if single, whereas it is not perceived in conditions of double simultaneous stimulation, that is when it is given in association with a concurrent stimulus addressed to unimpaired neural structures. The term 'unilateral neglect' describes the amazing behaviour shown by many individuals suffering from a unilateral brain lesion. Severely affected patients behave as if the side of egocentric space contralateral to the lesion had never existed (see Bisiach and Vallar 1988 for a recent review).

With few exceptions, early interpretations of extinction and unilateral neglect, whether couched in terms of disordered sensory interaction or in terms of attentional bias, were relatively peripheralist. (Peripheralist in the sense that it was thought that the dysfunction was located in 'hard-wired' neural mechanisms, below the level at which the so-called cognitive processes take place.) For many decades, and to some extent even today, 'extinction' and 'unilateral neglect' were therefore unproblematically used as synonyms (or more or less so). Just as an example, Denny-Brown (1962) maintained that unilateral neglect was a condition of global extinction of contralesional stimuli.

This view cannot account for representational aspects of unilateral neglect. Indeed, neglect patients not only fail to perceive one side of their body and environment: they seem to have lost the ability to *conceive* that side.

There have been times in which addressing issues such as cognitive representation from the standpoint of clinical neurology could have been considered a leap into darkness. Much of this wariness still lingers, despite the fact that the term 'representation' has even been used by neurophysiologists, such as Mountcastle (1981), when investigating single-cell activities. About 10 years ago, my associates and I started a programme of which the initial aim was to demonstrate the usefulness, and perhaps the indispensability, of notions such as 'space representation' for the understanding of unilateral neglect and related disorders.

We found that patients with right hemisphere lesions may omit left-side details while describing familiar surroundings seen from a fixed vantage point from memory. If the mental perspective is rotated so as to change the vantage point to a direction directly opposite the former, then previously neglected, left-side details—now located on the right side—are reported, whereas the previously reported right-side details—now located on the left, contralesional side—are neglected (Bisiach and Luzzatti 1978; Bisiach *et al.* 1981). Using a *same/different* task (Bisiach *et al.* 1979), we also found that neglect of the left side may not only affect the perception of stationary shapes in free-viewing conditions, so that shapes differing on that side are judged to be identical. Differences on the contralesional side may indeed be neglected, even if the shapes that the patient is asked to compare are moved left- or rightwards behind a vertical slit, so that *each* part can be adequately perceived in central vision at a given instant, but the whole *Gestalt* must be reconstructed, as it were, in an inner mental space; a space of which the left side appears therefore to be neglected much in the way as real, external space is neglected.

During the following years, several investigators provided further evidence of neglect phenomena in the representational domain (see Bisiach and Vallar 1988). Here, I will confine myself to a brief mention of a remarkable phenomenon reported by Baxter and Warrington (1983) and, subsequently, by Barbut and Gazzaniga (1987) in two patients suffering from neglect of the left side of space. Both patients were unable to spell the initial parts of short words correctly, as if spelling required reading with the mind's eye from an imaginary screen, the left side of which gradually faded into neglect. This interpretation is strengthened by the fact that Baxter and Warrington also asked their patient to spell words backwards and obtained the same result.

The hypothesis that the dysfunction underlying unilateral neglect might involve the topmost levels of neural activity is supported by the possible fractionation of the phenomenon as regards access to perceptual awareness. One of our patients (Bisiach *et al.* 1990) was asked to read 120 ten-letter words and non-words. Non-words were created by substituting the first half of words with a pronounceable or a non-pronounceable string of five letters. In reading words and pronounceable non-words such as *carnagione* (complexion) and *stomagione* (non-word), she consistently showed left neglect and pathological completion: for *carnagione*, for example, she read '*ragione*' (reason) and for *stomagione*, '*stagione*' (season). However, when non-pronounceable non-words were shown to her, she would name all or most other letters in the contralesional field. This difference was highly significant. It shows that access to perceptual awareness in the contralesional field was precluded after a very considerable amount of processing had taken place.

A similar conclusion is suggested by the singular behaviour of a patient described by Marshall and Halligan (1988). She insisted in denying the existence of any difference between the drawings of two houses, one of which had flames on its left side. However, asked to indicate in which house she would prefer to live, in a series of trials in which the picture of the burning house was randomly placed above or below the other, she would consistently indicate the latter.

At this point, one might wonder whether an elementary phenomenon, such as extinction on double simultaneous stimulation, and unilateral neglect are indeed different manifestations of a single, underlying dysfunction. Doubts have recently been raised by De Renzi and associates (De Renzi *et al.* 1984). They came to the conclusion that extinction is basically a *sensory* phenomenon (and that its inclusion in the sphere of neglect is problematical) on the grounds of three considerations: (a) extinction may be double-dissociated across sensory modalities; (b) no clear-cut left/right differences have been found as regards extinction, whereas it is widely admitted that hemi-neglect is more frequent and more severe among right brain-damaged patients; (c) three of their patients had severe visual neglect but no auditory extinction. None of these arguments, however, is decisive: minor forms of neglect are likely to be as frequent among left as among right brain-damaged patients, and very puzzling double dissociations may occur in neglect, even within *single* modalities (for example, there are patients who manifest severe visual neglect in reading but not in cancellation tasks, and vice versa). Nevertheless, well-known instances of extinction following spinal cord lesions seem indeed to call for an explanation in terms of relatively peripheral mechanisms.

Be that as it may, there are findings concerning extinction which can hardly, if at all, be explained by competition between concurrent stimulations, a competition the outcome of which is fully settled at a sensory level. Volpe *et al.* (1979) found that right brain-damaged patients, who denied perception of complex stimuli tachistoscopically projected in their left visual hemi-field if a concurrent stimulus was presented in the right hemi-field, were nonetheless able, on request, to make accurate *same/different* judgements relative to the extinguished and the extinguishing stimulus. Although infrequently, extinction of the left, contralesional stimulus may be observed even if both stimuli are delivered within the right, unaffected visual hemi-field of a right brain-damaged patient; this happens in spite of the fact that the extinguished stimulus lies nearer to the fovea than the stimulus that causes extinction. Furthermore, Bellas *et al.* (1988) have now found that patients with right parietal lesions may show left trigeminal *and* olfactory extinction on inhalation of volatile substances. As olfactory pathways do not cross in the nervous system, a relatively peripheral dysfunction should instead have caused left trigeminal but *right* olfactory extinction.

Bellas *et al.* have interpreted their findings in terms of a contralesional disorder of space representation.

There is a further point to be considered. My associates and I (Bisiach *et al.* 1989) have recently found that, in right brain-damaged patients, perceptual awareness of contralesional, elementary visual stimuli may be affected by the kind of required response (verbal versus motor). Stimuli were tachistoscopically projected, black dots: one either in the left or the right visual hemi-field, or one in each hemi-field. The explanation we offered for the decrement of correct responses found in patients with right brain damage in the motor-response as compared to the verbal-response condition is somewhat intricate and may or may not prove to be satisfactory. The essential point is that the results show how far factors affecting the reporting of very elementary stimuli can be removed from the sensory periphery.

Must we therefore conclude that, in spite of all surface resemblances, extinction phenomena are basically heterogeneous? A very interesting issue, one which so far nobody has tried to clarify, is whether brain lesions directly involving olfactory structures could cause ipsilesional extinction. If this were the case, the demonstration of a shift from ipsilesional to contralesional extinction in a single modality depending on the level of the lesion would indeed support the claim that there are at least two, radically different forms of extinction.

Although we are still largely in the realm of guesswork, I am rather inclined to believe that extinction, as well as neglect, can be due to dysfunctions at different levels of the central nervous system. The phenomena we observe may therefore be far from uniform: heterogeneity, however, is a relative concept and I suggest that an unitary interpretation of extinction and neglect is still possible and advisable.

As pointed out by Paillard (1987), the function subserving organism–environment interplay may be analysed, in evolved species, into two separate but interrelated and co-operating neuronal mappings of spatial relationship. The basic, 'hard-wired', sensorimotor apparatus subserves the primitive, externally driven *sensorimotor mode* of spatial information processing, relative to random searching for stimuli as well as to reflex-like orientation towards or away from such stimuli, as prescribed by the adaptive logic. The *representational mode* 'allows neural processing to step back from the immediate sensory input and to become progressively free from the environmental constraints under which sensorimotor analyzers have to work' so that 'spatial problems may be handled and solved by the interplay of the internal loops of cognitive operations' (Paillard 1987, p. 43).

Two notions must be borne in mind in order fully to appreciate the implications of this view for phenomena ranging from extinction to neglect.

First, the apparatus in which the representational mode of spatial information processing is implemented is not just grafted on top of the 'hard-wired', sensorimotor module. It has progressively evolved from the blueprint provided by the latter through the development of a growing quantity of internuncial network whose activity, though more and more versatile, bears the marks of its sensorimotor origins, from which it is not wholly independent and with which it is most likely to have some mechanisms in common. Secondly, the evolutionary derivation of the representational network from more elementary sensorimotor mechanisms suggests that the segregation of modality-specific channels which characterizes the latter is, to some extent, preserved in the former; this hypothesis is strengthened by the occurrence of modality-specific cognitive disorders such as those observed in the denial of cortical blindness, of cortical deafness, etc. (Bisiach and Geminiani, in press).

Mechanisms for sensory interaction apt to sharpen stimuli selectively through inhibition of neighbouring, concurring ones are already available at the level of the spinal cord, where axons of sensory cells, besides vertically connecting neighbouring segments, cross the midline to ensure co-operation between the two halves of the cord (Brodal 1981, p. 64). This allows peripheral processes of reciprocal control and of lateral inhibition which seem also to be possible—at that level—in virtue of 'top-down' modulation by cortico-fugal impulses (Brodal 1981, p. 81). Peripheral components of the central nervous system are thus already equipped with mechanisms able to prevent anarchy in organisms endowed with two relatively distinct sensorimotor apparatuses, each of which interfaced with one side of the corporeal and extra-corporeal environment. This function can be viewed as growing in sophistication in a 'bottom-up' direction, at various levels of bilateral, sub-cortical and cortical interaction, wherever commissural structures make the dialogue between the two sides of the nervous system possible.

Lesions of one side of this mechanism may impair active and reactive behaviour towards one side of the environment. However different the patterns of dysfunction resulting from lesions at different levels may be, they seem amenable to a basic paradigm of decline, in a weaker area of the mechanism, of activity that under normal circumstances would compete with activities in other areas of that mechanism. Extinction and neglect are manifestations of such a decline. Extinction may thus be expected to appear on the same or on the opposite side of the lesion, depending on its level. At any level, extinction and neglect phenomena may be expected to be global or circumscribed to—or even within—single modalities, depending on the extent of the lesion and on the kind of the activity during which they appear. Whether extinction and neglect phenomena can be more conveniently dealt with in sensory, attentional, or representational terms

also depends on the level of the dysfunction in a mechanism such as that
envisaged by Paillard (1987).

References

Barbut, D. and Gazzaniga, M. S. (1987). Disturbances in conceptual space involv-
ing language and speech. *Brain*, **110**, 1487–96.
Baxter, D. M. and Warrington, E. K. (1983). Neglect dysgraphia. *Journal of
Neurology, Neurosurgery and Psychiatry*, **46**, 1073–8.
Bellas, D. N., Eskenazi, B., and Wasserstein, J. (1988). The nature of unilateral
neglect in the olfactory sensory system. *Neuropsychologia*, **26**, 45–52.
Bisiach, E. and Geminiani, G. (1991). Anosognosia related to hemiplegia and
hemianopia. In *Awareness of deficit after brain injury* (ed. G. P. Prigatano and
D. L. Schacter). Oxford University Press, New York. (In press.)
Bisiach, E. and Luzzatti, C. (1978). Unilateral neglect of representational space.
Cortex, **14**, 129–33.
Bisiach, E. and Vallar, G. (1988). Hemineglect in humans. In *Handbook of
neuropsychology* (ed. F. Boller and J. Grafman), pp. 195–222. Elsevier, Amster-
dam.
Bisiach, E., Luzzatti, C., and Perani, D. (1979). Unilateral neglect, representational
schema and consciousness. *Brain*, **102**, 609–18.
Bisiach, E., Capitani, E., Luzzatti, C., and Perani, D. (1981). Brain and conscious
representation of outside reality. *Neuropsychologia*, **19**, 543–51.
Bisiach, E., Vallar, G., and Geminiani, G. (1989). Influence of response modality
on perceptual awareness of contralesional visual stimuli. *Brain*, **112**, 1627–36.
Bisiach, E., Meregalli, S., and Berti, A. (1990). Mechanisms of production control
and belief fixation in human visuospatial processing: Clinical evidence from
unilateral neglect and misrepresentation. In *Computational and clinical
approaches to pattern recognition and concept formation* (ed. M. L. Commons,
R. J. Herrstein, S. M. Kosslyn, and D. B. Mumford), pp. 3–21. Erlbaum, Hillsdale, NJ.
Brodal, A. (1981). *Neurological anatomy*. Oxford University Press.
Denny-Brown, D. (1962). Discussion fourth session: A. In *Interhemispheric
relations and cerebral dominance* (ed. V. B. Mountcastle), pp. 244–52. Johns
Hopkins Press, Baltimore.
De Renzi, E., Gentilini, M., and Pattacini, F. (1984). Auditory extinction following hemisphere damage. *Neuropsychologia*, **22**, 733–44.
Loeb, J. (1885). Die elementaren Störungen einfacher Funktionen nach ober-
flächlicher, umschriebener Verletzung des Grosshirns. *Pflüger's Archiv*, **37**,
51–6.
Marshall, J. C. and Halligan, P. W. (1988). Blindsight and insight in visuo-spatial
neglect. *Nature*, **336**, 766–7.
Mountcastle, V. B. (1981). Functional properties of the posterior parietal cortex
and their regulation by state controls: influence on excitability of interested
fixation and the angle of gaze. In *Brain mechanisms of perceptual awareness and*

purposeful behavior (ed. O. Pompeiano and C. Ajmone-Marsan), pp. 67–99. Raven, New York.

Paillard, J. (1987). Cognitive versus sensorimotor encoding of spatial information. In *Cognitive processes and spatial orientation in animal and man* (ed. P. Ellen and C. Thinus-Blanc), pp. 43–77. Martinus Nijhoff, Dordrecht.

Volpe, B. T., Le Doux, J. E., and Gazzaniga, M. S. (1979). Information processing in an 'extinguished' visual field. *Nature*, **282**, 722–4.

15

Self-motion and ocular motor disorders affect motion perception

T. BRANDT, M. DIETERICH, and T. PROBST

There is evidence that the perception of object motion is impaired by the perception of concurrent self-motion, by eye movements, or by ocular motor disorders (Dieterich and Brandt 1987; Brandt and Dieterich 1988; Sekuler *et al.* 1990). Under natural, environmental conditions one moves freely, with the two-fold perceptual task of controlling self-motion and perceiving object motion simultaneously. Experimental studies of motion perception, however, have a laboratory tradition in which thresholds for the detection of object motion are determined with the head stationary.

It was our incidental observation that one has considerable difficulty in seeing the tree-tops moving in the wind while driving a vehicle. This led us to perform experiments (described below) on thresholds for the detection of single-object motion under various stimulus conditions that simultaneously cause eye movements or induce the sensation of self-motion (Probst *et al.* 1986). The inhibitory interaction between self- and object-motion perception has practical implications when one is driving a vehicle because it impairs detection of critical changes in headway (Probst *et al.* 1984, 1987).

Independently, as also described below, we were able to demonstrate impaired perception of motion in patients with congenital and acquired, ocular motor disorders. Thresholds for detecting object motion were increased in these patients and consequently the detection of oscillopsia due to involuntary retinal slip was reduced. In fact, the angular displacement of perceived motion of the visual scene due to nystagmus or a defective vestibulo-ocular reflex did not quantitatively match the net retinal slip (Brandt 1982; Büchele *et al.* 1983; Wist *et al.* 1983). The amplitude of perceived motion (oscillopsia) was always smaller than would be expected from the amplitude of the nystagmus. We will demonstrate that the dissociation between the two can be explained by the combination of two separate mechanisms that involve motion perception:

- a physiological elevation of thresholds for detecting object motion on moving the eyes;

- a pathological elevation of thresholds for detecting object motion with either infra-nuclear ocular motor palsy or supra-nuclear ocular oscillations.

In a teleological sense, this 'adaptive suppression' of the detection of retinal-image motion is beneficial to the organism to the extent that it alleviates the distressing oscillopsia, but with the disadvantageous side-effect of impaired motion perception in general.

Eye movements impair object-motion perception

When Steinman and Collewijn (1980) considered how perceptually a stable world is deduced in the presence of considerable motion of the retinal image during head oscillation they were particularly intrigued 'by the possibility that vestibular signals are monitored by the visual system and used to compensate for retinal image motion that accompanies bodily movement'. We do not believe in such a mechanism but have experimental evidence (Fig. 15.1) for a different mechanism: a physiological impairment of the detection of retinal-image motion during eye movements. This contributes to the partial suppression of oscillopsia under perceptual conditions with inappropriate, compensatory eye movements. We have shown that the thresholds for egocentric perception of object motion are significantly raised during concurrent head oscillations of $\pm20°$ about the vertical Z-axis and fixation of the target (Degner and Brandt 1981; Brandt 1982). Subjects were exposed to a target that randomly moved either to the right or to the left at a constant angular velocity of 24' with a stepwise increase in exposure times from 0.25 to 10 s (20 repetitions of each stimulus condition). Conservative determination of the threshold was based on 18 out of 20 possible correct perceptions of movement as well as direction. Sinusoidal, active head oscillations raised the detection threshold for object motion by a factor of 2.9 at oscillations of 1 Hz and 6.4 at 2 Hz (Fig. 15.1), despite the intended stabilization of the target on the retina (vestibulo-ocular reflex). This effect increased disproportionately with increasing eccentricity of the image of the moving stimulus on the retina. Independently, Wertheim (1981) was able to demonstrate that during smooth pursuit of a target (head stationary) the threshold for detecting motion of a visual background increases in proportion to the ocular velocity, irrespective of whether the stimulus and the eyes move in the same or opposite directions.

The 'new' phenomenon of suppression of visual-motion perception during eye movements may reflect a basic sensorimotor mechanism because it has a somatosensory analogue. Coquery (1978) found elevated

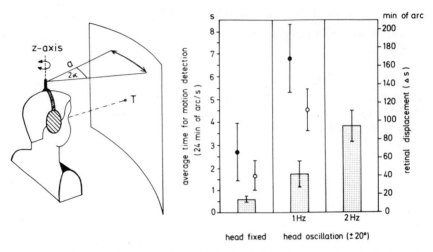

Fig. 15.1. Object-motion perception with horizontal head oscillations (vestibulo-ocular reflex). Thresholds for detection of object-motion (means ± SD) in 12 normal subjects (columns) as compared to 8 patients suffering from acquired peripheral ocular motor palsies (●: paretic eye; ○: unaffected eye). During the measurements the moving target (T; 24′ of arc/s; left or right) was fixated by the subject and the head was either fixed by a bite-board or voluntarily oscillated about the vertical Z-axis at 1 or 2 Hz with an amplitude α of ±20° (motion perception during vestibulo-ocular reflex). Physiologically, thresholds for object-motion detection significantly increase in normal subjects with increasing frequency of head oscillation (columns). With peripheral, ocular-motor palsies a further pathological elevation of thresholds can be obtained for both the head-fixed condition and head oscillation in both eyes, and is obviously more pronounced in the affected eye.

thresholds for the perception of electrical stimuli applied to a fingertip as well as partially suppressed, somatosensory-evoked potentials with simultaneous movement of the stimulated finger in man. The suppression of response activity in the medial lemniscus to contralateral electrical stimulation 100 ms before the onset of active movements in the cat (Ghez and Pisa 1972; Coulter 1973) seems to support the view of an efferent inhibition of sensory inflow. As suppression also occurs with passive movements of the limbs, 'afferent inhibition' must also be possible (Angel and Malenka 1982). Furthermore, analysis of electromyographic responses evoked by perturbations in the leg in man revealed that monosynaptic, stretch-reflex responses as well as supra-spinal pathways of group I afferents are suppressed during gait (Dietz 1986). Chapin and Woodward (1981) have speculated about an inhibitory interaction within the cortex itself (between motor area 4 and somatosensory area 3) because the reduction of afferent signals was more pronounced in cortex neurons than in corresponding nuclei within the spinal cord.

Self-motion perception impairs object-motion perception

That real motion of the eyes or the head is not the essential stimulus for suppressing object-motion perception was demonstrated by the effects of slow oscillations of the trunk (cervical stimulation) relative to the head, which was fixed by a bite-board (Probst *et al.* 1986), and by studies with 'circularvection' (explained below). In these experiments (Fig. 15.2 and 15.3), mean response times ($n = 20$) to the detection of motion of a projected object (5°/s) were determined instead of threshold measurements. The measured times indicating subjective onset of motion in a moving target are the sum of the reaction and the perception time. For cervical stimulation, the subjects sat on a rotary chair with the head firmly fixed in a helmet; the helmet itself was rigidly attached to the ceiling. The subject's trunk and legs were strapped on to the chair and sinusoidally oscillated at frequencies of 0.5 and 1 Hz with an amplitude of ±25°. The average time for detecting motion under 'static conditions' (no body motion: 436 ms) was significantly increased through body oscillation by a factor of 1.34

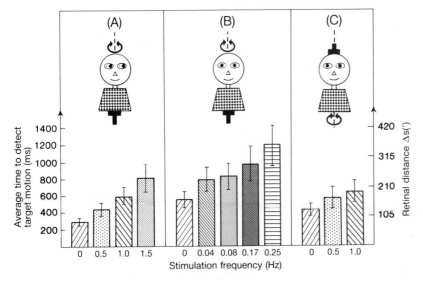

Fig. 15.2. Object-motion perception with head or trunk oscillations. Mean ± SD of the response times (in ms) or retinal distance (Δ s in min of arc), respectively, necessary to detect target motion (speed: 5°/s) during different modes of simultaneous body motion. The target was fixated during horizontal head oscillation by the vestibulo-ocular reflex (A), or with fixation suppression of that reflex (B) by use of an optokinetic helmet (laboratory model as used by astronauts in the Spacelab-1 mission), or (C) with the head fixed by the helmet and pure cervical stimulation provided by trunk oscillations. The response time to detect object-motion increased with increasing frequency of either head or trunk oscillations.

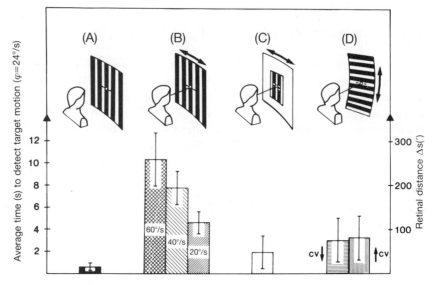

Fig. 15.3. Object-motion perception as affected by simultaneous pattern motion. Thresholds (means ± SD in s) or retinal distance (Δ s in min of arc), respectively, to detect motion of the 1° target moving horizontally with 24′ of arc/s φ during concurrent visually induced self-motion ('circularvection', CV) about the vertical Z-axis 'yawvection'; (B) or the horizontal Y-axis ('pitchvection', 60° s; (D) and during small-field, background motion, which does not induce the sensation of self-motion (C). Thresholds are significantly raised with CV (increasing with increasing CV velocity (B), as compared to the small-field condition without CV (C) and the stationary condition (A); CV perpendicular to object-motion also impairs object-motion perception (D).

(0.5 Hz) and 1.48 (1.0 Hz), respectively (Fig. 15.2). Thus, pure oscillation of the trunk with the head and the eyes fixed in space (cervical stimulation) significantly impairs detection of the motion of a fixated target.

Even stronger effects were seen with objectively stationary subjects for which apparent self-motion was visually induced by full-field, optokinetic stimulation with the head fixed, the subjects experiencing horizontal opto-kinetically induced circularvection (Fig. 15.3). The thresholds for perceiving horizontal motion of the target were raised by a factor of 5.5; here the target motion was perpendicular to the direction of the vertical-pattern motion, which induced 'pitchvection'. However, with concurrent horizontal motion of the target during horizontal-pattern motion, the thresholds were raised by a factor of 17.8. The physiological, inhibitory interaction between the perception of object motion and self-motion may reflect lack of specifity (or a side-effect) of a space-constancy mechanism (efference copy?) that provides us with a stable picture of the world during loco-motion. It has practical implications when one is driving a vehicle with the two-fold perceptual task of controlling self-motion (by 'linearvection') and

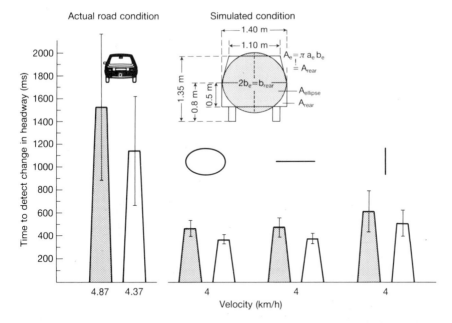

Fig. 15.4. Object-motion perception under real road and simulated conditions. Mean response times ($\pm$SD) were determined for the perception of changes in headway at distances of 20 (black column) and 40 m (white column) under real and simulated conditions without concurrent self-motion. An approximation of the perceptually affective area of the rear of the leading car was simulated by an ellipse of equivalent retinal size that was electronically generated by two, phase-displaced sine waves and an oscilloscope operating in the X, Y mode. Headway changes were simulated by adjusting the retinal ellipse area with a triangle-wave generator. The times taken to detect changes in headway were significantly greater for the actual road condition ('linearvection'). Under static conditions in the laboratory there was no difference between the detection of a gradual change in area of the ellipse and a horizontal bar with the same but one-dimensional movement. Detection times, however, significantly increase ($\alpha < 0.05$) if object movement occurred in the corresponding but vertical dimensions only (vertical bar).

perceiving object motion simultaneously. Authorities on road traffic accidents should consider an additional perceptual time of at least 300 ms for detecting critical changes in inter-car distances beyond the usual reaction time as expected from laboratory data with the subject's head fixed by a bite-board (Probst *et al.* 1984, 1987).

This hypothesis was proven in a field study (vehicle guidance under natural conditions), and in a corresponding simulation in the laboratory in which a stationary surround eliminated the perception of self-motion (Fig. 15.4). As demonstrated by comparing the results of the vehicle experiment with those of the corresponding laboratory simulation, object-motion perception is markedly impaired during a car ride. Typically, only the time between the subjective perception of a critical event in traffic and the start of braking is considered. The findings, however, indicate a hitherto unreported delay between the onset of the so-called objective stimulus situation (here the very beginning of the change in headway) and the perception of this event. The times for detecting a collision course, if thus corrected, lead to a change in our concept of the safe, inter-vehicular distance in a convoy. Fifty per cent of car accidents involving rear-end collisions occur at a relative velocity between the involved vehicles of only 19 km/h (HUK-Association 1975). Correspondingly, our findings suggest an increase in the total reaction time, which varies between 0.6 and 1.0 s, of at least 300 ms (inter-car distance 20 m; increasing with inter-car distance and disproportionally increasing at decreasing relative speed; Probst *et al.* 1984, 1987).

Binocular impairment of motion perception caused by monocular paresis of external eye muscles

The cause of apparent motion due to retinal-image motion in cases of infranuclear defects of eye movement is an inappropriate gain in the vestibulo-ocular reflex. This reflex normally serves to hold the direction of gaze in space constant during head movements by driving the eyes to move in their orbits in a direction opposite to that of head motion, and with a velocity and amplitude that 'compensates' for that motion. If the amplitude and/or velocity of eye movements are inappropriate, the result is a shift in the direction of gaze causing a displacement or slip of the retinal image, which may be perceived as an apparent motion of the fixated object (oscillopsia). As appealing and simple as this model is, it is not fully supported by recent studies. It has been shown that for healthy subjects, even under conditions of optimal fixation, either with a bite-board, with subjects sitting or standing as still as possible (Skavenski *et al.* 1979), or with head oscillations (Steinman and Collewijn 1980), appreciable displacements of retinal images result. The velocities of this retinal slip ranged between 20' with the head fixed by a bite-board to an average of 4°/s with head oscillations.

It was the amount of net retinal slip tolerated by the patients with infranuclear, ocular motor disorders making head movements without causing oscillopsia that led us to suspect an adaptive impairment of motion perception (Brandt 1982; Wist *et al.* 1983; Brandt and Dieterich 1986). This is dependent on the particular disease and distinct from the physiological phenomena described above.

Motion perception was investigated separately for the affected and unaffected eye while fixating a horizontally moving target (1° in diameter) with a constant velocity of 24′ in a total of 27 patients suffering from abducens ($n = 20$), oculomotor ($n = 4$), or trochlear nerve palsy ($n = 3$). Thresholds for the detection of object motion (8 patients) with the head fixed were significantly raised up to a factor of 5 for the paretic eye and a factor of 3.3 for the normal eye (see Fig. 15.1). With sinusoidal head oscillations at 1 Hz (which physiologically elevate thresholds), the ratio between thresholds in patients and normals was about 4 for the paretic eye and 2.7 for the unaffected eye (Fig. 15.1). This clearly suggests that in patients with acquired, peripheral, ocular motor palsies both the physiological and the adaptive (pathological) impairment of motion perception summate when the moving target is fixated during voluntary head motion. These effects are not restricted to the fovea but also apply to perception of motion within the peripheral retina. In normal subjects, thresholds increase with increasing eccentric location of the target on the retina (by a factor of 1.23 for 20° eccentricity); accordingly, pathological thresholds in patients are further elevated when a moving stimulus is viewed from the peripheral retina (by a factor of 1.7 for 20° eccentricity in the paretic eye; Brandt and Dieterich 1988).

A central mechanism must be assumed, which affects motion perception, because the perceptiveness of both eyes is involved, even though the paretic eye tends to perform more poorly. The raised thresholds for detection of object motion in these disorders are widely independent of the degree and acuteness of the paresis in the various palsies as compared to those of age-matched controls (Brandt and Dieterich 1986). The impairment seems independent of the direction of object motion in relation to the direction of malfunction of the particular eye muscle. They seem to last as long as the palsy lasts but may improve along with the recovery of the palsy (Dieterich and Brandt 1987).

Motion perception in acquired and congenital nystagmus

Oscillopsia is widely suppressed in congenital nystagmus, being usually absent in the primary position of gaze and in the null zone of the nystagmus, but still detectable by most sufferers as a subtle oscillation of fixated objects when eccentric gaze precipitates maximal amplitudes of the nystagmus. Ocular oscillation causes retinal-image slip, which degrades visual acuity when the angular velocity exceeds 4°/s (Westheimer and McKee 1975; Barnes and Smith 1981). Simultaneous, psychophysical and electro-oculographic measurements have been made by Büchele *et al.* (1983) in patients with acquired downbeat nystagmus in order to elucidate the relationship between retinal-image slip and oscillopsia. Oscillopsia is a permanent symptom in these patients, but illusory motion is always smaller,

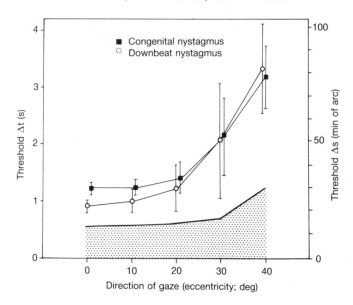

Fig. 15.5. Object-motion perception as a function of the eccentricity of horizontal gaze in patients with congenital nystagmus and acquired downbeat nystagmus. Thresholds for detection of object motion (24′ of arc/s; mean ± SD) as a function of the eccentricity of horizontal gaze (0–40°) in patients suffering from congenital nystagmus ($n = 5$) and acquired downbeat nystagmus ($n = 7$) as compared to normals ($n = 12$). Thresholds are indicated as Δt (exposure time in s) or Δs (displacement of stimulus in min of arc). Normals show only a slight increase in thresholds with eccentric gaze, which becomes more pronounced on lateral gaze of 40°. The thresholds for the patients are significantly raised, whether the ocular oscillation is congenital or acquired. There is a disproportionate increase on lateral gaze beyond 20°, which increases the amplitude of the nystagmus in both disorders.

with a ratio ranging from 0.13 to 0.61. According to this study, the mean amplitude of oscillopsia increases. Thus, there is a partial suppression of visual-motion perception for both the oscillation of the images of stationary objects upon the retina as well as for single objects moving within the visual scene. In the patients with downbeat nystagmus, detection of horizontal object motion was affected, although the direction of the nystagmus is vertical. This raises the question whether suppression of oscillopsia in congenital nystagmus is linked to impaired motion perception, as in acquired downbeat nystagmus. There is reason to believe that, in fact, there is an impairment of motion perception in general in these individuals (Figs 15.5 and 15.6). It remains a matter for further studies, however, whether this raised threshold also involves underestimation of objective velocity as well as dynamic visual orientation with respect to the predictability of changes in position of a moving target.

Oscillopsia, and therefore the sensitivity to retinal-image slip due to the

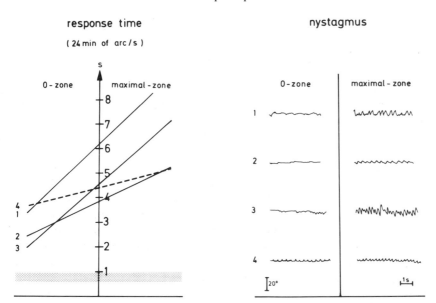

Fig. 15.6. Object-motion perception in patients with congenital nystagmus and manifest, latent nystagmus. Response times to horizontal object motion (means) in three patients with congenital nystagmus (1–3) and one patient with manifest, latent nystagmus (4) with fixation of the moving object in either the null (0) zone (not identical with gaze straight ahead) or the maximal zone of nystagmus (left). Shaded area represents SD of an age-matched control group (*n* = 40; 21–60 years old). For comparison see the original recordings of horizontal electro-oculography (right). Mean response times are pathologically prolonged at 2.0–3.7 s in the null zone with minimal involuntary ocular oscillation, and show a significant further increase to 5.0–9.0 s in the maximal zone with activated ocular oscillation in all four patients.

nystagmus, are obviously lower in congenital than in downbeat nystagmus, suggesting more powerful 'adaptation' in the congenital abnormality (Fig. 15.5). If patients with congenital nystagmus were able to subtract their current eye motion from the change in position of a viewed target on the retina (by an efference-copy mechanism), one would expect them to see an after-image oscillate in darkness according to their nystagmus. Surprisingly enough this was not observed by vom Hofe (1941), and particularly not by Goddé-Jolly and Larmande (1973), who reported on patients with congenital nystagmus who were able to fixate a stationary object with a foveal after-image without seeing either one oscillate. In contrast, Kommerell *et al.* (1986) found some patients with congenital nystagmus who did observe oscillation of an after-image in darkness with an amplitude of about half that of the nystagmus. This fits later observations by Leigh *et al.* (1988) in which oscillopsia (completely suppressed under natural conditions) was precipitated in some individuals by use of a combined lens device that enabled an approximate stabilization of vision of the real world despite the eyes moving. The powerful suppression of oscillopsia in chronic ocular oscillation, as well as the recurrence of oscillopsia with a stabilized retinal image (which interrupts continuous motion stimulation) is reminiscent of the well-known velocity habituation and motion after-effects that follow prolonged motion stimulation (Brandt *et al.* 1974). We do not believe that continuous evaluation of an extra-retinal 'efference copy signal' or an extra-retinal proprioceptive input are involved.

Conclusions

There is a physiological, inhibitory interaction between concurrent self-motion and object-motion perception that has been demonstrated for optokinetic as well as vestibular or somatosensory (cervical) stimulation.

Furthermore, there is a physiological mechanism of impaired motion perception with the eyes moving that contributes to the suppression of oscillopsia in ocular motor disorders but does not completely account for it. An additional, adaptive, binocular impairment of motion perception must be involved, which is separate from the physiological phenomenon and initiated by the particular ocular motor disorder (Fig. 15.7).

In all instances of ocular motor disorders investigated so far (either supra-nuclear or infra-nuclear; either congenital or acquired) the amplitude of the perceived motion of the visual scene was considerably smaller than

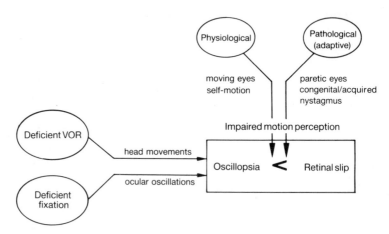

Fig. 15.7. Oscillopsia versus retinal slip: oscillopsia is either caused by inappropriate, compensatory eye movements (vestibulo-ocular reflex, VOR) during head motion or by ocular oscillations that override fixation. Oscillopsia amplitudes are always smaller than net retinal slip because of partial suppression of motion perception under these conditions. Suppression of motion perception is due to the summation of a physiological and a pathological ('adaptive') elevation of thresholds to detect retinal-image shifts of the viewed visual scene.

the calculated, net retinal slip. This partial suppression of distressing oscillopsia was inevitably linked to impaired motion perception in general.

References

Angel, R. W. and Malenka, R. C. (1982). Velocity dependent suppression of cutaneous sensitivity during movement. *Experimental Neurology*, **77**, 266–74.

Barnes, G. R. and Smith, R. (1981). The effects of visual discrimination of image movement across the stationary retina. *Aviation Space Environmental Medicine*, **52**, 466–72.

Brandt, T. (1982). The relationship between retinal image slip, oscillopsia and postural imbalance. In *Functional basis of ocular motility disorders* (ed. G. Lennerstrand, D. S. Zee, and E. L. Keller), pp. 379–85. Pergamon, Oxford.

Brandt, T. and Dieterich, M. (1986). Peripheral ocular motor palsy impairs motion perception. In *Adaptive processes in visual and oculomotor systems* (ed. E. L. Keller and D. S. Zee), pp. 457–63. Pergamon, Oxford.

Brandt, T. and Dieterich, M. (1988). Oscillopsia and motion perception. In *Physiological aspects of clinical neuro-ophthalmology* (ed. C. Kennard and F. Clifford Rose), pp. 321–39. Chapman and Hall, London.

Brandt, T., Dichgans, J., and Büchele, W. (1974). Motion habituation: inverted self-motion perception and optokinetic after-nystagmus. *Experimental Brain Research*, **21**, 337–52.

Büchele, W., Brandt, T., and Degner, D. (1983). Ataxia and oscillopsia in downbeat-nystagmus vertigo syndrome. *Advances in Oto-rhino-laryngology*, **30**, 291–7.

Chapin, J. K. and Woodward, D. J. (1981). Modulation of sensory responsiveness of single somatosensory cortical cells during movement and arousal behaviours. *Experimental Neurology*, **72**, 164–78.

Coquery, J.-M. (1978). Role of active movement in control of afferent input from skin in cat and man. In *Active touch—the mechanism of recognition of objects by manipulation* (ed. G. Gordon), pp. 161–9. Elmsford, New York.

Coulter, J. D. (1973). Sensory transmission through lemniscal pathway during voluntary movement in the cat. *Journal of Neurophysiology*, **37**, 831–45.

Degner, D. and Brandt, T. (1981). Interaction between self- and object-motion perception. *Pflügers Archiv* (suppl. 389, R.), **30**, 118.

Dieterich, M. and Brandt, T. (1987). Impaired motion perception in congenital nystagmus and acquired ocular motor palsy. *Clinical Visual Science*, **4**, 337–45.

Dietz, V. (1986). Afferent and efferent control of posture and gait. In *Disorders of posture and gait* (ed. W. Bles and T. Brandt), pp. 69–81. Elsevier, Amsterdam.

Ghez, G. and Pisa, M. (1972). Inhibition of afferent transmission in cuneate nuclear during voluntary movement in the cat. *Brain Research*, **40**, 145–51.

Goddé-Jolly, D. and Larmande, A. (1973). *Les nystagmus*. Masson, Paris.

HUK-Association (1975). A study by German motor traffic insurers on 28,936 car crashes with passenger injury. German Association of Third-Party Liability, Accident and Motor Traffic Insurers. Hamburg, Germany.

Kommerell, G. Horn, R., and Bach, M. (1986). Motion perception in congenital nystagmus. In *Adaptive processes in visual and oculomotor systems* (ed. E. L. Keller and D. S. Zee), pp. 485–91. Pergamon, Oxford.

Leigh, R. J., Dell Osso, L. F., Yaniglos, S. S., and Thurston, S. E. (1988). Oscillopsia, retinal image stabilisation and congenital nystagmus. *Investigative Ophthalmology and Visual Science*, **29**, 279–82.

Probst, T., Krafczyck, S., Brandt, T., and Wist, E. R. (1984). Interaction between perceived self-motion and object-motion impairs vehicle guidance. *Science*, **255**, 536–8.

Probst, T., Brandt, T., and Degner, D. (1986). Object-motion detection affected by concurrent self-motion perception: Psychophysics of a new phenomenon. *Behavioural Brain Research*, **22**, 1–11.

Probst, T., Krafczyk, S., and Brandt, T. (1987). Object-motion detection affected by concurrent self-motion perception: Applied aspects for vehicle guidance. *Journal of Ophthalmic and Physiological Optics*, **7**, 309–14.

Sekular, R., Anstis, S., Braddick, O. J., Brandt, T., Movshon, J. A., and Orban, G. (1990). The perception of motion. In *Visual perception. The neurophysiological foundations* (ed. L. Spillmann and J. S. Werner), pp. 205–30. Academic Press, New York.

Skavenski, A. A. Hansen, R. N., Steinman, R. M., and Winterson, B. J. (1979). Quality of retinal image stabilization during small natural and artificial body rotations in man. *Vision Research*, **19**, 675–83.

Steinman, R. M. and Collewijn, H. 1980). Binocular retinal image motion during active head rotation. *Vision Research*, **20**, 415–29.

vom Hofe, K. (1941). Untersuchungen über das Verhalten eines zentralen optischen Nachbildes bei und nach unwillkürlichen Bewegungen sowie mechanischen Verlagerungen des Auges. *Albrecht von Graefes Archiv für Klinische und Experimentelle Ophthalmologie*, **144**, 164–9.

Wertheim, A. H. (1981). On the relativity of perceived motion. *Acta Psychologica*, **48**, 97–110.

Westheimer, F. and McKee, S. P. (1975). Visual acuity in the presence of retinal-image motion. *Journal of the Optical Society of America*, **65**, 847–50.

Wist, E,. R., Brandt, T., and Krafczyk, S. (1983). Oscillopsia and retinal slip: Evidence supporting a clinical test. *Brain*, **106**, 153–68.

PART 4

The hippocampus and spatial memory

16

The hippocampal cognitive map and navigational strategies

JOHN O'KEEFE

Cognitive maps versus routes

In 1978, Nadel and I identified a set of spatial behaviours which, following Tolman, we suggested would require the existence of an allocentric mapping system (O'Keefe and Nadel 1978). In particular, we emphasized exploration of a novel environment, detection of changes (especially spatial alterations) of a familiar environment, navigation to a goal from different starting locations (in particular when these required movement in different directions), and detour behaviour—the adoption of a novel path when the usual route is blocked or otherwise unavailable. We suggested several properties of the mapping system, detailed evidence that the hippocampus was an important region of the brain involved in it, and sketched some ideas of how the map might be built from the known anatomy and physiology of this part of the limbic system. In particular, we emphasized the fact that the new information could be incorporated into the mapping system on the basis of single experiences, and that the motivation for originally constructing, and subsequently modifying, these spatial representations was not based on biological needs or desires but on the cognitive motivation of curiosity. Exploration was viewed as a purely cognitive activity, designed to keep the maps in register with the currently or most recently experienced configuration of the environment.

In particular, we wished to distinguish the mapping system from other strategies for moving from one part of an environment to another. These others were lumped together under the category of taxon strategies and likened to the route-like stimulus–response–stimulus (S–R–S) algorithms of the behaviourists. Those strategies, called guidances and orientations, were seen as based on purely egocentric information.

In the case of guidances, the strategy involves approaching or avoiding particular cues. This could be accomplished by any of several algorithms. For example, to approach a particular cue the animal might rotate within its egocentric framework (probably head- or body-based) until it had centralized the guidance cue at 0° on its body axis (straight ahead), and then move forward. Trying to keep the cue at 180° would lead to its avoidance.

Alternatively, the animal might move up or down a sensation gradient related to the cue. For example, it might act so as to increase (or decrease) the intensity or size of the cue. In this case, no spatial framework need be involved and it should be possible to train the animal to move in an arbitrary direction as long as there was a correlation between this movement and the size of the stimulus.

More than one cue could be used as a guidance at the same time and the resultant behaviour would be the resultant of these two independent strategies. For example, an animal might simultaneously approach one cue and avoid another. More interestingly, it might attempt to approach two spatially separated cues, and the behaviour would then be a compromise or resultant between the two independent strategies. Note that the strategies remain independent and there is no interaction between them.

Orientation strategies rely on the association of particular cues with particular responses. One such response strategy (see O'Keefe 1983) is the rotation of the direction of pointing by an angle within the body-centred, egocentric axis in the presence of a particular cue. For example, if a rat uses an orientation strategy to choose the right-hand arm in a T-maze problem, it might do so by turning 90° clockwise within a body-centred framework at the choice point. Notice, however, that any angle of rotation between 1° and 179° clockwise, given the apparatus constraint of a 90° clockwise or a 90° anticlockwise choice, will produce the correct response. Much of the control of behaviour in structured mazes might be provided by the apparatus and not by the organism. Evidence for this comes from a series of probe trials that was run on animals trained to make orientation strategies in T-mazes (O'Keefe 1983). On these trials the rats were transferred to an eight-arm, radial maze after they had learned the T-maze. This maze offered turns of 0°, 45° and 135°, as well as of 90°. While some animals had learned to execute a 90° turn, others chose 45° or 135° in preference to 90°. Rats with fornix lesions showed a similar pattern, emphasizing that this orientation strategy was independent of the hippocampal-based mapping system. Changes in this system were studied during reversal training. When the reward was shifted by 180° (e.g. from the left-hand to right-hand goal), the animals continued to choose the original (now non-rewarded) goal on the T-maze for a number of trials before switching to the new goal. During this time, probe trials in the eight-arm maze showed that, for some animals, the underlying angle of turn was changing in the absence of any apparent change on the T-maze. Particularly interesting were the systematic changes in the underlying angle of orientation that occurred in some animals. For example, in one lesioned rat, the underlying angle moved clockwise from L90° through L45° to 0° (straight ahead) in the eight-arm maze while the animal continued to turn left in the T-maze. At this point, it switched to the right-hand choice in the T-maze and the underlying angle continued to swing more positively clockwise as training proceeded (see Fig. 18 in O'Keefe 1983).

These findings illustrate several points about the orientation system. First, there may be a disparity between the surface behaviour and the underlying strategy. Any angle of turn between L1° and L179°, when combined with the forward motion in the start arm, leads to the choice of the left arm in the restricted set of choices offered by the T-maze. Second, changes in the underlying angle of orientation are incremental, although the surface behaviour in a particular task need not mirror this. Finally, the system is independent of the hippocampal map because fornix-lesioned rats, if anything, show its operation more clearly than controls.

Alternative navigational strategies

In the past 10 years, several alternative spatial strategies by which animals could find a goal have been proposed. Several have been based on an analysis of spatial behaviour while others have been derived from the spatial behaviour of neurons in the hippocampus and post-subiculum. In this section, I will describe briefly some of these and discuss their relationship to the above schema.

The models tend to fall into two classes, those that rely on simple, associative processes which combine the current sensory inputs with motor outputs in order to predict the resulting pattern of sensory inputs, and those that posit a goal location in an environment and attempt to identify mechanisms by which the organism might move to that location from any other location. The former have much in common with the S–R–S theories of the classical behaviourists and with what we have called orientation hypotheses, while some of the latter have properties related to what we have termed guidances.

The first model is that of McNaughton (1988). He proposed that the hippocampus acts as an association network that combines the sensory view at the current location with an intended movement to produce the expected view from the new location. The sensory view is essentially the snapshot of the sensory array in egocentric space, while movements are coded in terms of body turns in egocentric space (turn left, right, about face or continue straight). The S–R–S associations are learned as the animal moves around the environment. The generative power of the model derives from the motor equivalences coded in the response system, which can compute that, for example, two consecutive left turns are equivalent to an about turn in the same place. Another interesting feature of the model is that it suggests that the extensive collateral network in CA3, where each neuron contacts approximately 5 per cent of its neighbours, might form the basis of an auto-association system (see also Rolls 1989, and Chapter 19). Networks of this sort associate a pattern with itself and have the interesting property that part of the pattern is capable of retrieving the entire pattern.

The primary goal of McNaughton's model is to explain two findings about the hippocampal place cells. The first of these is that, in some testing situations, the majority of these cells are sensitive to the direction in which the animal is travelling. In the radial-arm maze, for example, a cell might fire in one of the arms as the animal moves away from the centre but not towards it (McNaughton *et al*. 1983). In an earlier paper (O'Keefe 1976), I had reported that, on elevated, three-arm mazes with broad arms, some place cells had directional fields while others fired in the field irrespective of direction. More recently it has been shown by Muller and his colleagues (Muller *et al*. 1987; Bostock *et al*. 1988; see also Chapter 17), that the cells have omnidirectional place fields in enclosed cylinders where the direction of movement is less constrained than in the mazes. If the cells were direction-specific under all circumstances, the idea that they were coding for some aspect of the egocentric sensory array would be strengthened.

The second finding about place cells which the McNaughton model is designed to account for is that of O'Keefe and Speakman (1987), namely, once the cell firing pattern for a part of an environment has been set up in the hippocampus, the spatial cues can be removed and the appropriate firing patterns are recorded as the rat continues to move around the environment (see Fig. 16.9 below). This is true even when it visits parts of the environment, after the cues have been removed, that it had not been allowed to visit in their presence on that trial. One explanation for this finding is that either in the hippocampus or in one of the structures afferent to it there exists a memory mechanism that uses the animal's movements either directly or indirectly to update the representation of the current location. Any theory of the hippocampus must take this into account. In a subsequent section, I will show how this is done in the cognitive map model.

One of the problems with the McNaughton model is that it does not provide a mechanism that accounts for the goal-directed aspects of spatial behaviour. In a familiar environment, animals can navigate from their current location to a desired location (such as one containing food or water) *or* move away from undesirable locations (such as those associated with danger or threat). The behaviourists attempted to incorporate this into their models by postulating an influence that propagated backwards through the chain of S–R–S links such that those S–R associations which eventuated in reward were selectively strengthened, even when they were distant from the reward in time and space. Perhaps the McNaughton model can be extended along these lines.

Other models of spatial behaviour, while not specifically designed to account for the role of the hippocampus, can shed light on different navigational strategies and their relation to mapping. They all share the notion that the goal in an environment has a privileged status and provides the point around which the representation is organized. They differ, in the main, in the type of information that they postulate can be extracted from the sensory array and the way it is used to get to the goal.

The first of these models is the ASN system of Barto and Sutton (1981). This postulates a matrix memory system which receives sensory inputs from cues in the environment and uses these to navigate to a goal. Each cue provides a gradient that falls off with a distance (e.g. as olfactory cues might), but no angular information is provided. The goal also provides a gradient of reinforcement and this is used to strengthen the synaptic weights of the connections in the memory matrix between each cue and movements towards the goal from a particular location. Movements are coded as directions in an abstract framework (north, south, east, west) that is postulated but not explained, but this does not appear to be an intrinsic component of the model. Computer simulations show that, during experience with an environment, the network generates a vector field where the unique pattern of input from the cues at each location is associated with a movement vector whose angle points in direction of the goal and whose magnitude is a reflection of the distance to the goal. The system solves the reinforcement problem by providing a gradient of reinforcement at every point in the environment, and by using a simple learning rule to strengthen connections, which climb this hill of reinforcement. The vector field is organized with the goal or peak of the reinforcement gradient as its focus; changing the location of the goal would change the vector field. As Barto and Sutton point out, the model seems appropriate for the description of the spatial behaviours of simple organisms such as bacteria (Koshland 1979).

The snapshot model of Cartwright and Collett (1983) was designed to explain the ability of bees to navigate to a goal on the basis of an object or small group of objects. They assumed that the behaviour was based on vision, and that the primary information available to the animal was the retinal size and angle of the objects. Their model proposes that the bee takes a snapshot of the visual array at the goal and stores this in memory. This array consists primarily of a circular distribution of dark and light segments which reflect the size and relative location of the objects in egocentric space. When the animal is at other points in the environment the visual array will vary from this canonical snapshot in systematic ways. By comparing the distribution of angles in the two pictures and, specifically, by calculating the angular differences between the two, the system generates a vector field across the environment, where, at each location in the environment, a vector points in the direction of the goal.

Similar goal-oriented models have been proposed by Wilkie and Palfrey (1987) and by Zipser (1986). These rely on the distance from the goal to a set of objects rather than the egocentric angles of the Cartwright–Collett model. The Wilkie–Palfrey model tries to account for the behaviour of rats in the Morris swimming task (Morris 1981). It assumes that the navigation is based on distal cues, and that the animal knows the distance to these cues at the goal and at other points in the swimming pool. The task is solved by storing in memory the distances to the cues from the goal platform and comparing these remembered values with those perceived at other locations in the pool. The rat moves in such a way as to reduce the difference between the two distances. If the remembered goal distance is greater, the rat moves away from the cue; if it is less, the rat moves towards it. The movement is the resultant of the independent action of each calculation of cue distance. Under the restricted conditions of the water maze, where the distant cues are outside of the pool, two cues will suffice for this model because the mirror-image locations, which might be confused with the 'real' locations, are outside the pool. No attempt is made to explain the animal's ability to compute the distances to the cues, but the existence of an environmentally based, Cartesian co-ordinate system appears to be a necessary assumption.

Zipser (1986) also proposed a model for moving to a goal from any location in an environment. His model also relies on a calculation of the distances of cues relative to the goal. It differs from the Wilkie–Palfrey model in that it uses an egocentric co-ordinate framework centred on the animal, and it does not require the animal to view the cues from the goal itself but only to know their distances at one location, where the distance to the goal is also known. Essentially, the idea is to solve for the transform matrix that maps the co-ordinates of the cues from the original location into the new location. Once this transform is found, the location of the goal within the animal's egocentric framework from any point where the cues are visible can be calculated using linear-matrix algebra.

A scheme that uses both the distance and the angle of objects has been put forward by Collett *et al.* (1986). They proposed that gerbils have information about the distance and angle of objects both from the goal and from its current location. These two vectors can be used to compute trajectories to the goal from the current location by vector subtraction. Animals were trained to search for seeds on the basis of nearby cylinders that served as landmarks. Several configurations of cylinders and starting positions were studied in different experiments. In one study, probe experiments in which the distance between two landmarks was increased found that the gerbils searched in two distinct locations, one relative to each landmark. This suggests that, at least under the specific conditions of this particular experiment, they were using the landmarks relatively independently and not performing a calculation as to the location of the goal based on the positions of both. The nature of the reference framework, or even whether the animals were consistently using the same framework, was left open. Some experiments showed that the relationship between a fixed starting point and an object could be used, as could the location of the object relative to a 'compass' direction, which might be derived from unknown distal cues. Finally, the framework could be supplied by the geometry of a set of land-marks themselves as the animals could learn goal location independently of the starting location and direction of approach to the landmark array. The latter two strategies would seem to imply some type of allocentric framework, whereas the first might be using a body-centred, egocentric one.

A neurocomputational model for the cognitive map

In our book (O'Keefe and Nadel 1978, pp. 217–30), we suggested that, in addition to the place information provided by the place cells, the mapping system required information about displacements resulting from movements, and also directional information, either in the form of a compass mechanism that measured angles relative to external landmarks such as geomagnetic north or in the form of a system for integrating the changes of angle in an egocentric framework. We already had evidence that the frequency of theta during jumping was correlated with the distance jumped (Morris *et al.* 1976; O'Keefe and Nadel 1978, pp. 179–82) but there was no physiological evidence for the directional component. Taube *et al.* (1990; see also Chapter 17) have now found cells in the post-subiculum that code for the direction of the rat's head. The ingredients for a mapping system, then, are the place cells of the hippocampus, the head-direction cells of the post-subiculum, and the theta system of the hippocampal formation. I have suggested that the place cells are involved in the calculation of the centroid of the cue configuration, the head-direction cells in the calculation of the overall slope of the cue configuration, and the theta system in the coding of movement displacements and in vector calculations (O'Keefe 1990). In the next section, I will briefly describe this proposal and show how the theta system might operate.

The centroid and the slope

Figure 16.1 shows the environmental information available to the mapping system. I assume that cues in the environment are represented within the neocortical sensoria as a bundle of qualities (proximal size, modality,

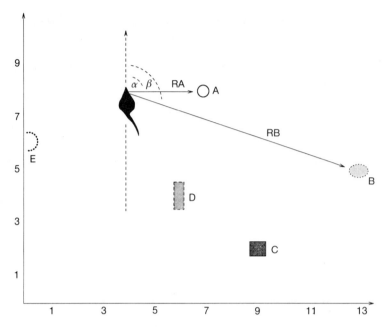

Fig. 16.1. A rat in an environment consisting of five cues A–E. A Cartesian framework with an arbitrary metric has been superimposed upon the environment but is not available to the animal. The dashed line through the animal's head represents the axis of an egocentric, polar co-ordinate framework centred on the head (E-space). This moves with the animal as it moves through the environment. Each cue is identified by its sensory attributes and its location in the E-space by a vector. Cue vector A has length RA and angle α; cue vector B has length RB and angle β.

intensity, etc.), and are set within an egocentric framework centred on the rat's head (or body). Each cue is represented independently of all the others and there is no interaction (except where one occludes the other).

Before these data arrive at the mapping system, they need to be operated upon by a system that uses the movement parallax generated by each cue as the animal moves around an environment as a clue to its veridical distance in egocentric space (henceforth called E space in contrast to the allocentric space generated in the cognitive mapping system: A space). In O'Keefe (1988), there is a suggestion for one way that the coefficient relating a proximal attribute of a cue, such as size or intensity, to distance could be calculated. The data presented to the mapping system, then, consist of a set of cues, each located in E space by a distance and angle. The mapping system computes two pieces of information from these data: the geometrical centroid of the set of cues, and the slope of the distribution of the same cues. The first is used as the centre of a polar, A space framework, while the second provides a direction that can be used as a

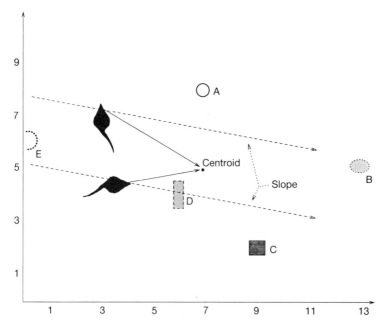

Fig. 16.2. The centroid and the overall slope for the set of five cues shown from two locations in the environment. The centroid is a location in the environment that does not change with the animal's movements and is calculated by the vector summation of the cue vectors at any point in the environment. The second parameter, the overall slope, is also derived from the cues at any point in the environment and represents the average slopes of all the cue pairs in E-space. The magnitude or distance measure of the centroid from the animal's location does not change with an in-place, pure rotational movement. In contrast, the animal's orientation with respect to the slope axis does vary with rotations but is insensitive to translations.

reference from which angles in A space can be measured. An example of these two parameters for the cue set of Fig. 16.1 for two orientations and two locations of the rat in the environment is shown in Fig. 16.2. In the remainder of this section I will set out a concrete proposal about the method by which these parameters are calculated. Note that the length of the centroid vector does not change as the animal rotates in a fixed location but that both its length and angle vary with translation movements, regardless of whether or not these are associated with rotations (Fig. 16.2). In contrast, the angle that the animal's head makes with the slope varies with rotation but is invariant with translations.

Computation of the overall slope and centroid of an environment

The first measure derived from the distribution of cues in an environment is the slope. This is defined as the deviation from symmetry or isotropism

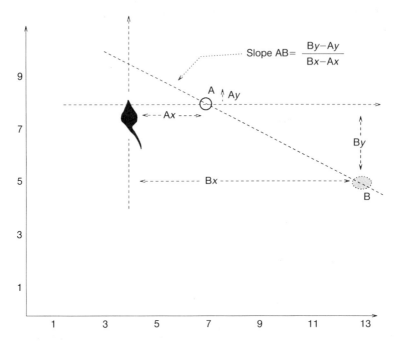

Fig. 16.3. Method for computing the slope of a pair of cues in E-space. The x and y co-ordinates of each cue are calculated. The slope is defined as the difference between the y co-ordinates divided by the difference between x co-ordinates. This ratio is the same for all locations at which cues A and B can be sensed as long as the animal maintains the same orientation relative to the environment.

of the cue configuration in different directions. It can be measured as follows: at any given location in an environment a line drawn between two cues has a slope in E space defined as the difference between the y co-ordinates divided by the difference between the x co-ordinates. Fig. 16.3 shows this computation for two of the cues in Fig. 16.1. Notice that this measure depends on having previously assigned veridical distance coefficients to the cues A and B. Now, as pointed out above, one of the interesting properties of this measure of slope is that although it varies as a function of rotational movements it is invariant with translation movements, i.e. it is identical at all locations in the environment for identical headings or directions of pointing. It follows that it can be used as a measure of direction: averaging across the slopes for all of the cue pairs in an environment gives the overall slope, which can serve as a measure of the asymmetry of the cue distribution in a particular environment. The overall slope for the set of cues A–E is drawn on the diagram of Fig. 16.2. The calculation of overall slope could be carried out in several stages. Instead of taking all of the cue pairs at once, small sub-sets could be used to

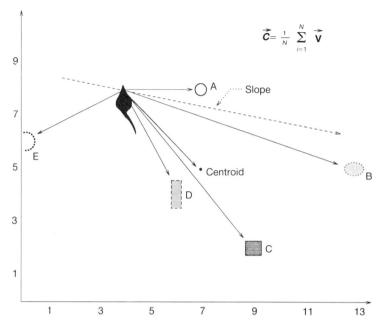

$$\vec{c} = \frac{1}{N} \sum_{i=1}^{N} \vec{v}$$

Fig. 16.4. The centroid ($\vec{c}$) is the geometric mean of the cue locations which is calculated by taking the vector average of all of the cues.

produce different estimates of the overall slope and these in turn could be averaged to get the overall slope. It is suggested that the post subicular direction cells encode these calculations of partial slope.

The centroid of the environment is defined as the geometric centre or centre of mass of the cues in the environment. This is calculated by taking the grand mean vector of the cue vectors in either A space or E space. In E space, each cue angle would be calculated from the egocentric head direction; in A space the angle would be taken relative to the allocentric direction of slope. This latter option would require that the cue vectors be rotated from the head-centred, E-space framework into alignment with the slope before the centroid calculation, whereas in the former option the rotations would be performed after the centroid calculations. Fig. 16.4 shows the vectors to each cue and the overall centroid vector based on the average. In a fashion analogous to the partial computations of the slope, it is assumed that the overall centroid vector is estimated by different neurons on the basis of subsets of the total cue set. Fig. 16.5 illustrates two partial centroid vectors based on three cues. It is suggested that the place cells are encoding some aspect of the centroid vector information, perhaps the reciprocal of the partial centroid vectors.

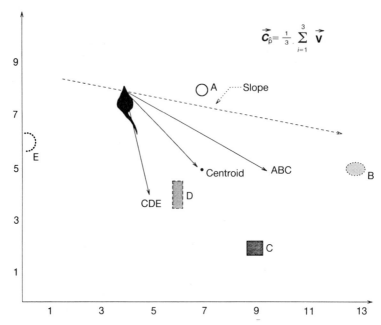

Fig. 16.5. Partial estimates of the centroid ($\vec{c}\hat{p}$) vector are given by the vector averages of sub-sets of cues. The centroid estimates based on cue sub-sets ABC and CDE are shown in addition to the overall centroid. Note that these vectors are different from the centroid and from each other.

Phasor mechanism for vector calculations

The vector calculations postulated for this system could be achieved by networks of neurons. I have previously suggested that they might rely on the sinusoidal properties of the theta system. The basic idea is the opposite of the phasor representation of sinusoids. In this representation a set of sinusoids of the same frequency but different amplitudes and phases is represented by a set of vectors where the length and angle of each corresponds to the amplitude and phase of the respective sinusoid. Addition or subtraction of sinusoids can be done in the vector domain.

The present scheme suggests the opposite move, i.e., the representation of spatial vectors by neuronal sinusoids. Fig. 16.6 shows an example of this. Cue vectors A and B with lengths RA and RB and angles α and β are represented in a polar co-ordinate space in the top part of the figure. Their vector average is shown as vector C with length RC and angle γ. The corresponding sinusoidal representations are shown in the lower half of the figure. The clock signal marks the reference from which the $0°$ angle and the unit amplitude are measured but does not itself enter the calculation. Linear addition of the A and B sinusoids gives the C sinusoid, which has the

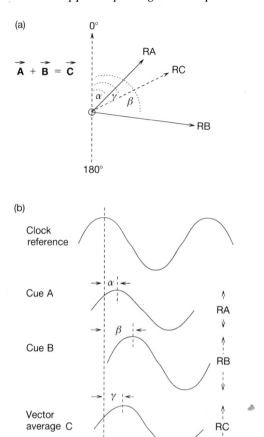

Fig. 16.6. Use of sinusoids to represent vectors: (a) shows the vector addition of a vector of length RA and angle α to a vector of length RB and angle β to obtain a vector of length RC and angle γ; (b) shows the representation of these vectors by sinusoids where the amplitude corresponds to the vector length and the phase shift corresponds to the vector angle. Summing the sine waves sums the vectors.

correct amplitude and phase to represent the C vector. Subtraction of vectors can be accomplished by the 180° phase shifting of one, followed by addition.

Uses of the mapping system.

I. Exploration

It is assumed that the representation of an environment is originally constructed during exploration. When an animal first enters an environment, the mapping system searches for a representation with the correct set of cue-distance coefficients, partial slopes, and partial centroids to match the in-coming sensory data. During the first few movements there will be numerous possible representations that might fit but these will be rapidly selected amongst in favour of the one that is most successful in predicting the succession of inputs to match the internal translation computations. As it is unlikely that the sensory input will fit exactly any stored representation, a decision rule will need to be applied to assess the 'closeness of fit' to the best representation. Once this has been selected, deviations from the stored representations will be corrected. This model predicts that exploration will only be elicited by changes in the stored, cue-distance coefficients, the slope, or the centroid. In particular, it predicts that symmetrical changes in the location of objects in an environment, such as the uniform enlargement or compression of the geometrical configuration of the cues, will not elicit exploration. Thinus-Blanc and her colleagues have carried out an elegant set of experiments in which they systematically studied the amount and direction of exploratory activity by changes in an environment consisting of four distinct objects, usually originally in a square configuration (Poucet *et al.* 1986; Thinus-Blanc *et al.* 1987, and Chapter 18). They found that movement of one object or the interchange of objects elicited exploration directed in some cases at the displaced object and in others at the remaining, unmoved objects as well. Most interesting, for the present discussion, is that the enlargement of the square by the simultaneous movement of the objects away from the centre did not elicit exploration, as predicted by the model. It is one of the goals of the model to predict the pattern of exploration elicited in these experiments. Notice that none of the goal-centric models that relies on a privileged goal location can predict the exploration of a non-rewarded environment.

II. Prediction of the next location on the basis of the current location plus movement

The model treats movement as a translocation vector that is represented as a sinusoid where the distance of the displacement is represented as the amplitude of the sinusoid and the angle of turn as the phase of the sinusoid relative to the clock reference. Consequently, the expected location can be calculated by the addition of the vector array representing the current location and this movement vector (Fig. 16.7). Vanderwolf (1969, 1971) originally reported that electro-encephalographic theta activity from the hippocampus was correlated with movements which he called 'voluntary' but which Nadel and I suggested might more aptly be characterized as those that change the animal's position in the environment (O'Keefe and Nadel 1978). In a series of experiments in collaboration with the late Abe

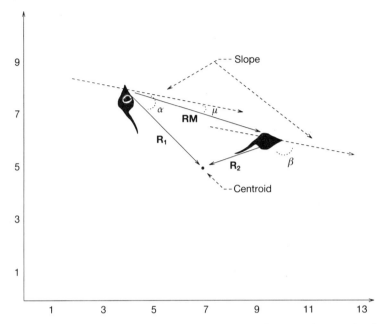

Fig. 16.7. Schema showing the movement from one location (on the left) to another (on the right) as a vector with amplitude **RM** and angle relative to the axis of slope μ. The centroid vectors R_1 and R_2 from the start and finish location are also shown. Their angles relative to the axis of eccentricity are labelled α and β respectively. The location vectors and the movement vector form a vector triangle so that, given any two, the third can be computed.

Black, and with Richard Morris and his colleagues (Morris *et al.* 1976; O'Keefe and Nadel 1978, pp. 179–82; Morris and Hagan 1983), it was found that the frequency of theta (but not the amplitude) was a function of the distance jumped. Changes in the weight carried by the rat during the jump had no effect, ruling out factors such as force exerted as the relevant variable. As this finding does not conform in detail to the predictions of the present model, which would lead one to expect that the amplitude and not the wavelength of theta reflect the distance or speed of movement, we intend re-investigating this phenomenon to ascertain whether there is anything peculiar about vertical jumping that would account for the findings. In particular, there has been little exploration of the way in which the third dimension might be represented in the map.

The model predicts that once the correct representation of an environment has been set up, the sensory cues can be removed and the system can update the current representation as the animal moves around the environment on the basis of the movements involved. Andrew Speakman and I tested this prediction in a cue-controlled environment (see Fig. 16.8, taken

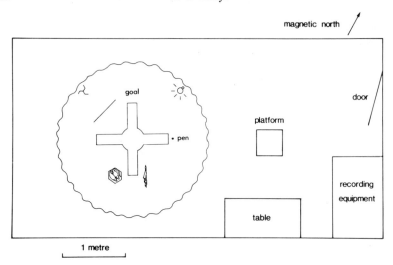

Fig. 16.8. Layout of the cue-controlled environment for studying the memory- and goal-related properties of the hippocampal place cells. The elevated +-maze is isolated from the rest of the laboratory by a set of black curtains. Six cues provide spatial information by which the rat can locate the goal. Clockwise, they are a light, an odour source such as a pen, a towel, a rat cage, a fan, and a large, white card. Usually the goal was located between the card and fan on one side and the light on the other. Between trials the constellation of cues was rotated by multiples of 90° in a pseudo-random fashion. On perceptual trials the cues were present throughout the entire trial and the rat was trained to go to the goal regardless of the arm from which it was started. On memory trials the cues were only present for the first part of each trial, during which the rat was confined to the start arm. After this the cues were removed and the rat remained in the start arm for an additional period during which the memory capacity of both the rat and the place cells could be assessed. During goal-shift experiments the location of the goal relative to the cues was moved after the cell-field locations had been mapped in order to test whether the fields would move with the goal or stay constant relative to the spatial cues. Usually the goal was moved by 180°, which in the configuration shown would have relocated it to the arm between the towel and the rat cage. Between trials the rat was held on the platform outside the cue-controlled environment.

from O'Keefe and Speakman 1987). In this environment, rats are taught both reference-memory and working-memory versions of a place-learning task. Cues to the location of the goal arm of a four-arm maze are spread around the environment. Rotation of the cues and the goal by steps of 90°, 180°, or 270° from trial to trial forces the rat to use the controlled spatial cues to solve the task. When they have learned to approach the goal with the cues present throughout the trial, a working-memory version of the task is run. Here the cues are available for the first part of each trial but are then removed so that choice of the goal must be made in their absence and hence based on memory for their location on that trial. Rats that performed at a high success rate were implanted with micro-drives and CA1

UNIT FIRING RATE

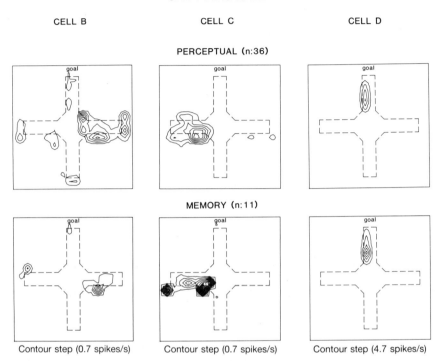

Fig. 16.9. Place fields of three, simultaneously recorded, CA1 complex-spike cells in the cue-controlled environment. Each picture is a montage constructed from a number of trials in which the cues have different orientations to the experimental room. The data have been rotated so that all of the trials are orientated with the goal at the top. The firing rate in different parts of the maze is shown as a contour plot that represents the number of action potentials in that spot divided by the amount of time the animal spent there. The top row of pictures show the firing fields derived from 36 trials when the cues were present during the recording. Each cell has a different, preferred patch of the maze. The lower row shows the firing fields of the same cells during those parts of 12 trials after the cues had been removed. The fields in these and the large majority of cells tested continued to identify the same locations on the maze, demonstrating their memory capacity. (From O'Keefe and Speakman 1987.)

and CA3 hippocampal neurons recorded during the task. It was found that 27 of 30 units that were recorded in the working-memory version of this task maintained their place fields after cue removal (see Fig 16.9 for examples of this result). One interpretation of this finding is that the internal representation of the animal's location on maze, in combination with the information about the rat's movements, were sufficient to update the place-field representation. An alternative interpretation is that on each trial the representation of the controlled spatial cues and the representation of the remaining cues (including the maze and background cues) are brought into correspondence, and that these latter cues are sufficient to support correct place-cell firing during the memory period.

III. Generation of the movement transform necessary to go from the current location to a desired (goal) location

The vector operation shown above in Fig. 16.7 can be performed in reverse. That is, given two vectors—one representing the current location and the other a desired location—the system can subtract the two and calculate the movement vector required. This, in turn, would be sent to an egocentric, motor-generating structure, which would translate it into muscle movements. The subtraction requires that the vector for current location be shifted by 180° before being added to the vector for stored location. The system allows the animal to cope with detours in which it is necessary to find a different route to the goal when the direct or usual route has been blocked or is otherwise unavailable. There have been many demonstrations of this ability in the published record on animal behaviour since the classic one by Tolman *et al.* (1946) (see Chapuis 1987 for a recent summary).

In the spatial, working-memory task described above, Speakman and I included detour trials in which the animal was not allowed to run directly to the goal at the end of the memory period but instead was first forced into one of the two non-start, non-goal arms and then allowed to choose. They did so accurately, and valuable unit recording was obtained from one of these animals. We found that the appropriate place units fired in these 'detour' arms. This means that not only the representation for the start arm but also for the rest of the maze is activated and maintained during each trial.

Several conclusions relevant to the present model can be drawn from these observations. Firstly, the system must be capable of computing the updated, current location after a move the animal had not made before. I have suggested elsewhere (O'Keefe 1990) that this and similar detour abilities of the spatial system place severe constraints on the properties of the component for movement translation, such that it needs to be capable of calculating the equivalence of, for example, two right turns and a straight in the plus-maze, or the diagonal of the triangle in the triangulation detour. Secondly, the absence of any evidence for an influence of the goal destination on the firing of the non-goal place cells in this and other experiments suggests that this component of the system is not located in the CA3 or CA1 fields of the hippocampus but might be located in an area very close to them anatomically (see below).

IV. The role of the goal in the spatial representation

The present model suggests that the spatial representation of an environment does not rely on the preferred view from the goal nor does it give this location a greater representation than any other. The storage of these incentive locations takes place outside the hippocampus proper and should be sought in regions that receive inputs both from there and from either the motivational centres of the hypothalamus or incentive areas such as the amygdala. The lateral septum is a clear possibility, as are the retro-hippocampal regions such as the subicular region.

As pointed out earlier (O'Keefe 1979), several observations on the hippocampal place cells support this notion. The distribution of place fields in an environment does not show a preferential representation of the goal (O'Keefe and Speakman 1987). A more direct test of the hypothesis involves the mapping of place fields in an environment before and after movement of the goal. Speakman and O'Keefe (1990) did this experiment in the cue-controlled environment during a spatial-reference memory task (with the cues rotated between trials but available throughout each trial) and found that 16 of 19 cells remained in their location relative to the spatial cues and did not show any tendency to orient to the goal when it was removed. Figure 16.10 shows an example of this phenomenon. A different result was found by Breese *et al.* (1989) in a formally similar experiment. They found that the place fields tended to concentrate around one or more

UNIT FIRING RATE

BEFORE (n:12)　　　　　　　**AFTER** (n:12)

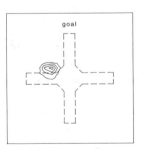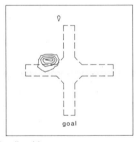

Contour step (3.0 spikes/s)

Fig. 16.10. An example of the constancy of the place-field firing with respect to the controlled spatial cues following the shift of goal location: The left-hand picture shows the field firing during 12 trials before the goal shift when the goal was the arm at the top while the right-hand picture shows the results from 12 trials after the animal had learned to stop approaching this arm but had instead learned to go to the 180° opposite arm, the one at the bottom (see Fig. 16.8).

of the water-reward locations in their task and that the fields shifted
location when the goal location was shifted. We have suggested that these
differences in results might be due to the number of spatial location cues
available to the animal in the two experiments. In our experiment there
were six cues in addition to the food in the goal whereas in Breese's
experiment there was only a single polarizing stimulus in addition to the
reward. We have previously pointed out that rewards have cue properties
and can function as spatial cues as well as reinforcers. They would be more
likely to do so in conditions where the number of non-reward cues is small.
However, when the reward and the remaining spatial cues provide conflicting information, the reward enjoys no particular privileged status.

Mapping the cognitive map onto the hippocampal system

At this stage in our knowledge of the physiology of the hippocampus any
attempt to assign specific roles to its different regions must be counted as
extremely speculative. Nevertheless, some clues exist and the exercise may
prove useful if it encourages experimentation.

The phasor theory gives a large role in the vector computations to the
sinusoidal theta rhythm. It suggests that each granule and pyramidal cell
acts as an harmonic oscillator which sums its sinusoidal inputs and produces an output that sets up an oscillation in its projection targets. The
extra-cellular, electro-encephalographic theta would reflect the activity
of a large number of such oscillators. Where there is a high degree of
synchronization between these underlying oscillators, the amplitude of
the electro-encephalographic theta will be large and regular; as the phases
of the oscillators become shifted relative to the clock reference and to
each other, the theta amplitude drops and the rhythm becomes irregular.
This suggests that the absence of extra-cellular theta in the CA3 region
may reflect extensive or even total desynchrony of the underlying CA3
pyramids.

The medial septum and diagonal band of Broca appear to act as a
pacemaker for the hippocampal theta rhythm. Vanderwolf and his colleagues (Vanderwolf et al. 1975) have shown that there are at least two
theta systems, one sensitive to atropine and the other not. The second
correlates with some aspect of the animal's movements (see above) and,
according to the present model, broadcasts the translation vector to the
hippocampus. The non-movement theta is, on the present model, the
reference clock.

Upper layers of the entorhinal cortex contain place-coded neurons, and
it is proposed that this is the route of entry of the sensory information into
the mapping system. It is plausible to assume that the veridical distances

have been assigned to the cue vectors before this stage in the circuit. The direct projection of the perforant path to the CA3 pyramids provides the basis for the calculation of the partial centroid estimates. On this view, each CA3 pyramid calculates the vector average of the cue-vector inputs impinging on its dendrites. Each pyramid has a pre-wired set of possible cue inputs and can only respond to the sub-set of this set that it actually encounters in a particular environment. The summed vectors on the dendrites of the CA are turned into an average when they are divided by the activity of the basket cells, which we assume to be the theta cells. After McNaughton (1988), I assume that one of the functions of this network is to count the number of active inputs to a group of pyramidal cells and to divide their activity by this number through their inhibitory action at the soma.

The CA1 pyramids receive a direct input from the upper layers of the entorhinal cortex and an equally powerful input from the CA3 pyramids via the Schaffer collaterals. Recordings from the CA1 and CA3 pyramidal cells have failed to reveal major differences in their firing rates, place-field characteristics, etc. This may simply mean that the present recording techniques are not sensitive enough to pick up such differences or more probably that the transformation is one at the cross-fibre level. I have suggested (O'Keefe 1988, 1990) that this transformation may have something to do with the necessity to invert the centroid representation in order to allow it to be combined with a stored representation of a goal location to yield the movement vector necessary to go to that location. In the present model, this operation would involve the phase shift of the centroid representations by $180°$ to compute the negative of the CA3 representation.

This negative of the current representation, when added to a stored goal vector, gives the movement vector necessary to get to that location (see above). A major projection target of the CA1 region is the neighbouring subiculum. The subiculum also receives inputs from neural areas associated with incentives, such as the amygdala and perhaps the anterior thalamus, and projects to motor programming structures such as the nucleus accumbens. As such it is a good candidate for the structure performing the addition of the incentive location and the negative of the current to derive the movement vector.

Acknowledgements

The research reported here was supported by the Medical Research Council of Britain. I would like to thank Andrew Speakman who collaborated in that research.

References

Barto, A. G. and Sutton, R. S. (1981). Landmark learning: An illustration of associative search. *Biological Cybernetics*, **42**, 1–8.

Bostock, E., Taube, J., and Muller, R. U. (1988). The effects of head orientation on the firing of hippocampal place cells. *Society for Neuroscience Abstracts*, **13**, 127.

Breese, C. R., Hampson, R. E., and Deadwyler, S. A. (1989). Hippocampal place cells: stereotypy and plasticity. *Journal of Neuroscience*, **9**, 1097–111.

Cartwright, B. A. and Collett, T. S. (1982). How honey bees use landmarks to guide their return to a good source. *Nature*, **295**, 560–4.

Chapuis, N. (1987). Detour and shortcut abilities in several species of mammals. In *Cognitive processes and spatial orientation in animals and man*, Vol. 2 (ed. P. Ellen and C. Thinus-Blanc), pp. 97–106. Martinus Nijhoff, Dordrecht.

Collett, T. S., Cartwright, B. A., and Smith, B. A. (1986). Landmark learning and visuo-spatial memories in gerbils. *Journal of Comparative Physiology*, **158**, 835–51.

Koshland, D. E. (1979). A model regulatory system: bacterial chemotaxis. *Physiology Review*, **59**, 811–62.

McNaughton, B. L. (1988). Neural mechanisms for spatial computation and information storage. In *Neural connections and mental computations* (ed. L. Nadel, L. A. Cooper, P. Culicover, and R. M. Harnish), pp. 285–350. MIT Press, Cambridge, Mass.

McNaughton, B. L., Barnes, C. A., and O'Keefe, J. (1983). The contributions of position, direction and velocity to single unit activity in the hippocampus of freely-moving rats. *Experimental Brain Research*, **52**, 41–9.

Morris, R. C. (1981). Spatial localization does not depend on the presence of local cues. *Learning and Motivation*, **12**, 239–60.

Morris, R. G. M., Black, A. B., and O'Keefe, J. (1976). Hippocampal EEG during a ballistic movement. *Neuroscience Letters*, **3**, 102.

Morris, R. G. M. and Hagan J. J. (1983). Hippocampal electrical activity and ballistic movement. In *Neurobiology of the hippocampus* (ed. W. Seifert), pp. 321–31. Academic Press.

Muller, R. U. and Kubie, J. L. (1987). The effects of changes in the environment on the spatial firing of hippocampal complex-spike cells. *Journal of Neuroscience*, **7**, 1951–68.

Muller, R. U., Kubie, J. L., and Ranck, J. B. (1987). Spatial firing patterns of hippocampal complex-spike cells in a fixed environment. *Journal of Neuroscience*, **7**, 1935–50.

O'Keefe, J. (1976). Place units in the hippocampus of the freely moving rat. *Experimental Neurology*, **51**, 78–109.

O'Keefe, J. (1979). A review of the hippocampal place cells. *Progress in Neurobiology*, **13**, 419–39.

O'Keefe, J. (1983). Spatial memory within and without the hippocampal system. In *Neurobiology of the hippocampus* (ed. W. Seifert), pp. 375–403. Academic Press, London.

O'Keefe, J. (1988). Computations the hippocampus might perform. In *Neural connections and mental computations* (ed. L. Nadel, L. A. Cooper, P. Culicover, and R. M. Harnish), p. 225–84. MIT Press, Cambridge, Mass.

O'Keefe, J. (1990). A computational theory of the hippocampal cognitive map. *Progress in brain research*, Vol. 83 (ed. J. Storm-Mathisen, J. Zimmer, and O. P. Ottersen), pp. 301–12. Elsevier, Amsterdam.

O'Keefe, J. and Conway, D. H. (1978). Hippocampal place units in the freely moving rat: why they fire where they fire. *Experimental Brain Research*, **31**, 573–90.

O'Keefe, J. and Nadel, L. (1978). *The hippocampus as a cognitive map*. Clarendon, Oxford.

O'Keefe, J. and Speakman, A. (1987). Single unit activity in the rat hippocampus during a spatial memory task. *Experimental Brain Research*, **68**, 1–27.

Poucet, B., Chapuis, N., Durup, M., and Thinus-Blanc, C. (1986). A study of exploratory behaviour as an index of spatial knowledge in hamsters. *Animal Learning and Behaviour*, **14**, 93–100.

Rolls, E. T. (1989). Functions of neuronal networks in the hippocampus and neocortex in memory. In *Neural models of plasticity: experimental and theoretical approaches* (ed. J. H. Byrne, and W. O. Berry), pp. 240–65. Academic Press, San Diego.

Speakman, A. S. and O'Keefe, J. (1990). Hippocampal complex spike cells do not change their place fields if the goal is moved within a cue controlled environment. *European Journal of Neuroscience*, **2**, 544–55.

Taube, J. S., Muller, R. U., and Ranck, J. B. Jr. (1990). Head-direction cells recorded from the post-subiculum in freely moving rats. I. Description and quantitative analysis. *Journal of Neuroscience*, **10**, 420–35.

Thinus-Blanc, C., Bouzouba, L., Chaix, K., Chapuis, N., Durup, M., and Poucet, B. (1987). A study of spatial parameters encoded during exploration in hamsters. *Journal of Experimental Psychology: Animal Behaviour Processes*, **13**, 418–27.

Tolman, E. C., Ritchie, B. F., and Kalish, D. (1946). Studies in spatial learning I. Orientation and the short-cut. *Journal of Experimental Psychology*, **36**, 13–24.

Vanderwolf, C. H. (1969). Hippocampal electrical activity and voluntary movement in the rat. *EEG and Clinical Neurophysiology*, **26**, 407–18.

Vanderwolf, C. H. (1971). Limbic–diencephalic mechanisms of voluntary movement. *Psychology Review*, **78**, 83–113.

Vanderwolf, C. H., Kramis, R., Gillcpsic, L. A., and Bland, B. H. (1975). Hippocampal slow activity and neocortical low voltage fast activity: relations to behavior. In *The hippocampus; a comprehensive treatise* (ed. R. L. Isaacson and K. Pribram) pp. 101–28. Plenum, New York.

Wilkie, D. M. and Palfrey, R. (1987). A computer simulation model of rats' place navigation in the Morris water maze. *Behavioral Research Methods, Instruments and Computers*, **19**, 400–3.

Zipser, D. (1986). Biologically plausible models of place recognition and place location. In *Parallel distributed processing* (ed. J. L. McClelland and D. E. Rumelhart), pp. 432–70. MIT Press, Cambridge, Mass.

17

Spatial firing correlates of neurons in the hippocampal formation of freely moving rats

R. U. MULLER, J. L. KUBIE, E. M. BOSTOCK,
J. S. TAUBE, and G. J. QUIRK

Navigation and mapping

A large fraction of the behaviour of rats consists of translocational move-ments that solve the problem of getting to a goal from a starting point. In solving this sort of spatial problem, the rat must follow a specific path that is somehow selected from the set of possible paths. For convenience, we will say that the task of path selection is accomplished by a neural 'naviga-tional system'. Our research is aimed at understanding the organization and operation of this system.

The starting point for our approach is the 'cognitive mapping' theory of O'Keefe and Nadel (1978). According to this theory, the navigational system uses two very different methods to compute paths. The 'taxon' method is based on stimulus–response association learning, and solutions take the form of 'routes'. A route is a chain of locomotor responses to an ordered series of specific stimulus configurations, such that the vector sum of the responses connects the initial position to the goal. Each response to a stimulus configuration carries the rat to the position where the next con-figuration in the series is available. The penultimate response brings the rat to a place from which the goal can be sensed, and the final response gets the rat to the goal. The locations of critical stimulus configurations can be thought of as intermediate goals. In short, a route is a sequence of independent loco-motor responses associated in stimulus–response–stimulus (S–R–S) fashion, with local stimulus configurations, and does not depend on a repre-sentation of the spatial framework in which locomotion takes place. The chain-like nature of routes allows for paths that cross themselves. This is possible if the two views from the crossing point are not associated with each other so that the same physical locus is treated as two different places.

The second, 'locale' method postulates the ability to learn a map-like representation of the environment, and solutions take the form of straight lines in unobstructed space. More generally, locale solutions are geodesics (shortest paths) that are optimized with respect to the structure of the entire mapped region, taking into account barriers. As stated by O'Keefe and Nadel, it is crucial that 'no object or place on the map is a goal' (p. 89).

The map is a cohesive representation that can be used to compute geodesics which connect every pair of points in the territory. This means that the rat can go to different goals from a single starting point or can get to a fixed goal from an arbitrary starting point without the need to build enormous numbers of routes.

The existence of a map-like component of the navigational system is inferred from the ability of rats to solve spatial problems that are apparently too complex to be solved with a taxon method (Tolman 1948). Given the power of stimulus–response association learning to explain a wide range of problem solving, it is unwise to expect that a crucial experiment will prove the necessity of a neural map (Terrace 1984). Nevertheless, the case for maps is strengthened by evidence that the navigational system can use the large-scale structure of the environment in path selection. Currently, performance in the Morris swimming task (Morris 1981) is considered the best example of a spatial problem that cannot be solved without an abstract representation of the surroundings. Morris demonstrated that rats learn to swim directly to an unmarked goal (an underwater platform) from a fixed starting position, and go directly to the same hidden platform the first time they leave from a novel starting position. In the cognitive mapping theory, the ability to swim directly to a hidden goal from a new starting position is interpreted as an example of the ability to find geodesics between arbitrary pairs of points.

The Morris experiment is subject to the criticism that the path from the novel starting position to the hidden platform may have previously been taken as the rat learned the initial task. A clever variant done by Sutherland and Rudy (1988) shows, however, that rats can indeed solve the novel path problem. Rats were first trained in the presence of a visible escape platform. The rats were seen reliably to swim directly from the fixed starting point to the goal, and never experienced a wide range of routes. Nevertheless, they were able to swim to the hidden platform the first time they were released from a new starting point. This result is extremely hard to explain in terms of taxon schemes, and is perhaps the clearest example of why it seems necessary to infer the existence of a map-like representation of the environment.

The hippocampus is postulated to be the neural locus of the cognitive map

Although the systematic treatment of the behavioural origins of Tolman's mapping hypothesis by O'Keefe and Nadel (1978) is a valuable contribution, the heart of their theory is the concept that the mapping capacity of the navigational system is localized to the hippocampus. O'Keefe and Nadel marshalled three lines of evidence in favour of the spatial hypothesis of hippocampal function. First, they reviewed the published record on lesions of the hippocampus and argued that all the effects of such lesions are secondary to the loss of spatial mapping abilities. There are now reasons to believe that the functions of the rat hippocampus are not exclusively spatial in nature (Olton *et al.* 1979; Berger *et al.* 1983; Wiener *et al.* 1989), but later work has corroborated the idea that hippocampal lesions play havoc with the ability to learn complex spatial problems. For example, Morris *et al.* (1982) showed that hippocampal damage greatly impairs the ability of rats to swim to the hidden platform, but does not affect performance with a visible platform.

The second line of evidence for the spatial theory comes from the work of Vanderwolf and his colleagues, who have shown that the state of the hippocampal electro-encephalogram (EEG) is reliably correlated with the concurrent behavioural state of the rat. Vanderwolf (1969) demonstrated that large-amplitude, irregular EEG activity (LIA) is associated with quiet alertness and with repetitive, 'housekeeping' activities such as grooming, chewing, and licking. In contrast, the 5–8 Hz, sine-like 'theta' rhythm was seen when the rat walked, jumped or made postural adjustments. O'Keefe and Nadel interpreted these findings to mean that LIA occurs when the rat is stationary relative to its surroundings, as it is during quiet alertness or when movement is averaged for a cycle of a repetitive activity, and that theta occurs when the rat makes a net movement relative to its surroundings. The notion that changes in hippocampal EEG state are correlated with changes in locomotor state summarizes most, if not all, of Vanderwolf's observations, and makes a great deal of sense if the hippocampus is involved in path selection.

The third and most convincing line of evidence for the spatial theory arises from correlations observed between the state of the rat and activity of individual hippocampal neurons. Ranck (1973) classified hippocampal neurons as either 'theta' or 'complex-spike' cells according to electrophysiological properties. Later work (Fox and Ranck 1975, 1981) established that theta cells are local, inhibitory inter-neurons and that complex-spike cells are hippocampal pyramidal cells in both the CA1 (regio superior) and CA3/4 (regio inferior). It is important to add that all single-cell recordings in freely moving rats up to the present have been made from the dorsal (septal) portion of the hippocampus; the ventral (temporal) portion is *terra incognita*.

Theta cells were named for the reliable correlation between their firing rate and the presence and absence of the theta EEG pattern; their rate approximately doubles when the EEG state switches from LIA to theta. At the behavioural level, it is expected and experimentally confirmed that theta cells fire faster during locomotion than otherwise (Ranck 1973). Later work has revealed additional properties of theta cells that pertain to the spatial theory, some of which are considered below.

Place cells and maps

Before complex-spike cells were identified as a class, O'Keefe and Dostrovsky (1971) described the 'place cell' phenomenon that lies at the centre of the mapping theory. It is now clear that place cells are a large (and perhaps complete) sub-set of complex-spike cells (Thompson and Best 1989). Place cells were named for their property 'location-specific' firing: under many conditions, their firing rate varies strongly with the head position of a freely moving rat in the environment. A place cell is intensely active only when the head is inside a bounded region that will be referred to as the cell's 'firing field'. Outside the firing field, the cell is virtually silent, so that the position of the firing field is easily detected, even by naive observers (Best and Ranck 1982).

The place-cell phenomenon was taken as direct evidence that the hippocampus is involved in mapping. In the theory, the conjoint firing of place cells signals the position of the rat in its environment; as the rat moves, the set of cells that is most active changes accordingly. This picture is reasonable in that the number of place cells is very large, firing fields are homogeneously scattered over the surface of the environment, and the average field size is an appreciable fraction of the area of the environment. Taken together, these facts suggest that the rat's position can be represented with high resolution by the place-cell population. The theory did not specify how the rat's position on the map could be read.

Assessment of the cognitive mapping theory

The cognitive mapping theory of O'Keefe and Nadel is subject to criticism on several grounds. A fundamental objection is raised by reports that complex-spike cells are not well described as place cells, but instead fire in relation to specific aspects of the rat's behaviour. For example, Ranck (1973) divided complex-spike cells into sub-classes according to correlations between their firing and behavioural sequences in which goal-directed and consummatory segments were of major importance. Using quantitative methods, Eichenbaum and his colleagues (Eichenbaum *et al* 1987; Wiener *et al*. 1989) have also reported relationships between complex-cell activity and behavioural sequence. Breese *et al*. (1989) showed a correlation between firing and the location where a water reward is available. It seems clear that such strong associations between behaviour and complex-spike cell activity do not fit the spatial theory as originally stated. It is nevertheless our contention that the firing of complex-spike cells can approach ideal location-specificity in a reduced environment (Muller *et al*.

1987; Bostock *et al*. 1990) and that the place-cell phenomenon must be part of any complete explanation of hippocampal function. We also note that the same investigators who reported behaviour-specific firing of complex-spike cells also have reported location-specific firing.

A second kind of objection accepts that the empirical bases of the theory are correct, but that the mapping interpretation is wrong. This position has been taken by McNaughton and his collegues (McNaughton 1989, McNaughton *et al*. 1989), who suggest that the hippocampus solves spatial problems with taxon rather than locale methods. In their view, each place cell signals the rat's arrival at a critical locus in a route; the cell fires because the cue configuration matches a cell-specific template. In turn, the place-cell discharge activates the motion necessary for the rat to go to the next critical cue locus.

McNaughton thus proposes that the current cue configuration triggers place-cell discharge in a sensory-like fashion. In this way, McNaughton's model resembles the computational model of Zipser (1985). The major difference concerns the directional selectivity of place cells. In Zipser's scheme, place cell firing within the field is independent of head direction because the sensory surface is a 360° retina. McNaughton (1989) points out that the effective cue configuration ('local view') depends on head orienta-tion as well as head position. In his model, place cells are expected to show direction-specific as well as location-specific firing because each cell is activated by a certain local view. The empirical basis for the local-view model is the tendency for place cells to fire more rapidly as a rat walks in or out a specific arm of an eight-arm maze (McNaughton *et al*. 1983; Mizu-mori *et al*. 1989; Bostock *et al*. 1988). We will refer to the hypothesis expressed by Zipser and modified by McNaughton as the 'sensory model' of place-cell firing. It is important to note that the local-view model can be falsified by finding circumstances in which place-cell firing is omnidirectional. One purpose of this chapter is to present some of our evidence on the directional firing properties of place cells.

In our current understanding, we accept both the empirical bases of the mapping theory and the general idea that the hippocampal representation is map-like. In particular, we agree that the hippocampus can compute arbitrary paths through the environment, and imagine that the paths will prove to be geodesic in nature. We also agree that the ability to compute arbitrary paths implies that the representation must take the entire en-vironment into account, so that the representation is not a list of local views.

Our major disagreement with the theory of O'Keefe and Nadel concerns the extent to which the cohesive representation literally resembles a map. O'Keefe and Nadel (1978) assumed that the representation is Euclidean, and that it explicitly calculates the distance and angle between arbitrary pairs of points (see O'Keefe 1990, and Chapter 16). It is our view that the computations made by the hippocampus are better described as topological than metric. We will mention some arguments against the metric hypothesis in the results, and propose an alternative interpretation in the discussion.

The assumption that the hippocampus implements an abstract representation of the environment leads naturally to the question of how associated brain structures contribute to the representation. The main purpose of this chapter is to summarize our evidence that the firing of cells in other portions of the hippocampal formation is correlated with aspects of the rat's spatial state (head position and/or head direction); in some cases the correlation is as clear as it is for place cells. We believe, in other words, that the locale component of the navigational system is subserved by a much larger cortical region than the hippocampus alone.

Behavioural methods

Our studies of place cells and related neuronal classes have been done under the same reduced behavioural conditions, so that comparisons among cell classes are facilitated. Before recordings are made, hungry rats are trained to retrieve small food pellets scattered into a cylindrical recording chamber. As a result, the rats spend almost all their time walking, and visit all parts of the chamber (Muller *et al.* 1987; Bostock *et al.* 1986). The cylinder is 76 cm in diameter and is uniformly grey except for a single white cardboard sheet that occupies 100° of arc of the wall. The cylinder is surrounded by a circular curtain that creates a controlled cue environment. To investigate the properties of place cells, the visual appearance of the cylinder can be modified or a different chamber can be substituted.

In our opinion, the pellet-chasing task is too simple to imagine that it requires a locale (mapping) solution, and it is unlikely that hippocampal lesions would cause very much reduction in the efficiency of pellet finding. Our primary finding is that location-specific firing is robust under these circumstances, in which the reward can be obtained merely by walking to it (Muller *et al.* 1987). Regardless of its nature, the representation is clearly active even though it is apparently unnecessary. What is not clear is if the hippocampus controls behaviour during pellet chasing or if it is in some sort of 'tracking' mode.

The pellet-chasing task has several properties that are worth making explicit. First, it transfers easily when the environment is modified. This means that the spatial firing properties of individual cells can be compared with behaviour held constant and only the surroundings changed. Second, it makes behaviour quite homogeneous in time and space. A numerical analysis of behaviour during pellet chasing indicates that rats spend 90 per cent of the time moving around, 7 per cent in quiet alertness and the remaining 3 per cent in grooming or rearing. Finally, the open floor of the cylinder contains no set starting point or set goal, so that the behavioural space shares with the putative map the property that there are no preferred points. It is our belief that the properties of place cells and of the hippocampal representation are more easily interpreted when the space is 'behaviourally isotropic'.

Recording methods

To measure automatically the spatial firing correlates of place cells and other neuronal types, we measure, in parallel, unitary activity and the position of one or two lights attached to the rat's head at 60 Hz. Unitary activity is recorded with a movable array of 10 electrodes (Kubie 1984). Candidate waveforms are passed through a series of three, time-and-amplitude window discriminators; the acceptance pulse of the third discriminator is counted as an action potential. The time of occurrence of each spike is not saved. Instead, the number of spikes fired during each 1/60th s interval is counted and sent to a computer along with the digitized head-light positions. The combined spike and position information is referred to as a 'sample'; 3600 samples are obtained per minute.

In earlier work, only head position was measured by tracking the position of a white light mounted on the electrode carrier. Position was measured to 1 part in 64 (6-bit resolution) for the X and Y co-ordinates. Each small pixel in the 64 by 64 grid was about 3 cm on a side, so that the area of the cylinder contained about 500 pixels; the size of each pixel is approximately the size of the rat's head. When only one spot is tracked, 16 min of recording time are enough to get a clear picture of spatial firing distributions as the average time spent in a pixel is about 2 s.

More recently, we have measured both head position and orientation by independently tracking a red and a green, light-emitting diode (LED) arranged fore and aft on the rat's head. To achieve adequate angular resolution for head direction, the linear resolution for locating the individual LEDs must be increased. With the two-spot tracker, linear resolution was increased eight-fold by detecting light position to 1 part in 256 and by zooming the TV camera view in two-fold. With a linear resolution of about 4 mm and an 8 cm separation between the LEDs, the angular resolution is about 3°. When firing is treated as a function of position, the three low-order bits for X and Y are discarded to bring the linear resolution back to about 3.0 cm; if the full spatial resolution is used, the total recording time to get a good estimate of the spatial rate distribution becomes prohibitive.

Numerical and display methods

For one-spot data, the serial spike/position samples are sorted according to position by accumulating light-detections and spikes into two 64 by 64 arrays. When the head is detected in a pixel, the corresponding element of a time-in-location array is incremented by one, and the corresponding element of a spike array is incremented by the number of spikes fired during the 16.7 ms interval. When all the samples have been sorted into pixels, the spatial firing-rate distribution is gotten by dividing the spike array by the time array on a pixel-by-pixel basis. Numerical methods can then be used to characterize the spatial firing pattern. For example, the local smoothness of firing fields can be estimated by calculating a two-dimensional auto-correlation (Muller and Kubie 1989; Kubie *et al.* 1990b).

Colour-coded, firing-rate maps are used to visualize positional firing patterns. To make such a map, pixel firing rates are divided into six categories that are each represented by a different colour. Pixels in which the rate was exactly zero are coded yellow and increasing firing rates are coded in the order orange, red, green, blue and purple. In this way, a firing field appears as a dark patch on a yellow background; the firing field in Plate 1A is near the cylinder wall at 10 o'clock. In figure legends, numeric values for the rank-scaled categories are the firing rate in the median pixel for each category. Regions that were never visited are shown as white. If all pixels in the apparatus were visited, the floors appears as a coloured region on a white background. Pixels in the apparatus that were not visited are also coded white.

For two-spot data, serial samples are sorted according to position and head orientation. Generally, angular sorting is done at two resolutions. To describe how firing rate varies only with head direction, we divided the circle into either forty 9° bins or sixty 6° bins. When head position and direction are dealt with together, only eight 45° bins are used and much longer recordings are made. For example, with eight angular bins and 500 pixels for each bin, the sampling time for each of the 4000 possible position–direction combinations is about 1 s if the total recording time is 64 min. With the two-spot tracker, it is often of interest to make a direction-independent rate map and also eight direction-specific maps. When direction-specific maps are colour-coded, the same rank ordering applies to all of the eight maps and not each map separately.

Results

Up to now, we have measured the spatial firing in four parts of the hippocampal formation. We have recorded from theta cells and place cells in the hippocampus proper. All the data for theta cells and much of the data for place cells were obtained with the one-spot system; the two-spot system was used to test our subjective impression that place cells show little if any direction-specificity during pellet chasing (Muller *et al.* 1987). We also recorded from units in the medial entorhinal cortex (MEC), the subiculum and the postsubiculum. The MEC was studied because it is the major source of cortical input to the hippocampus; cells in MEC were investigated with the one-spot tracker. Recordings from the subiculum were initiated because it is a major target for axons of CA1, hippocampal, pyramidal cells. The postsubiculum is not strongly connected with the hippocampus proper, but was studied (Taube *et al.* 1990a,b) because exploratory work revealed that many postsubicular neurons show nearly ideal direction-specific firing (Ranck 1984). Postsubicular and subicular units were studied with the two-spot tracker.

Basic properties of place cells

The spatial firing patterns for four complex-spike cells are shown as colour-coded rate maps in Plate 1. Three of the cells have distinct firing fields, whereas the positional pattern of the fourth (Plate 1D) is 'null'; the nearly uniform yellow appearance of the map indicates that the cell was virtually silent everywhere in the cylinder. It is also possible for a single place cell to have two (or more) firing fields (Muller *et al.* 1987). The shapes of firing field in Plate 1A, B and C representative of all fields seen in the cylinder. Fields vary according to angular location, size, and peak firing rate, but each field is either elliptic (Plates 1A and 1B) or crescent-like (Plate 1C); circular fields are taken as ellipses with zero eccentricity. Elliptic fields are usually found away from the cylinder wall, whereas the peak of crescent fields is generally next to the wall. The concavity of crescent fields makes it impossible to describe all fields as two-dimensional, Gaussian distributions. Note that the existence of qualitatively different field shapes suggests that cues must be combined in at least two different ways if they act to trigger place-cell firing in the manner of the sensory model.

In a grey rectangular apparatus with one, white, short wall, there are linear analogues of crescent fields that may occupy the entire length of one of the long walls (Muller *et al.* 1987). Such a linear field therefore encompasses a diverse set of total stimulus configurations or local views. It is hard to understand why the stimulus configurations at distant points trigger the same unit if each place cell signals a position in a route. The existence of linear and crescent fields is also unexpected from the Euclidean mapping model in which distance between points is represented by the distance between firing field centres.

A second argument against Euclidean mapping has more fundamental origins. In the Euclidean model, the rat's position is represented by the discharge of all cells whose fields contain the rat's real-world locus. Presumably, the computed position is an average of the positions of the field centres of the active units, weighted by the discharge rate of each cell. The difficulty with this scheme is that it produces systematic errors as the rat approaches the wall, even though fields are evenly distributed across the surface of the cylinder (Muller *et al.* 1987). The computed position near the wall lies closer to the centre than it should because there are no cells whose field centres lie outside the wall. In other words, the accuracy of the calculation is compromised by symmetry considerations; the computed position is veridical only when the rat's true position is surrounded by the same number of field centres in all directions (see Figures 11 and 12 in Muller *et al.* 1987).

One of the more puzzling aspects of the place-cell phenomenon is the great similarity of the firing patterns of cells in CA1 and CA3/4, despite well-known differences of connectivity and biochemistry in the two regions. Recently, however, two distinctions between CA1 and CA3/4 cells have been reported. Mizumori *et al.* (1989) found greater positional selectivity greater for CA3/4 than CA1 units on an eight-arm maze. They also found that the firing of CA3/4 units is more strongly disrupted by injections of tetracaine into the medial septum (the theta rhythm pacemaker). Muller and Kubie (1989) showed that place-cell firing predicts the future position of rats on a short (~100 ms) time-scale. Interestingly, the prediction interval is longer for CA1 cells than for CA3/4 cells. It is nevertheless clear that a full understanding of spatial information processing requires more precise differentiation of CA12 and CA3/4 place cells. It is also essential to explain how differences arise in terms of hippocampal circuitry.

Directional firing properties of place cells

The essential question of whether place-cell discharge depends on head direction as well as head position has received a good deal of attention but is still unresolved. Most recordings have been made on radial mazes. O'Keefe (1976) found that some cells were omnidirectional and others were directionally selective on a Y maze. Olton *et al.* (1978) reported clear location specificity but little directional specificity on an eight-arm maze. Using the same apparatus, McNaughton *et al.* (1983) and Mizumori *et al.* (1989) found that the in-field discharge rate depends strongly on whether the rat runs inward or outward on the appropriate arm. Qualitative observations during pellet chasing in the cylinder revealed little variation of place-cell firing with head direction (Muller *et al.* 1987).

As noted above, we used a two-spot tracker to assess quantitatively the directional specificity of place cells during pellet chasing (Bostock *et al.* 1988). Under the stated circumstances, we find that place-cell discharge is almost completely independent of head direction. Angle-specific rate maps at 45° resolution are shown for two typical place cells in Plates 2 and 3. The angle-specific maps are arranged in an octagon around an angle-independent map for the cell, such that the vector that connects the centre of the angle-independent map to the centre of each of the angle-specific maps is parallel to the middle of the relevant, 45°, head-direction range. The black outline around each map indicates the limits of the angle-independent map, or in other words the set of pixels visited from at least one head direction.

The lack of directional tuning for the central field in Plate 2 is evident from the angle-specific rate maps; each map has nearly the same colour-coding and each is a reasonbly good replica of the angle-independent map. If there were significant tuning for head direction, the field region would be coded mostly in orange and red for low-rate directions and mostly in blue and purple for high-rate directions. The lack of directional selectivity may be further appreciated by comparing Plate 2 to Plates 8, 9, and 10, which are for a post-subicular, head-direction cell, a subicular, head-direction cell, and a subicular, position-by-direction cell.

A conspicuous feature of each angle-specific map is the unsampled (white) crescent between the wall and the cylinder centre. The angular position of the unsampled region rotates systematically with the head-direction range such that the centre of the unsampled region lies at the tail of the diametric vector that points to the middle of the appropriate direction range. The unsampled region is a strictly mechanical effect that arises because the rat's head cannot point towards the cylinder centre when the head is at the wall without severe damage to the rat's body. In general, there must be a region that cannot be entered at all head directions adjacent to any boundary that the rat cannot cross. The unsampled region has no strong effect on the central field in Plate 2 because the unsampled region has little overlap with the field in any head-direction field. In contrast, it is clear that the unsampled region must affect the firing of cells with fields near the boundary.

The interaction between the unsampled region and an edge field is illustrated in Plate 3 for a field at 2:30 o'clock. The intensity and area of discharge is nearly constant at head directions for which the unsampled region does not overlap the field and is reduced to the extent that the unsampled region and the field intersect. It is our contention that the place cell of Plate 3 has no intrinsic directional selectivity and that the unsampled region fully accounts for the apparent deviation from directional invariance.

The lack of directional tuning for place cells in the small cylinder implies that the local view model is not a general explanation of location-specific firing. The constancy of firing rate with head orientation occurs even though different head orientations must be associated with different views of the white cue card, an object of known salience (Muller and Kubie 1987). In a more positive vein, the omnidirectional nature of firing fields is compatible with the original idea of O'Keefe and Nadel (1978) that place cells signal place in an abstract representation.

In contrast to the negligible directional selectivity of place-cell firing in the cylinder, McNaughton *et al.* (1983) and Mizumori *et al.* (1989) report that fields are directional on an eight-arm maze. Bostock *et al.* (1988) also saw fields on the maze with significant directional tuning, but found that other cells discharge about equally when the rat ran in or out on the appropriate arm. In addition, fields on the centre platform of the maze were omnidirectional. Recently, Leonard *et al.* (1990) have confirmed the omnidirectionality of place-cell firing in the cylinder which was reported by Bostock *et al.* (1988).

The variable directional selectivity of place cells has implications beyond the adequacy of the local-view model. In our opinion, the directional firing differences in the cylinder and the eight-arm maze are probably due to the restriction of trajectories in that maze. In other words, we expect that place cells in rats trained to run only in straight lines from the centre of the cylinder to eight equally spaced goals around the circumference will also show significant directional-firing specificity. This expectation is based on the notion that place-cell activity reflects kinematic properties of the rat's environment (Muller and Kubie 1987).

Variations in place-cell firing caused by changing the cue configuration

One way to explore the properties and significance of place cells is to see how their activity is affected by well-defined changes in the environment. For this purpose, it is critical to isolate the recording apparatus by putting it in a controlled cue environment (O'Keefe and Conway 1978). It is easy to limit visual stimuli by surrounding the apparatus with curtains (O'Keefe and Conway 1978; Muller *et al.* 1987), but more complete isolation would be valuable. Once the controlled environment is created, it is possible to introduce a set of experimenter-selected stimuli that can be tested for their ability to affect place cells.

The simplest manipulation is to co-rotate the experimenter-selected stimuli. If firing fields rotate equally, it can be concluded that the stimuli are salient for the place cells and that the importance of the rotated stimuli outweighs the contributions of stationary stimuli. O'Keefe and Conway (1978) found that rotations of a set of four complex stimuli cause equal rotations of firing fields on a four-arm radial maze (O'Keefe and Conway

1978). Field rotations were also caused by rotations of the white cue card attached to the cylinder wall (Muller and Kubie 1987).

Once the salience of a set of stimuli is established by rotation experiments, the importance of members of the set can be determined by deleting sub-sets. O'Keefe and Conway (1978) found that removing any one or two of the four stimuli did not affect location-specific firing. It follows that each place cell is partially controlled by all four stimuli; individual cells are not selectively responsive to particular sub-sets of the available stimuli. In addition, because the stimuli were adequate for different sense modalities, O'Keefe and Conway concluded that location-specific firing can be supported by visual, auditory, tactile, and olfactory information.

In the O'Keefe and Conway experiment, removing all four of experimenter-selected stimuli caused location-specific firing to break down; individual cells ceased to discharge or discharged in a spatially homogeneous fashion. In contrast, deleting the single white card in the cylinder left positional firing mainly intact (Muller and Kubie 1987); the shape, size, peak firing rate and radial position of fields were unchanged, although the crispness of the fields was somewhat reduced. For many cells, the angular position of the field was also unchanged, but for others the field rotated by an unpredictable amount in the absence of the card. Newer work on the four-arm maze by O'Keefe and Speakman (1987) confirms that all intentional polarizing stimuli can be removed without affecting firing fields. In our view, the results of cue-deletion experiments provide strong evidence against the sensory model. The sensory model supposes that the firing rate decreases in all directions from a maximum because the driving of the cell by the local stimulus configuration weakens away from the field centre. Since removing cues of known salience does not alter the shape, size, position, or intensity of firing fields, it seems incorrect to treat place cells as high-order, multi-sensory units.

An interesting modification of the sensory model assumes that place-cell discharge reflects the processing of sensory information by a neural network that can do 'pattern completion' (see, for example, Grossberg 1980; Kohonen 1984). Such a network classifies input patterns (total stimulus configurations or local views) into output patterns (firing fields). The ability to do pattern completion means that a partial input pattern (reduced cue set) causes the corresponding output pattern to be reproduced at lower resolution, precisely the effect seen for place cells after cue removal (Muller and Kubie 1987).

Sharp *et al.* (1988, 1990) tested the pattern completion idea by adding instead of removing stimuli. Specifically, a second white card was attached to the cylinder wall, 180° away from the first to make the cylinder visually symmetrical. The simplest form of pattern completion predicts that place cells should have symmetrical firing patterns under these circumstances.

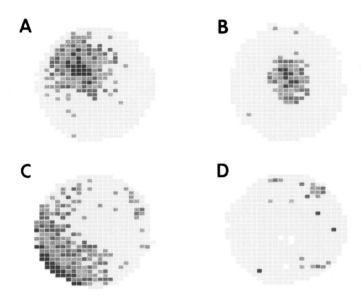

Plate 1. Four examples of the firing patterns of hippocampal complex-spike cells in 16-min recording sessions. Cells A and B displayed round fields, and the field of cell C is crescent shaped. Cell D showed no firing field in the cylinder. Median firing rates are as follows (from lowest to highest, yellow, orange, red, green, blue, purple in AP/s): cell A—0.0, 0.9, 3.0, 6.7, 11.0, 16.5; Cell B—0.0, 1.0, 2.2, 5.6, 11.6, 17.6; cell C—0.0, 0.4, 1.4, 3.3, 6.3, 15.3; cell D—0.0, 0.1, 0.3, 0.4, 0.7, 1.3.

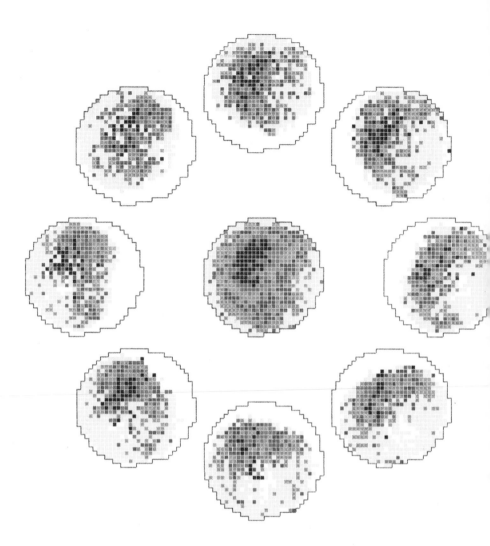

Plate 2. Head-direction independent (centre) and direction-specific firing rate maps for a hippocampal place cell whose firing field is away from the cylinder wall. Note that the spatial firing pattern in each direction-specific map is a reasonable reproduction of the direction-independent pattern, indicating that there is little or no firing rate modulation by head direction. Median firing rates for centre map: 0.0, 0.4, 1.2, 2.8, 5.6, 10.6 AP/s. Median rates for direction-specific maps: 0.0, 1.1, 3.5, 6.7, 11.5, 21.0 AP/s.

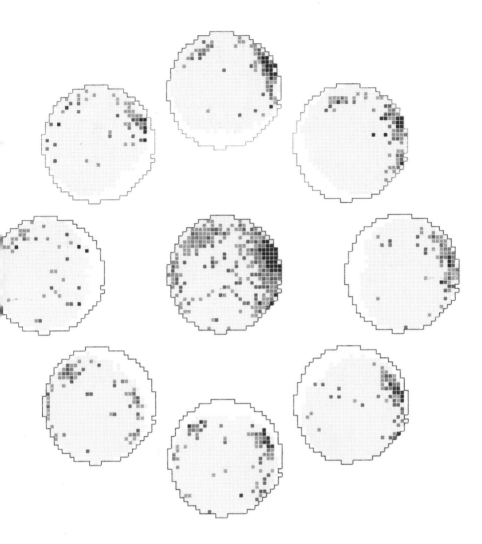

Plate 3. Head-direction independent (centre) and direction-specific firing rate maps for a hippocampal place cell whose firing field is next to the cylinder wall. Note that the spatial firing pattern in each direction-specific map is a reasonable reproduction of the direction-independent pattern except for head directions at which the unsampled (white) region encroaches on the field. The apparent directional selectivity arises because of this interaction. Median firing rates for centre map: 0.0, 0.1, 0.2, 0.4, 0.7, 2.9 AP/s. Median rates for direction-specific maps: 0.0, 0.3, 0.8, 1.4, 2.4, 4.8 AP/s.

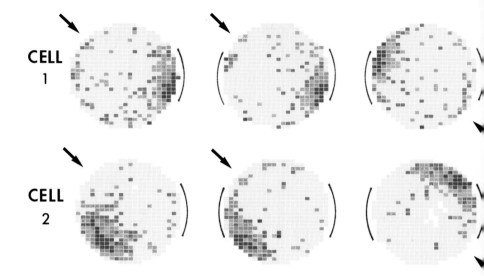

Plate 4. Two examples of the effects of adding a second cue-card to the recording chamber. The arrows indicate the angle of entry of the rat for each session. In both cells, the addition of a second card had no effect on the firing pattern (left and middle), but when the angle of entry was rotated 180°, the field also rotated (right). Median firing rates: cell 1—left, 0.0, 0.4, 0.8, 1.5, 3.2, 12.0; middle, 0.0, 0.4, 0.8, 2.2, 6.1; right, 0.0, 0.4, 0.9, 2.2, 6.9: cell 2—left, 0.0, 0.9, 2.6, 6.9, 12.0, 21.0; middle, 0.0, 0.4, 2.5, 5.7, 9.7, 15.0; right, 0.0, 0.9, 2.7, 7.1, 12.0, 15.3 AP/s.

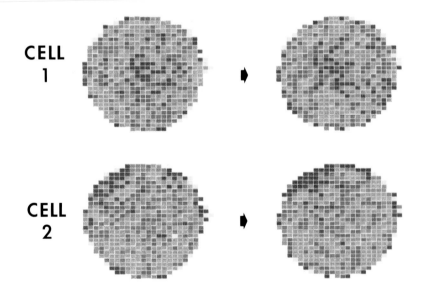

Plate 5. Two simultaneously recorded hippocampal theta cells recorded in consecutive 16-min recording sessions (replications). Note that the firing patterns of the two cell, while quite reproducible, differ markedly from each other. Median firing rates: cell 1—left, 0.0, 16.7, 20.6, 23.4, 26.1, 31.3; right, 0.0, 16.1, 19.6, 22.1, 24.4, 30.0; cell 2—left, 0.0, 8.1, 11.7, 13.8, 16.5, 21.5; right, 0.0, 9.5, 13.0 15.7, 19.2, 27.0 AP/s.

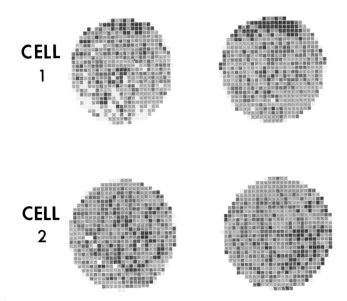

Plate 6. Two medial entorhinal cells (MEC), each recorded for 16 min (left) and 48 min (right). The improvement in the spatial selectivity of the firing patterns with sampling times indicates that the entorhinal firing patterns are stationary. Median firing rates: cell 1—left, 0.0, 2.3, 4.9, 7.7, 10.6, 16.0; right, 0.0, 2.2, 4.6, 7.1, 9.7, 13.6; cell 2—left, 0.0, 11.8, 16.5, 20.2, 23.4, 30.0; right, 0.0, 13.7, 18.1, 20.8, 23.3, 26.6 AP/s.

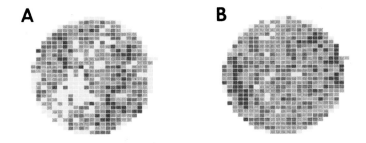

Plate 7. Spatial firing patterns of unidentified cells in the dentate gyrus. Median firing rates: cell A—0.0, 1.0, 2.6, 4.3, 6.3, 10.8; cell B—0.0, 3.0, 7.3, 11.7, 18.9, 29.1 AP/s.

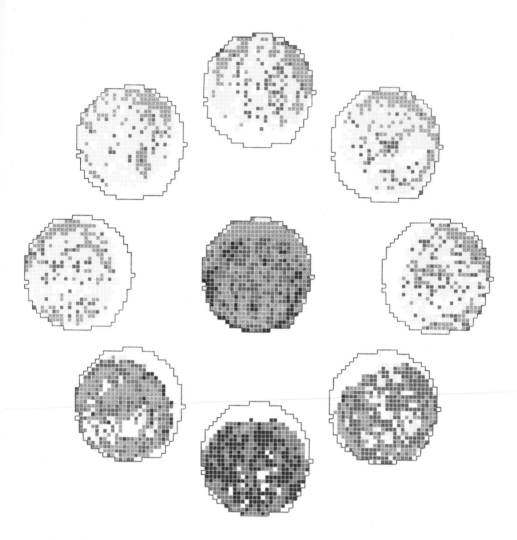

Plate 8. Head-direction independent (centre) and direction-specific firing rate maps for a post-subicular head-direction cell. The directional selectivity is easily seen in the surrounding maps, where intense firing is mainly confined to the 45° bin centred on 270°. The apparent location specficity seen in the centre map is due to the fact that the rat's head cannot point in the preferred direction when the rat is near the top of the cylinder. Median firing rates for centre map: 0.0, 7.1, 24.6, 38.5, 55.2, 81.5—median rates for direction-specific maps: 0.0, 2.7, 15.0, 51.4, 105.0, 144.0 AP/s.

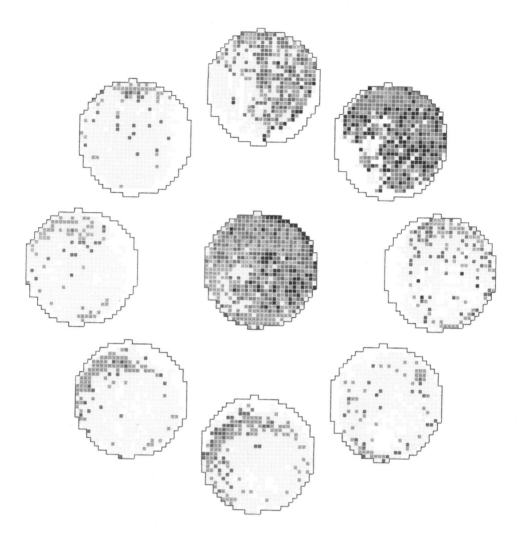

Plate 9. Head-direction independent (centre) and direction-specific firing rate maps for a subicular head-direction cell. The directional selectivity is seen in the surrounding maps, where intense firing is mainly confined to the 45° bin centred on 45°. The apparent location specficity in the centre map is due to the fact that the rat's head cannot point in the preferred direction when the rat at the cylinder wall near 225°. Median firing rates for centre map: 0.0, 0.6, 1.5, 2.4, 3.5, 6.5—median rates for direction-specific maps: 0.0, 0.9, 3.5, 10.9, 18.8, 27.7 AP/s.

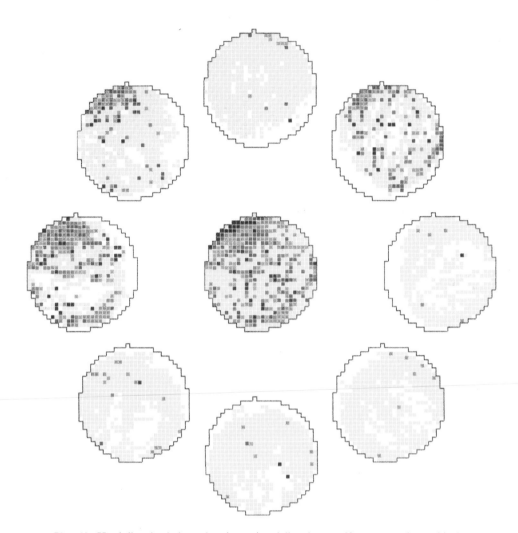

Plate 10. Head-direction independent (centre) and direction-specific rate maps for a subicular cell whose firing is modulated by both position and head direction. The firing field is near 11 o'clock. While the rat's head is within the field, intense firing occurs when the head direction is in the 45° bin centred on 180° (9 o'clock). Weaker firing is also seen when the head direction is in the 45° bin centred on 45°. Median firing rates for centre map: 0.0, 0.3, 0.7, 1.2, 2.2, 3.8—median rates for direction-specific maps: 0.0, 1.2, 3.1, 5.1, 8.8, 18.8 AP/s.

This prediction is incorrect; the spatial firing patterns of most cells were unaffected by adding the second card as shown in Plate 4. The maps in the first column illustrate one-card fields. The maps in the second column show that the two-card field of both cells is the same as the one-card field.

In principle, the asymmetrical firing patterns could depend on unintentional differences between the two cards. To test this possibility, the rat's entry position into the cylinder was rotated by 180°. As shown in the third column, field positions also rotated 180°. Thus, the cards were equivalent to each other with regard to place-cell discharge, whether or not they could be distinguished by the rats. Additional experiments showed that the cards were salient when both were present. A minority of place cells (3 out of 18) had symmetrical field pairs in the presence of the two cards, but long-term recording from these cells showed that even their positional firing patterns did not conform to expectations from the simple pattern-completion hypothesis (Sharp *et al.* 1990). For example, one cell developed a second field diametrically opposite the first after several two-card exposures and then retained both fields when only one card was present.

It is important to note that a more sophisticated version of the pattern-completion scheme is able to account for most of the two-card results. In this modified version, the rat's entry position is treated as cue that is combined with fixed sensory cues during pattern completion (Sharp 1989). The visual environment can be rendered unambiguous if the rat can remember its starting location over the 16 min of a typical session. The ability to use starting location as a 'trace' cue to allow for firing in only one or two equivalent locations could come about in several ways. For example, the rat could use path integration to distinguish two halves of the cylinder (Sharp 1989; McNaughton 1989). Alternatively, an association could be made between entry position and an uncontrolled stimulus asymmetry at the start of the session (O'Keefe 1983) or the rat could mark the environment. Regardless of the mechanism, several independent demonstrations of the control of place-cell firing by earlier events (O'Keefe and Speakman 1987; Quirk *et al.* 1990) suggest it is reasonable to allow trace cues in the pattern completion scheme. It therefore becomes a critical issue whether the invariant shape of the spatial firing pattern can be accommodated by pattern completion.

How does the place-cell population represent the environment?

In fixed surroundings, a fraction of complex-spike cells are known to be place cells because they have firing fields. In the same conditions, however, other cells with well-isolated waveforms are nearly silent. Silent cells are classified as place cells when they have a field in at least one other environment (Kubie and Ranck 1984; Muller and Kubie 1987). A study by Thompson and Best (1989) indicates that only about 15 per cent of complex-spike cells that are spontaneously active during light barbiturate anaesthesia or slow-wave sleep have fields in a particular environment. It therefore seems that spatial information processing in a given apparatus is done by a relatively small fraction of the complex-spike cell population; the small fraction will be referred to as the 'active sub-set'. The active sub-set is characteristic for a fixed environment; the same cells are active each time the rat is returned to the same surroundings.

If a cell is recorded in two 'sufficiently different' environments, for example the cylinder and a rectangle of similar size and visual appearance, it may have fields in both, only one, or neither environment (Muller and Kubie 1987). In addition, if the cell has a field in both apparatuses, the positions and other characteristics of the fields are apparently unrelated (O'Keefe and Conway 1978; Kubie and Ranck 1984; Muller and Kubie 1987; Thompson and Best 1989). Major changes occur in spatial firing pattern even though the apparatuses are simple topological variants of each other.

At the population level, it can be said that spatial information processing is done by two different active sub-sets. The two sub-sets overlap because some cells have fields in both apparatuses. Nevertheless, because the fields in the cylinder and rectangle are unrelated, it appears that the overlap of the active sub-sets is a combinatorial feature of the network that results from random assignment of place cells into the active sub-sets. In our view, it is proper to think of the active sub-sets as independent or as orthogonal to each other; each is characteristic for one of the environments.

In one sense, the structural basis of the map is the entire hippocampus and all of its neurons. Nevertheless, to the extent that it proves correct to divide place cells into active and silent sub-sets in fixed surroundings, it is useful to equate the map with the currently active sub-set because no processing is done by silent cells. In this case, the cylinder and rectangle each has its own map, and one may be considered a 'remapping' of the other onto the place-cell population.

For the cylinder and rectangle, it is useful to say that the remapping is 'complete' because the active sub-sets are independent. In contrast, cue rotations may be said to produce a 'null' remapping because the active sub-sets are the same under standard and rotated conditions. More precisely, cue rotations affect the angular position of all firing fields to the same extent and leave all other properties unchanged. The standard and rotated maps are therefore identical if the card is taken as the angular reference, and one may be viewed as a null remapping of the other. Bostock *et al.* (1988) have found that substitution of a black card for the white card in the cylinder is associated with a complete remapping in some rats and a null remapping in others.

Between null and complete remappings we have found several examples of 'partial remappings' (Muller and Kubie 1987). For instance, when individual cells are recorded in the cylinder and in a version that is scaled up by a factor of two in height and diameter, it is found that about half the active place cells in one cylinder become silent or develop new fields in the other. In contrast, the fields of the other half of the cells scale in a manner that mimics the scaling of the cylinders; if size is ignored, the fields of these cells are unchanged by the scaling manipulation (see Figures 6 and 7 in Muller and Kubie 1987). The partial remapping suggests that the population reflects both the similarity in shape and visual appearance of the two cylinders and also their difference in size; it is unclear if this information can be used by the rat. Different partial remappings are seen when all visual cues are deleted by turning off the lights (Quirk *et al.* 1990). If the lights are turned off when the rat is already in the recording chamber, the remapping is minor; the fields of most cells persist from light to dark conditions. In contrast, if the rat is put into the recording chamber in the dark, the remapping is about 75 per cent complete. Interestingly, if the room lights are turned on after the rat is introduced to the chamber in the dark, the fields of many cells do not revert to their initial light configurations, but instead persist in the form seen during initial darkness. Partial remappings are also seen when an opaque barrier is placed onto the otherwise open floor of the cylinder (Muller and Kubie 1987). The firing of cells with fields distant from the cylinder is unchanged. The firing of most cells with fields near the barrier is strongly suppressed, although an example was seen in which a small field expanded around the barrier. It therefore appears that the remapping is local without a loss of information in the region of the barrier. A transparent barrier is as effective as the opaque barrier in suppressing firing. In contrast, the lead base used to anchor the barriers has little effect.

In our view, the nature of the changes in the place-cell population associated with remappings argue strongly against the sensory hypothesis. The positional firing patterns of individual cells do not stretch to mimic the topologically different but visually similar cylinder and rectangle, as might be expected if each cell is triggered only by the local stimulus configuration or local view. As shown below, topological stretching is seen for cells in the MEC, an area that contributes a major portion of the neo-cortical input to the hippocampus). Similarly, alterations in firing caused by barriers seem to be organized in terms of a region and not in terms of changes in stimulus configuration caused by the barriers. In summary, remappings appear to take the structure of the environment into account. Positional firing patterns change in cohesive ways and not independently for individual place cells.

Hippocampal theta cells

Hippocampal theta cells recorded from freely moving rats are inhibitory inter-neurons (Fox and Ranck 1975). They are crucial for regulating the overall excitability of the hippocampal network, as has been elegantly demonstrated experimentally and with computational models by Miles, Traub, Wong, and their colleagues (see, for example, Traub *et al.* 1989). In addition, as noted above, the time-averaged firing of theta cells is tightly coupled to the state of the hippocampal EEG and to the locomotor state of the rat. These effects are mediated by inputs from the medial septum, which is considered to be the pacemaker for the theta rhythm (Petsche *et al.* 1962; Stewart and Fox 1989). This drive is clear in freely moving rats where theta-cell firing increases during walking and slows during quiet immobility.

Theta cells also receive excitatory input from pyramidal cells. As theta cells inhibit pyramidal cells, the pyramidal cells are subject to both feedforward inhibition (from the septum) and feedback inhibition. In addition, if the convergence of pyramidal cells onto theta cells is not too great, it is possible that the location-specific firing of the pyramidal cells will drive location-specific firing of theta cells. (If the convergence is very high, spatial firing variations would be averaged out unless each theta cell preferentially receives input from place cells with overlapping fields.)

Weak spatial variations of theta-cells discharge on an eight-arm maze were reported by McNaughton *et al.* (1983). A recent paper from McNaughton's laboratory described only locomotor firing correlates for theta cells (Mizumori *et al.* 1989), in agreement with Christian and Deadwyler (1989). In contrast, Kubie *et al.* (1990b) found that the spatial and locomotor modulations of theta cell discharge rate were both around 2:1. Plate 5 shows firing rate maps from a pair of simultaneously recorded theta cells. Several features of the maps are worth noting. First, the zero-rate regions characteristic of place cells are absent; theta cells are active over the entire surface of the apparatus. Second, rate variations are rather large in scale; regions of rapid firing are about the same size as place-cell firing fields. Third, the spatial firing pattern of each cell is reproducible. Finally, the two spatial firing patterns are distinguishable from each. If the locomotor correlate were pre-potent, the spatial firing patterns would be expected to look the same as there is only one locomotor sequence during a simultaneous recording.

Kubie *et al.* (1990b) stated that there are about three high firing-rate regions for the typical theta cell. If each such region is assumed to reflect excitatory drive from a single place cell, the effective convergence is also about three. This is considerably lower than estimates of about 15 to 20 from analyses of EPSP amplitude (Miles and Wong 1984; Lecaille *et al.* 1987). The two estimates can be brought closely into line, however, by taking silent place cells into account. If the active sub-set is about 15 per cent of the pyramidal cell population, the corrected convergence from the spatial analysis is also on the order of 20.

Clearly, theta cells must be considered in any full treatment of information processing by the hippocampus; at the least, they must be functionally connected to pyramidal cells to prevent runaway activity in the hippocampus (Traub *et al.* 1989). The fact that theta cells show significant spatial-firing variations hints at a more interesting role. Along these lines, Thompson and Best (1989) raise the fascinating notion that the integrity of the active place-cell sub-set is maintained by the pattern of inhibition across place cells produced by theta-cell discharge.

In transition to considering the spatial firing properties of cells in other parts of the hippocampal formation, we note that neurons that share characteristics of the theta cells of CA1 and CA3/4 have been described in the dentate gyrus (Rose 1986), the post-subiculum (Taube *et al.* 1990a), and medial entorhinal cortex (Quirk 1990), as well in the medial septum, which is the theta-rhythm pacemaker. The fact that cells with theta-modulated firing occur in many parts of the hippocampal formation indicates that these cortical regions are functionally related, and provides additional motivation for analysing the spatial firing properties of their neurons.

Spatial firing properties of neurons in other regions of the hippocampal formation

The major connections of several parts of the hippocampal formation are summarized in Fig. 17.1. Most of the indicated connections are taken from the excellent review paper by Amaral and Witter (1989). The exception is the pathway that runs from the post-subiculum to the subiculum. The boundaries of the post-subiculum are not currently well defined (see Taube *et al.* 1990a), and the pathway is inferred from the functional properties of cells in the post-subiculum and subiculum rather than from anatomical findings.

Superimposed on the connectivity diagram of Fig. 17.1 are brief descriptions of the spatial firing characteristics of neurons in the cortical areas. Broadly speaking, all the cell types found during pellet chasing in the cylinder fall into three classes. Neurons that show location-specific firing are seen in the hippocampus, dentate gyrus, medial entorhinal cortex, and the subiculum. Neurons that show head direction-specific firing are found

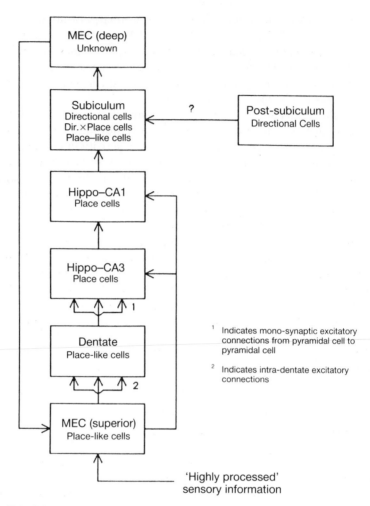

Fig. 17.1. Schematic diagram of connections among portions of the hippocampal (hippo) formation, including brief descriptions of neuronal spatial-firing correlates—MEC, medial entorhinal cortex.

in the post-subiculum and subiculum. Finally, cells whose firing is correlated with both head position and direction are found in the subiculum. It is worth remembering that this classification must be modified to include hippocampal place cells whose location-specific firing on an eight-arm maze is modulated by head direction. The remainder of the results section summarizes the spatial firing properties of neurons in the relevant areas; separate papers are cited for more complete descriptions.

Medial entorhinal cortex

The MEC is the major source of cortical input to the dentate gyrus and hippocampus (Swanson and Cowan 1977; Kohler 1986); fibres to the hippocampus arise from layers II and III (Steward and Scoville 1976). The MEC is in turn the target of 'highly processed' sensory information from polymodal sensory cortical regions (Jones and Powell 1970; Deacon *et al.* 1983). Thus, there are anatomical reasons to believe that the ability of place cells to show location-specific firing depends on the integrity of connections from MEC. This presumption is supported by the finding that lesions of entorhinal cortex also impair performance in complex spatial tasks (e.g. Schenck and Morris 1985) and by interesting changes in place-cell firing after similar lesions (Miller and Best 1980).

Recordings from neurons in superficial layers of the MEC reveal that many of the cells show location-specific firing that is reminiscent of, but noisier than that of place cells (Quirk 1990). Firing-rate maps for two MEC cells are shown in the left column of Plate 6 after 16 min and in the right column after 48 min of recording. The notion that the spatial firing variations seen with the briefer recording time represent true location-specific firing is supported by the increased clarity of the firing-rate contours seen after additional recording time; the location-specific firing is noisy but stationary.

The idea that the firing of cells in the MEC is directly associated with place cells is reinforced by the effects of cue rotation and removal experiments, whose outcomes parallel those for place cells. In particular, card rotations cause equal rotations of the positional firing patterns of MEC cells and card removals do not greatly disrupt the patterns. In contrast, recordings of individual MEC cells in the cylinder and a square chamber of similar size and visual appearance reveal major differences from place cells. First, no MEC cell became silent in either apparatus, although this commonly happened for place cells. Second, the positional firing patterns of MEC cells in the cylinder and square often appeared to be related. More precisely, the patterns in the two apparatuses seemed to be topological transforms of each other, such that the position of the region of rapid firing bore the same relationship to the white card in each apparatus. In other words, changes in the location-specific firing of MEC cells but not place cells commonly mimic the shape change of the apparatus (see Quirk *et al.* 1989, 1990).

Given that cells in superficial layers of the MEC supply direct and relayed information to place cells, the observation that their spatial firing patterns undergo a topological transformation makes it tempting to conclude that MEC cells are more 'sensory-like'. Additional anatomical considerations make it clear, however, that the superficial-layer neurons receive information that has been processed by the hippocampus (Amaral and Witter 1989). Until the functional significance of the cyclic pathways in the hippocampal formations is better understood, conclusions about the main direction of spatial information flow must be considered tentative. Nevertheless, it is hard to understand how the spatial firing patterns of superficial MEC cells could undergo a topological transformation after the same manipulation that causes a complete remapping in the hippocampus if the MEC cells are driven by the hippocampus.

Dentate gyrus

It is commonly agreed that the discharge of cells in the dentate gyrus is modulated by the state of the hippocampal EEG and is correspondingly correlated to locomotor activity (Rose 1983; Mizumori *et al.* 1989). According to Mizumori *et al.*, stratum granulosum inter-neurons generally show this sort of correlation, whereas identified granule cells are generally silent. We have not made systematic recordings from cells of the dentate gyrus, but have obtained several examples of the spatial firing patterns of unclassified cells in the upper blade of the dentate while moving the electrode array from CA1 to CA3/4. Two examples of firing-rate maps are shown in Plate 7, where it is seen that the cells were active over the entire surface of the apparatus. The firing-rate contours of dentate gyrus cells were smoother than those of hippocampal theta cells or MEC cells. Clearly, the dentate gyrus is an important target for a full study.

Head-direction cells in the post-subiculum

During preliminary explorations of the spatial firing of cells in retro-hippocampal areas, Ranck (1984) described head direction (or directional) cells in the post-subiculum. The properties of these cells were quantitatively characterized by Taube *et al.* (1990a,b). Directional cells fire only when the rat's head points in an approximately 90° range of angles in the horizontal plane. Their firing increases linearly from a near-zero baseline to a maximum at the 'preferred direction' as the head rotates either clockwise or counter-clockwise towards the preferred direction (Fig. 17.2A). Firing depends on the angle that the midline of the rat's head makes with a reference direction in the environment, and is independent of neck position. Preferred directions for individual cells occur with equal frequency in each of the four quadrants, so that no there is no overall preferred direction in the laboratory frame for the population. Directional firing is remarkably independent of behaviour; it persists even if the rat is carried by and around the apparatus.

The basic properties of a post-subicular directional cells are visible in the

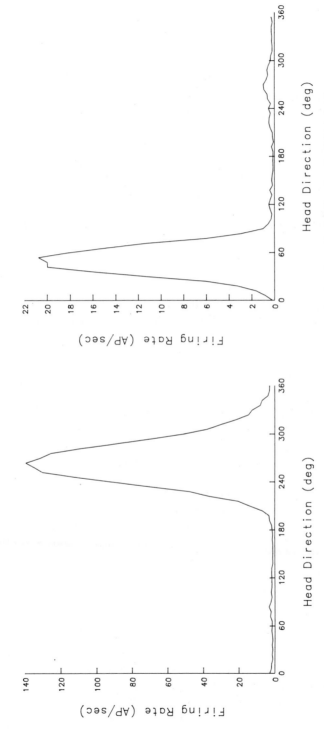

Fig. 17.2. Firing rate as a function of head direction for a post-subicular directional cell (left) and a subicular directional cell (right). The two rate-direction functions are quite similar: for both, rate increases linearly as the head turns to the preferred direction either clockwise or counter-clockwise.

rate maps of Plate 8. The strong correlation between head direction and firing rate is evident from the direction-specific maps, where firing is almost entirely confined to the three, 45° angular bins centred on 225, 270, and 315°. The direction-independent map gives the impression that firing rate also depends on position, but in fact the positional-rate gradients arise from the interaction between nearly ideal, azimuth-specific firing and the unsampled region at each head direction. In particular, the low rate associated with the region at the tail of the diametric vector that points in the preferred direction comes about because the head cannot point in the preferred direction in that region. The homogeneous appearance of the direction-specific map centred on 270° (near the preferred direction) indicates that the preferred direction is constant over the surface of the apparatus or, in other words, that preferred-direction is constant over the surface of the apparatus or, in other words, that preferred-direction vectors are parallel. It can be concluded that head-direction cells are not triggered when the head points to some critical feature local to the cylinder; if the cell is tuned to a critical stimulus source, the source must lie far outside the cylinder. In short, directional-cell firing is not correlated with local view.

Head-direction cells were tested with several of the manipulations previously used for place cells (Taube *et al.* 1990b). It was found that rotations of the white cue card reliably caused nearly equal rotations of preferred direction, even if the card rotation was done with the rat still in the cylinder. The strong control exerted by the card eliminates the possibility that directional cells fire when the head points to a distant stimulus source, and shows that directional cells are no better described in simple sensory terms than are place cells. The same observation also indicates that preferred direction co-rotates along with the angular position of place-cell firing fields and the angular position of MEC-cell firing patterns after card rotations. The common effects of cue rotations suggest that the three regions act together in a system with a single angular reference. Also in parallel with the results obtained from the hippocampus and MEC, card removal leaves directional firing intact except for a possible rotation of preferred direction. When pairs of directional cells are simultaneously recorded, card removal may cause the preferred direction of both cells to rotate, but the amount of rotation is equal, indicating that all cells use a common angular reference even when the most obvious choice is no longer present.

Individual directional cells were also recorded in the cylinder, rectangle, and square. Such changes in shape never caused directional cells to become silent or to undergo major changes in peak firing rate at the preferred direction. As was true for card removal, shape change was associated only with rotation of preferred direction. In addition, the extent of preferred-direction shift was the same for both members of simultaneously recorded cell pairs.

Overall, the effects of shape changes imply that there is no analogue of the complete remapping seen for the place-cell population. More formally, the active sub-set of head-direction cells is constant and identical to the entire directional-cell population. It seems that the mapping of preferred directions on to the azimuth is fixed, so that the angular distance between the preferred directions of arbitrary cell pairs is the same in all environments. In this sense, the contribution of the post-subiculum to the navigational system is simpler than the contribution of the hippocampus. Preliminary work (Taube *et al.* 1989) indicates that performance on the three-arm maze is disrupted by post-subicular lesions, suggesting that directional cells play a direct role in navigation. Further work along these lines will be most profitable if behavioural means are found to differentiate the effects of post-subicular and hippocampal lesions.

Spatial firing properties of cells in the subiculum

The subiculum is the main target of axons from CA1 pyramidal/place cells. In addition, it is a source of input to a remarkably diverse set of structures including the MEC, lateral septum, pre-subiculum, para-subiculum, retrosplenial cortex and nucleus accumbens. As expected from the extensive subicular connections, lesions of the subiculum damage performance in complex navigational tasks. Of great significance is the finding by Morris *et al.* (1989) that subicular lesions are associated with qualitatively different deviations of trajectory away from geodesics (optimally efficient paths) as compared to hippocampal lesions.

We have now completed a quantitative study of the spatial firing correlates of subicular cells. In our current understanding, subicular cells can be divided into three classes during pellet chasing in the cylinder. Some subicular neurons are directional cells with properties similar to those in the post-subiculum, as shown in Fig. 17.2B and Plate 9. The preferred direction of subicular directional cells is controlled by the angular position of the white card, and card removal does not disrupt directional firing. Subicular directional cells do not seem to cease firing after the shape of the apparatus is changed, although their preferred directions may rotate.

The second class of subicular cells signal both head position and head direction. More precisely, direction-independent firing-rate show firing fields reminiscent of those for place cells, but direction-specific maps show that the firing rate is modulated to varying extents by head direction. An example of the spatial firing properties of a subicular place-by-direction cells is shown in Plate 10. Note that firing is rapid in a restricted, crescent-like region near 11 o'clock in the direction-independent map, but that the rate varies strongly with head direction, being maximal in the 45° bin centred on 270°. Interestingly, the firing rate is also elevated at a second head direction (45°), with a clear minimum between the two preferred directions; we never saw an example of a post-subicular directional cell with two preferred directions. In parallel with other cell classes, the angular position of the firing field and the preferred direction of firing rotate equally with rotations of the white card. Finally, we have also seen examples of non-directional, location-specific firing that is somewhat noisier than that of place cells but smoother than that of MEC cells.

The distribution of positional and directional, firing correlates among cell types in parts of the hippocampal formation can be interpreted in terms of connections among the regions. In our opinion, the simplest interpretation is that there is functional convergence in the subiculum of positional influences from CA1 of the hippocampus and directional influences from the post-subiculum. If this view is accepted, it is easy to explain the variations in directional firing range of subicular head-direction cells in terms of surround inhibition or summation of signals from post-subicular head-direction cells as well as the existence of place-by-direction or pure place cells.

An interesting aspect of the proposed, subicular, convergence scheme concerns the difficulties it presents for falsification by anatomical methods, since the difficulties arise from the strength of the signal transmitted by each post-subicular directional cell. The strong signal implies that it would not take input from many post-subicular cells to explain the directional firing properties of subicular cells; only a hundred or so axons would suffice if their divergence in the subiculum were great enough. It would therefore be necessary to show that the number of fibres from the post-subiculum to the subiculum is extremely small or zero; the proposed convergence scheme cannot be falsified by finding that the post-subiculum to subiculum projection is weak relative to other projections.

Discussion

As noted in the introduction, lesion experiments suggest that the rat hippocampus is not exclusively involved in navigation (Tonkiss *et al.* 1988). In addition, under some circumstances, knowing what the rat is doing may better predict neuronal firing rates than knowing the rat's spatial relationship to the environment (Ranck 1973; Wiener *et al.* 1989). It is therefore important to entertain first the hypothesis that behavioural firing correlations are always primary, and that spatial correlates arise only because rats tend to do certain things in certain places or when they face in certain directions.

In addressing this issue, we consider only the pellet-chasing task, even though place cells have most often been observed during performance of complex spatial tasks in which the hippocampal formation plays a role in guiding locomotion (see, for example, O'Keefe and Speakman 1987). It is our claim that direct observation and objective measurements leave little room for the hypothesis that the spatial-firing correlates of cells in the hippocampal formation are secondary to the location- or direction-specific emission of behaviours that are themselves correlated with firing.

The main basis for our contention is that the rat's behaviour during pellet chasing is almost completely limited to locomotion; other activities simply do not occur often enough to account for more than a small fraction of the total number of action potentials generated during a session. If firing is nevertheless correlated with behavioural state, the correlations must therefore be with details of locomotion such as gait, trajectory, or running speed.

In our experience, none of these explanations bears up under close scrutiny. For example, place cells usually discharge whenever the rat's head enters the firing field, independent of the path through the relevant region. In-field firing occurs just as well when the rat moves around or is stationary, regardless of whether the head is scanning or is still (Kubie *et al.* 1985). Furthermore, many place cells (Muller *et al.* 1987) and all head-direction cells (Taube *et al.* 1990a) show their characteristic discharge pattern when the rat is carried by hand around the cylinder. The lack of directional firing specificity for place cells is also out of line with the notion that the details of the locomotor state are critical firing correlates. Finally, we have found that the local smoothness of the spatial firing patterns of MEC cells (Quirk 1990) and hippocampal theta cells (Kubie *et al.* 1990b) increases when only samples obtained during rapid locomotion are used, with no parallel decreases in spatial firing-rate variations; walking speed is thus unlikely to be the major activity correlate of MEC or theta cells. We conclude that neurons of the hippocampal formation discharge in association with spatial variables under some circumstances, and that at least hippocampal complex-spike cells discharge in association with behavioural variables under other circumstances. In our view, the context sensitivity of the predominant firing correlate for complex-spike cells suggests that spatial and behavioural correlates are special cases of a more general information-handling process (see Eichenbaum and Cohen 1988). In any event, the additional, context sensitivity implies an extraordinary flexibility for the role of the hippocampus.

The related notion that the hippocampus is essential for sophisticated navigation is challenged by work which shows that impaired performance in the Morris swimming task varies with the interval between training and the time at which hippocampal lesions are made (Sutherland *et al.* 1987). If lesions are made 12 weeks after training to the hidden platform, their effects are much less than at shorter intervals, although performance is not quite as good as with normals; intervals longer than 12 weeks produce no further sparing. This result is reminiscent of the gradient of retrograde amnesia seen in humans (Scoville and Milner 1957; Squire 1982) and other primates (Mishkin 1982) after hippocampal lesions, although the time-scale is considerably shorter. It is useful to add that anterograde amnesia, a second component of the human hippocampal syndrome, can also be demonstrated in rats. Kubie *et al.* (1989, 1990a) found that performance is spared with long, training–lesion intervals in a dry, appetitive version of the swimming task. In addition, they showed that the same rats were incapable of learning to go to a new hidden location in the same apparatus. The conclusion that the hippocampus is not essential for performance in well-established spatial problems has been shown in two other ways by McNaughton *et al.* (1986) and by Butcher *et al.* (1989).

If the navigational computations performed by the hippocampal forma-tion are a special case of a more general function, and locale solutions can be generated in the absence of the hippocampus, it may be asked if it is appropriate to continue to focus on spatial firing correlates. In our opinion, a spatial analysis will be fruitful for three main reasons. First, the flexibility of processing by the hippocampus proper is apparently not shared by the post-subiculum; head-direction cells are apparently dedicated to the single function of signalling orientation under all circumstances. Thus, at least one part of the hippocampal formation appears to be mainly concerned with spatial information processing. Second, the place-cell signal is ex-tremely strong and stable in fixed conditions; it provides an excellent baseline for additional work that may shed light on the significance of long-term potentiation and issues related to learning and memory. Finally, even if the location-specific firing is just one mode of complex-cell activity, we believe it provides the best opportunity for a particular solution about information processing by the hippocampus. The study of spatial informa-tion processing is preferred because the geometry and sensory features of the accessible space can be manipulated in precise ways. We have found that the effects of such manipulations are relatively easy to characterize for place cells and other spatial cell types; in many cases, the nature of the manipulation is directly mimicked by the changes in positional and direc-tional, firing patterns. The ease of categorization of effect in turn makes it easy to compare the effects of specific manipulations for different cell classes.

At the present time, the best example of the power of this method is the differential effect that changing the shape of the apparatus has on the positional firing patterns of place cells and cells in the superficial layers of the MEC. The fact that the firing patterns of MEC cells undergoes a topological transformation that mimics the shape change whereas the patterns of place cells changes much more drastically is evidence that the main flow of information is from MEC to Ammon's horn. The same conclusion has been drawn from anatomical work (Steward and Scoville 1976), but the functional evidence helps eliminate the return pathways from the hippocampus to superficial layers of MEC as the carriers of the most detailed information. More importantly, it is now possible to formulate hypotheses to explain the transformation that occurs between entorhinal cortex and the hippocampus.

Spatial functions of the hippocampal formation

A major finding of the work summarized here is the occurrence of cells with spatial firing correlates in all the parts of the hippocampal formation we have so far studied. At the present time, our understanding of how the portions of the hippocampal formation co-operate to generate a spatial representation is very limited. Moreover, little can be said about how the connectivity of the hippocampal formation explains observed transformations of spatial firing patterns. Nevertheless, the fact that all of the known cell classes are affected in the same way by card rotations and (except for theta cells, which were not tested) by card removals strongly implies that the hippocampal formation acts as a coherent spatial system.

At the present time, two models have been proposed to explain how the hippocampal formation guides navigation. We first consider the pattern-completion model of McNaughton (1989, 1990). We then turn to the Euclidean mapping model of O'Keefe (1989, 1990). Finally, we present the outlines of a third scheme that we believe avoids some of the difficulties presented by the others and at the same time address the critical question of how the environment is represented by activity of the place cell population.

McNaughton's pattern-completion theory

McNaughton's model (1989; see also McNaughton and Nadel 1990) avoids the notion of a global representation of the environment and postulates that each place cell is triggered by a certain local view. In this scheme, a given local view is associated with other local views according to the movements necessary to carry the rat from its original head location and orientation to the new position and head orientation. Navigational guidance is presumably achieved by linking sets of local views into linear lists, where the local views are interpreted as critical positions in a route. The route could then be followed by sequentially making the motions that cause the local views in the list to appear in order. Additional flexibility is incorporated into the model by suggesting that the links between successive local views are not fixed motions, but rather the output of an extra-hippocampal system that can calculate motion equivalency (e.g. two 90° right turns result in the same orientation as two 90° left turns). McNaughton (1989) argues that 'the ability to compute movement equivalences' allows the rat to calculate novel routes to a goal.

O'Keefe (1990) raises two objections to this stimulus–response association scheme. First, he imagines that the amount of memory needed to store a large number of local views and the motions that connect local-view pairs would be excessive. Whether this difficulty is valid depends on the granularity of the local views and the combinatorial problem of storing paths between pairs of local views. Second, O'Keefe challenges the idea that McNaughton's scheme is rich enough to explain the ability of rats to take short cuts or take detours, and the ability to get to a goal from a new starting point (Sutherland and Rudy 1988). The cogency of this objection can be decided by implementing McNaughton's scheme as a computer model and resting its capabilities.

We have three additional difficulties with McNaughton's model. The first has to do with the local-view concept. During pellet chasing in the cylinder, there is little or no indication that place-cell firing is direction- as well as location-specific. We argue that this evidence falsifies local view as a necessary element in theories of spatial information processing by the hippocampus. On the other hand, local view may play a role during navigation in the eight-arm maze. In other words, McNaughton's model is not generally applicable, but is predictive of place cells properties in radial mazes. At the navigational level, the existence of directionally selective place cells might mean that the hippocampus can generate taxon as well as locale solutions to spatial problems. This is not a far-fetched idea if the hippocampus is already known to be flexible enough to represent both spatial and behavioural variables.

Our second disagreement with McNaughton's (1989) theory concerns his proposition that the invariance of place-cell firing after removing a sub-set of the cues implies the operation of a pattern-completion associator (Marr 1969; Kohonen 1984). When the full set of stimuli is available, the firing rate of each place cell is determined by the closeness of the match between the local view and a cell-specific template. When cues are removed, each cell continues to fire in the same region because inhibitory inter-neurons (theta cells) perform an operation that approximates integer division of the activity of the principal cells (place cells). In this scheme, the discharge of the inhibitory inter-neurons should be proportional to the number of input (from entorhinal cortex) cells that are active and should be insensitive to which input cells are active. After Marr (1969), McNaughton stresses that the inhibitory inter-neuron discharge should not be modulated in parallel with the signal carried by the principal cells, and so should not show location-specific firing.

In our opinion, the pattern-completion scheme proposed by McNaughton (1989) is incorrect in two ways. First, our data from the MEC suggest that the number of active input cells does not change after card removal (Quirk 1990). For this reason, the theta cells do not receive the right sort of signal to allow the integer division approximation. Second, we find that the strength of the spatial signal carried by theta cells is somewhat greater than the strength of the behavioural signal. We disagree with the statement that 'intensive application of statistics can sometimes reveal a small degree of spatial selectivity in these interneurons' (McNaughton 1989, p. 330). It is true that 'this selectivity is many-fold less than for the principal cells', but the modulation is nevertheless appreciable and is visible in firing rate maps without *any* application of statistics.

Our final disagreement with McNaughton's theory arises from the invariance of the shapes of firing fields after cue deletion or addition (Muller and Kubie 1987; Quirk *et al.* 1990; Sharp *et al.* 1990). If place-cell firing is sensory-like in the sense that it is triggered by cell-specific combinations of stimulus features, changes in the local view or total stimulus configuration should, in general, distort the shapes of firing fields. In our view, the uncoupling of spatial firing patterns from the stimulus configuration is so strong as to preclude the general applicability of sensory models, even if they incorporate the powerful idea of pattern completion. We believe that pattern completion of the stimulus constellation serves to select the active sub-set of place cells. Once the active sub-set is selected, the firing of individual cells is remarkably refractory to changes in the sensory environment.

O'Keefe's Euclidian mapping theory

For theoretical reasons, as stated by O'Keefe and Nadel (1978, Chapter 1), O'Keefe (1989, 1990) maintains that the hippocampus implements a Euclidian (and therefore metric) representation of the environment. The metric representation is assumed to include both the hippocampus and the post-subiculum. The place cells calculate the rat's distance from a point; the origin point (centroid) is calculated with respect to the available cue constellation. The representation is therefore polar, such that radius is signalled by the place cells and angle is signalled by post-subicular, head-direction cells. (Taube *et al.* 1990a,b) suggested an alternative interpretation of the coexistence of place cells and directional cells, in which the directional system is mainly responsible for navigation over large distances, and the place-cell system is mainly responsible for navigation

within a restricted region. This notion follows the work of Bingman *et al.*
(1984).

In the results, we indicated two difficulties with a metric theory. First, we
showed that the calculated position is systematically in error when the rat is
near an impenetrable boundary. A more serious error appears when the
rat is allowed to move behind one or more of the cues, in which case the
centroid becomes undefined. Second, we argued that the existence of
extended (crescent or linear) firing fields suggests that spatial firing distributions do not generally reflect the distance between the rat's head and a
point of most rapid firing. The variation in firing-field shapes is hard to
explain with a metric theory, as the computations would have to 'know
about' field shape and could not operate strictly on current place-cell
activity.

A major objection to the Euclidean theory concerns the variable directional selectivity of place cells. It is hard to understand why an elementary
property of firing fields depends on external conditions if the hippocampus
makes explicit Euclidean computations. If the representation is metric,
place-cell discharge should or should not take head direction into account;
it is not in the scope of the theory that two entirely different mapping
algorithms should be used in different environments. It is also hard to
imagine how event-correlated firing could arise if the hippocampus is
specialized for metric computations.

Elements of a topological theory of the hippocampal spatial representation

We conclude this chapter by showing that a topological representation of
the environment can be generated by taking advantage of known properties of the CA3 pyramidal cells. We emphasize that this theory is incomplete in many ways. For example, it ignores the directional cells of the
post-subiculum as well as the place cells of CA1. It also assumes that
the CA3 pyramidal cells function as place cells without attempting to
explain how their firing is organized in terms of inputs from entorhinal
cortex. At this stage of its development, the main value of the theory is to
show that the CA3 place-cell population can come to reflect the connectivity
of the environment in a holistic manner, and so potentially permit geodesic
calculations.

The first step in the theory assumes that a pattern-completion process
takes place when a rat is put into a recording chamber. If the chamber is
familiar, the appropriate, active sub-set of place cells is selected, possibly
by imposing a chamber-specific, synaptic drive pattern on the theta cells.
The key difference from McNaughton's theory is that pattern completion
operates at the level of the entire place-cell population and not for each
place cell independently. The active sub-set is an ensemble that has a form

of permanency. A cell in the active sub-set will not be triggered by a cue configuration that strongly resembles the configuration available to the rat within the cell's firing field in a different chamber.

If the recording chamber is sufficiently different from chambers familiar to the rat, the pattern-completion process does not result in the selection of an established, active sub-set. Instead, a new active sub-set is generated by unknown combinatorial rules. The notion that a new active sub-set (map) can be generated very soon after the rat is put into new surroundings is supported by the findings of Hill (1978). Hill showed that most place cells fire the first time the rat passes through the region of the steady-state firing field. Additional support comes from the black-card substitution experiment of Bostock *et al.* (1990), where it was found that a switch from a null to a complete remapping took place very rapidly.

The theory focuses on two known properties of CA3 pyramidal cells. First, the CA3 cells make excitatory, monosynaptic contacts with each other (Miles and Wong 1986). For a pair of randomly chosen cells, the probability that one excites the other is only about 2 per cent, but the probability of contact is constant over large fractions of the septo-temporal extent of CA3/4. Second, the strength of the synapses increases when the pre-and post-synaptic cells fire in close temporal association (Miles and Wong 1987). In our first-order model, the modifiable synapses do not affect spatial firing patterns; the synapses only change in strength.

Given these assumptions, it is not hard to see that the pattern of synaptic strengths can come to reflect the connectivity of the space accessible to the rat, producing a topological representation of the space. Initially all synaptic strengths are zero. It is also convenient to imagine that the maximal synaptic strength is unity. As the rat moves around the environment, CA3 place cells will fire within their fields. The critical point is that only synapses that connect cells with overlapping firing fields will increase in strength; synapses that connect cells with widely separated fields will remain weak. The encoding of distance by synaptic strength arises as a direct consequence of exploratory movements, and from the inability of rats to move fast enough to make cells with widely separated fields fire in close, temporal order. It is an interesting consequence of this scheme that the encoding of distance depends in part on the rat's running speed.

In addition to storing a representation of the local connectivity of the environment, the intra-CA3, modifiable synapses may contain enough information to allow geodesics between widely separated points to be calculated. The representation of indirect trajectories will in general involve larger numbers of place cells than the representation of optimal paths, so that the product of the synaptic strengths is greater for short than for long paths.

It is clear that this simple model does not speak to the issue of how the connections can be used to guide the rat's behaviour. To go further, it is necessary to relax the restriction that the modifiable synapses within CA3 do not affect firing rates, and to propose a mechanism by which the goal position as well as the starting position can be represented in the set of place cells. It is also necessary to explain how possible trajectories can be read out of CA3. Nevertheless, we believe that this scheme is promising for spatial computations, and that it has the additional advantage that it can be used for non-spatial computations so long as the firing correlates of the pyramidal cells are suitably altered; the lateral synaptic network in CA3 may be able to calculate the equivalents of geodesics in general problem space.

Acknowledgments

We would like to thank Dr James B. Ranck Jr. and Dr Pat E. Sharp for conceptual and experimental contributions that are continully referred to in this chapter. R.U.M. would also like to thank Mr Mario Scavello and Mr Peter Gustas for valuable conversations. Our research was supported by NIH grants NS20686 (J.L.K and R.U.M) and NS14497 (J.B.R Jr. and R.U.M).

References

Amaral, D. G. and Witter, M. P. (1989). The three dimensional organization of the hippocampal formation: a review of anatomical data. *Neuroscience*, **31**, 571–91.
Berger, T. W., Rinaldi, P. C., Weisz, D. J., and Thompson, R. F. (1983). Single-unit analysis of different hippocampal cell types during classical conditioning of the nictitating membrane response. *Journal of Neurophysiology*, **50**, 1197–219.
Best, P. J. and Ranck, J. R., Jr. (1982). The reliability of the relationship between hippocampal unit activity and sensory-behavioral events in the rat. *Experimental Neurology*, **75**, 652–64.
Bingman, V., Bagnoli, P., Ioale, P., and Casini, J. (1984). Homing behavior of pigeons after telencephalic ablations. *Brain Behavior and Evolution*, **24**, 94–108.
Bostock, E. M., Muller, R. U., and Kubie, J. L. (1986). Firing fields of hippocampal neurons: A stimulus manipulation that alters place cell mapping of the environment. *Society for Neuroscience Abstracts*, **12**, 522.
Bostock, E., Taube, J., and Muller, R. U. (1988). The effects of head orientation on the firing of hippocampal place cells. *Neuroscience Abstracts*, **18**, 127.
Breese, C. R. Hampson, R. E., and Deadwyler, S. A. (1989). Hippocampal place cells: stereotypy and plasticity. *Journal of Neuroscience*, **9**, 1097–111.
Butcher, S. P., Hendry, R., and Morris, R. G. M. (1989). NMDA receptors and memory: parallels between their role in learning and memory. *Society for Neuroscience Abstracts*, **15**, 463.
Christian, E. P. and Deadwyler, S. A. (1986). Behavioral functions of hippocampal

subtypes: evidence for two non-overlapping populations in the rat. *Journal of Neurophysiology*, **55**, 331–48.

Deacon, T. W. Eichenbaum, H. Rosenberg, P., and Eckmann, K. W. (1983). Afferent connections of the perirhinal cortex in the rat. *Journal of Comparative Neurology*, **220**, 168–190.

Eichenbaum, H. and Cohen, N. J. (1988). Representation in the hippocampus. What do hippocampal neurons code? *Trends in Neuroscience*, **11**, 244–8.

Eichenbaum, H., Kuperstein, M., Fagan, A., and Nagode, J. (1987). Cue-sampling and goal approach correlates of hippocampal unit activity in rats performing an odor discrimination task. *Journal of Neuroscience*, **7**, 716–32.

Fox, S. E. and Ranck, J. B. Jr. (1975). Localization and anatomical identification of theta and complex spike cells in the dorsal hippocampal formation of rats. *Experimental Neurology*, **49**, 299–313.

Fox, S. E. and Ranck, J. B. Jr. (1981). Electrophysiological characteristics of hippocampal complex-spike cells and theta cells. *Experimental Brain Research*, **41**, 399–410.

Grossberg, S. (1980). How does a brain build a cognitive code? *Psychology Review*, **87**, 1–51.

Hill, A. J. (1978). First occurence of hippocampal spatial firing in a new environment. *Experimental Neurology*, **62**, 282–97.

Jones, E. G. and Powell, T. P. S. (1970). An anatomical study of converging sensory pathways within the cerebral cortex of the monkey. *Brain*, **93**, 793–820.

Kohonen, T. (1984). *Self organization and associative memory* (2nd edn). Springer-Verlag, Berlin.

Kohler, C. (1986). Intrinsic connections of the retrohippocampal region in the rat brain: II. The medial entorhinal area. *Journal of Comparative Neurology*, **246**, 146–9.

Kubie, J. L. (1984). A drivable bundle of microwires for collecting single unit data from freely moving rats. *Physiology and Behavior*, **32**, 115–18.

Kubie, J. L. and Ranck, J. B. Jr. (1984). Hippocampal neuronal firing, context, and learning. In *Neuropsychology of memory* (ed. L. R. Squire and N. Butters). Guilford Press, New York.

Kubie, J. L., Muller, R. U., and Fox, S. E. (1985). Firing fields of place cells: interim report. In *Electrical activity of the archichortex* (ed. G. Buzsaki and C. H. Vanderwolf). Hungarian Academy of Sciences, Budapest.

Kubie, J. L., Dayyani, S., Sutherland, R. J., and Muller, R. U. (1989). Hippocampal lesions disrupt acquisition but not retention of navigational behaviour in a highly familiar environment. *Society for Neuroscience Abstracts*, **15**, 609.

Kubie, J. L., Dayyani, S., Muller, R. U., Cohen, B., Major, E., and Sutherland, R. J. (1990a). Hippocampal lesions in rats produce a temporarily graded amnesia on a spatial memory task. *Society for Neuroscience Abstracts*, **16**, 737.

Kubie, J. L., Muller, R. U., and Bostock, E. M. (1990b). Spatial firing properties of hippocampal theta cells. *Journal of Neuroscience*, **10**, 1110–23.

Lacaille, J.-C., Mueller, A. L., Kunkel, D. D., and Scwartzkroin, P. A. (1987). Local circuit interactions between oriens/alveus interneurons and CA1 pyramidal cells in hippocampal slices: electrophysioloy and morphology. *Journal of Neuroscience*, **7**, 1979–93.

Leonard, B. W., McNaughton, B. L., Barnes, C. A., and Marquis, M. (1990). The contribution of proximal and distal complexity to the discharge of hippocampal 'place' cells. *Society for Neuroscience Abstracts*, **16**, 441.

Marr, D. (1969). A theory of cerebellar cortex. *Journal of Physiology* (Lond), **202**, 437–70.

McNaughton, B. L. 1989). Neuronal mechanisms for spatial computation and information storage. In *Neural connections, mental computation* (ed. L. Nadel, L. A. Cooper, P. Culicover, and R. M. Harnish), pp. 285–350. MIT Press, Cambridge, MA.

McNaughton, B. L. and Nadel, L. (1990). Hebb–Marr networks and the neuro-biological representation of action in space. In *Neuroscience and Connection Theory* (ed. M. A. Gluck and D. E. Rumelhart) pp. 1–64. Lawrence Erlbaum Associates, Hillsdale, New Jersey.

McNaughton, B. L., Barnes, C. A., and O'Keefe, J. O. (1983). The contribution of position, direction, and velocity to single unit activity in the hippocampus of freely moving rats. *Experimental Brain Research*, **52**, 41–9.

McNaughton, B. L., Barnes, C. A., Rao, G., Baldwin, J., and Rasmussen, M. (1986). Long-term enhancement of hippocampal synaptic transmission and the aquisition of spatial information. *Journal of Neuroscience*, **6**, 563–71.

McNaughton, B. L., Leonard, B., and Chen, L. (1989). Cortical–hippocampal interactions and cognitive mapping: A hypothesis based on reintegration of the parietal and inferotemporal pathways for visual processing. *Psychobiology*, **17**, 236–46.

Miles, R. and Wong, R. K. S. (1984). Unitary inhibitory synaptic potentials in the guinea-pig hippocampus. *Journal of Physiology*, **356**, 97–113.

Miles, R. and Wong, R. K. S. (1986). Excitatory synaptic connections between CA3 neurones in the guinea pig hippocampus. *Journal of Physiology*, **373**, 397–418.

Miles, R. and Wong, R. K. S. (1987). Latent synaptic pathways revealed after tetanic stimulation in the hippocampus. *Nature*, **329**, 724–6.

Miller, V. M. and Best, P. J. (1980). Spatial correlates of hippocampal unit activity are altered by lesions of the fornix and entorhinal cortex. *Brain Research*, **194**, 311–23.

Mishkin, M. (1982). A memory system in the monkey. *Philosophical Transactions of the Royal Society London*, **298**, 85–95.

Mizumori, S. J. Y., McNaughton, B. L., and Barnes, C. A. (1989). Preserved spatial coding in hippocampal CA1 pyramids during reversible suppression of CA3c output: evidence for pattern completion in the hippocampus. *Journal of Neuroscience*, **9**, 3915–28.

Morris, R. G. M. (1981). Spatial localization does not require the presence of local cues. *Learning and Motivation*, **12**, 239–60.

Morris, R. G. M., Garrud, P., Rawlins, J. N. P., and O'Keefe, J. (1982). Place navigation impaired in rats with hippocampal lesions. *Nature*, **297**, 681–3.

Morris, R. G. M., Schenk, F. Tweedie, F., and Jarrard, L. E. (1989). Dissociation between components of spatial memory after ibotenate lesions of the hippocampus. *Society for Neuroscience Abstracts*, **15**, 609.

Muller, R. U. and Kubie, J. L. (1987). The effects of changes in the environment on the spatial firing of hippocampal complex-spike cells. *Journal of Neuroscience*, **7**, 1951–68.

Muller, R. U. and Kubie, J. L. (1989). The firing of hippocampal place cells predicts the future position of freely moving rats. *Journal of Neuroscience*, **9**, 4101–10.

Muller, R. U., Kubie, J. L. and Ranck, J. B. Jr. (1987). Spatial firing patterns for hippocampal complex-spike cells in a fixed environment. *Journal of Neuroscience*, **7**, 1935–50.

O'Keefe, J. (1976). Place units in the hippocampus of the freely moving rat. *Experimental Neurology*, **51**, 78–109.

O'Keefe, J. (1983). Spatial memory within and without the hippocampal system. In *Neurobiology of the hippocampus* (ed. W. Seifert), pp. 375–403. Academic Press, London.

O'Keefe, J. (1989). Computations the hippocampus might perform. In *Neural connections, mental computation* (ed. L. Nadel., L. A. Cooper, P. Culicover, and R. M. Harnish), pp. 225–84. MIT Press, Cambridge, MA.

O'Keefe, J. (1990). A computational model of the hippocampal cognitive map. In *Understanding the brain through the hippocampus: the hippocampal region as a model for studying brain structure and function* (ed. J. Storm-Mathisen, J. Zimmer, and O. P. Ottersen), *Progress in Brain Research*. Elsevier, Amsterdam.

O'Keefe, J. and Conway, D. H. (1978). Hippocampal place cells in the freely moving rat: Why they fire, where they fire? *Experimental Brain Research*, **31**, 573–90.

O'Keefe, J. and Dostrovsky, J. (1971). The hippocampus as spatial map. Preliminary evidence from unit activity in the freely moving rat. *Brain Research*, **34**, 171–5.

O'Keefe, J. and Nadel, L. (1978). *The hippocampus as a cognitive map*. Clarendon, London.

O'Keefe, J. and Speakman, A. (1987). Single unit activity in the rat hippocampus during a spatial memory task. *Experimental Brain Research*, **68**, 1–27.

Olton, D. S., Branch, M., and Best, P. (1978). Spatial correlates of hippocampal unit activity. *Experimental Neurology*, **58**, 387–409.

Olton, D. S., Becker, J. T., and Handelmann, G. E. (1979). Hippocampus, space and memory. *Behavioral and Brain Science*, **2**, 313–65.

Petsche, H., Stumpf, C., and Gogolak, G. (1962). The significance of the rabbit's septum as a relay station between the midbrain and the hippocampus. I. The control of hippocampus arousal activity by the septum cells. *Electroencephalography Clinical Neurophysiology*, **14**, 202–11.

Quirk, G. J. (1990). A spatial analysis of the firing of neurons in the medial entorhinal cortex of the rat. Doctoral dissertation. State University of New York.

Quirk, G. J., Muller, R. U., and Kubie, J. L. (1989). The firing of entorhinal place cells is more sensory-bound than that of hippocampal place cells. *Society for Neuroscience Abstracts*, **15**, 404.

Quirk, G. J., Muller, R. U., and Kubie, J. L. (1990). The firing of hippocampal place cells in the dark depends on the rat's recent experience. *Journal of Neuroscience*, **10**, 2008–17.

Ranck, J. B., Jr. (1973). Studies on single neurons in dorsal hippocampal formation and septum in unrestrained rats. *Experimental Neurology*, **41**, 461–555.

Ranck, J. B., Jr. (1984). Head-direction cells in the deep layers of dorsal presubiculum in freely moving rats. *Society for Neuroscience Abstracts*, **10**, 599.

Rose, G. (1983). Physiological and behavioral characteristics of Dentate granule cells. In *Neurobiology of the hippocampus* (ed. W. Seifert) pp. 449–72. Academic Press, London.

Rose, G., Diamond, D., and Lynch, G. S. (1983). Dentate granule cells in the rat hippocampal formation have the behavioral characteristics of theta neurons. *Brain research*, **266**, 29–37.

Schenck, F. and Morris, R. G. M. (1985). Dissociation between components of spatial memory in rats after recovery from the effects of retrohippocampal lesions. *Experimental Brain Research*, **58**, 11–28.

Scoville, W. B. and Milner, B. (1957). Loss of recent memory after bilateral hippo-campal lesions. *Journal of Neurological Psychiatry*, **20**, 11–21.

Sharp, P. E. (1989). Computer simulation of hippocampal place cells. *Society for Neuroscience Abstracts*, **15**, 403.

Sharp, P. E., Kubie, J. L., and Muller, R. U. (1988). Hippocampal place cells can fire differently in two visually identical locations in a symmetrical chamber. *Society for Neuroscience Abstracts*, **14**, 127.

Sharp, P. E., Kubie, J. L., and Muller, R. U. (1990). Firing properties of hippo-campal neurons in a visually-symmetric stimulus environment: contributions of multiple sensory cues and mnemonic processes. *Journal of Neuroscience*, (in press).

Steward, O. and Scoville, S. (1976). Cells of origin of entorhinal cortical afferents to the hippocampus and fascia dentata of the rat. *Journal of Comparative Neurology*, **169**, 347–70.

Squire, L. R. (1982). The neuropsychology of human memory. *Annual Review of Neuroscience*, **5**, 241–73.

Stewart, M. and Fox, S. E. (1989). Two populations of rhythmically bursting neurons in rat medial septum are revealed by atropine. *Journal of Neurophysiology*, **61**, 982–93.

Sutherland, R. J. and Rudy, J. W. (1988). Place learning in the Morris place task is impaired by damage to the hippocampal formation even if the temporal demands are reduced. *Psychobiology*, **6**, 157–63.

Sutherland, R. J., Arnold, K. A., and Rodriguez, A. R. (1987). Anterograde and retrograde effects on place memory after limbic or diencephalic damage. *Society for Neuroscience Abstracts*, **13**, 1066.

Swanson, L. W. and Cowan, W. M. (1977). An autoradiographic study of the organization of the efferent connections of the hippocampal formation in the rat. *Journal of Comparative Neurology*, **172**, 49–84.

Taube, J. S., Kesslak, J. P., and Cotman, C. W. (1989). Lesions of the rat post-subiculum impair performance on spatial tasks. *Society for Neuroscience Abstracts*, **15**, 607.

Taube, J. S., Muller, R. U., and Ranck, J. B. Jr. (1990a). Head direction cells recorded from the postsubiculum in freely moving rats. I. Description and quantitative analysis. *Journal of Neuroscience*, **10**, 420–35.

Taube, J. S., Muller, R. U., and Ranck, J. B. Jr. (1990b). Head direction cells recorded from the postsubiculum in freely moving rats. II. The effects of environmental manipulations. *Journal of Neuroscience*, **10**, 436–47.

Terrace, H. S. (1984). Animal cognition. In *Animal cognition* (ed. H. L. Roitblat, T. G. Bever and H. S. Terrace), pp. 7–28. Erlbaum, Hillsdale, NJ.

Thompson, L. T. and Best, P. J. (1989). Place cells and silent cells in the hippocampus of freely-behaving rats. *Journal of Neuroscience*, **9**, 2382–90.

Tolman, E. C. (1948). Cognitive maps in rats and men. *Psychology Review*, **40**, 60–70.

Tonkiss, J., Morris, R. G. M., and Rawlins, J. N. P. (1988). Intraventricular infusion of the NMDA antagonist AP5 impairs performance on a non-spatial operant DRL task in the rat. *Experimental Brain Research*, **73**, 181–8.

Traub, R. D., Miles, R., and Wong, R. K. S. (1989). A model of the origin of rhythmic population oscillations in the hippocampal slice. *Science*, **243**, 1319–26.

Vanderwolf, C. H. (1969). Hippocampal electrical activity and voluntary movement in the rat. *Electroencephalography, and Clinical Neurophysiology*, **26**, 407–18.

Wiener, S. L., Paul, C. A., and Eichenbaum, H. (1989). Spatial and behavioral correlates of hippocampal neuronal activity. *Journal of Neuroscience*, **9**, 2737–63.

Zipser, P. (1985). A comutational model of hippocampal place fields. *Behavioral Neuroscience*, **99**, 283–98.

18

The hippocampus, exploratory activity, and spatial memory

C. THINUS-BLANC, E. SAVE, M.-C. BUHOT, and
B. POUCET

Introduction

There is now an impressive set of data which supports the prominent role
of the hippocampus in spatial memory. But the hippocampal formation is
also involved in exploratory activity, although this function is supported by
a much smaller body of studies. Recent psychological studies have now
provided direct evidence that exploration and spatial knowledge are closely
related to each other by functional, reciprocal links. Hence, it is somewhat
surprising that these three poles of interest, the hippocampus, exploration,
and spatial knowledge, have not been integrated into a unified, conceptual
framework since O'Keefe and Nadel's classic book was published in 1978.
It is true that this task is far from easy. In the case of the functional
relationship between the hippocampus and spatial cognition, awkward
problems may be raised, such as those related to the processing and
transformation of information acquired during exploratory activity into
spatial knowledge. Exploration is a sensorimotor activity, organized along
a body-centred referent, entailing the position of the sensory receptors, the
direction of the displacement, gravitational forces, and so on. At the brain
level, visual information is projected topographically. In contrast, by their
very nature, spatial representations such as cognitive maps must be independent of the subject's current position at a given time; the information is
said to be allocentrically organized. So far, a topographical distribution of
spatial information has not been discovered in any higher level associative
structure involved in spatial mapping and memory. The different levels
of brain functioning roughly correspond, at both the psychological and
behavioural levels, to the processes involved, respectively, in visually
guided behaviours and in oriented displacements relying upon some environmental representation.

In this chapter we will illustrate in brief, using recent findings, the
functional paired relationships between the hippocampus, exploratory
behaviour, and spatial memory. Special emphasis will be placed on the
questions and problems relating to an overall neural and psychological

conception of the spatial processes. Finally, we will attempt to provide a broader definition of the spatial representations.

Exploration and spatial knowledge

Exploratory activity is displayed by most mammalian species in the presence of novelty. This reaction can take several forms, depending both on the nature of the new event and on the species under study. However, the easily observable, feverish activity of a small rodent sniffing objects, walking around in an unfamiliar experimental apparatus, and the discreet, sweeping glance of a human being entering a café appear to be different manifestations of an identical process. Both kinds of behaviour are induced by curiosity; both are aimed at reducing the uncertainty related to novelty (Berlyne 1966). Although the motivation triggering investigatory reactions has been the subject of intense debate, the overall interpretation of the result of this activity is straightforward: the asymptotic level of exploration reached after habituation corresponds to the stage when processing, integration, and storage of some characteristics of the initially unfamiliar situation are more or less completed. These characteristics can be related to the intrinsic features of the objects contained in a considered space. More interestingly, some of the spatial relationships between objects are also spontaneously processed during exploration.

Accordingly, evidence has accumulated which shows that exploratory activity in response to novelty leads to spatial knowledge. This assertion is illustrated by the beneficial effects of a period of exploration on the performance scores of animals solving spatial tasks such as the Maier three-table test. This experimental paradigm has been successfully used since the pioneering experiments of Maier (1929). Three platforms are linked to each other by a runway system. After a period of exploration on this apparatus, animals are then required to return to a table where they have just been fed. If the period of exploration is removed, rats fail to solve the problem (Ellen *et al.* 1982). The conclusion of these studies is that, during exploration, animals build up a cognitive representation of the problem space that is necessary to solve the problem (see also Renner 1988). Exploration has also been found to play a crucial role in spatial orientation in hamsters, cats, and dogs subjected to short-cut and detour tasks (Chapuis *et al.* 1983, 1987; Poucet *et al.* 1983).

There is very little direct evidence of the cognitive nature of exploration, though the number of studies is increasing. Some relevant data are provided by experiments using a procedure based on the decrease in exploratory activity over time (habituation) and its reactivation following a change. In this procedure, animals are first allowed to explore an open field

336 C. Thinus-Blanc, E. Save, M.-C. Buhot, and B. Poucet

containing one or several objects. The number as well as the duration of contacts with these objects are recorded. Although this measure of exploratory activity is not exhaustive, it is a valid index of object investigation which can be easily contrasted with more diffuse locomotor activity (Buhot et al. 1989a,b). After habituation, a novel situation is created by modifying the spatial arrangement of the object set. This novelty is exclusively spatial because the objects themselves are not changed. Usually, a renewal of exploration is then observed. This renewal may sometimes be as intense as if the whole situation had been changed or one of the objects was totally new. The intensity of the renewed exploration has been found to depend largely on the spatial parameters that are affected by the change. Such findings have come not only in tests on primates (Joubert and Vauclair 1986) but also in tests on several species of rodents: rats (Sutherland 1985; Poucet 1989) gerbils (Thinus-Blanc and Ingle 1985) and hamsters (Poucet et al. 1986; Thinus-Blanc et al. 1987). In the latter experiments it has been shown, for example, that hamsters are more likely to encode geometrical relationships (i.e. the shape defined by the object set) than absolute distances between the objects. A recent study (see Note 1) has shown that the behaviour in response to a spatial change would depend, to some extent, on the animal starting its exploration from a particular place which could be used as a point of reference associated with a specific perspective of the arrangement of the objects.

Such data tend to upset the classical conception of spatial representations in terms of accurate cartographic maps. For instance, one cannot rule out the possibility that the knowledge of the geometrical relationships between objects could take the form of stored images, or 'snapshots', of an array of landmarks as seen from a particular location. These snapshots have been found to guide the orientation performance of both honey bees (Cartwright and Collett 1983) and gerbils (Collett et al. 1986), which, in order to locate a hidden goal, appear to search the best match between the retinal and stored images of the layout.

Whatever the hypotheses likely to account for spatial orientation, exploratory activity and habituation **do** appear to be of considerable methodological interest in the study of spatial memory. The renewal of investigative activity after habituation implies that a change bearing exclusively upon the spatial features of the situation has been detected. Such a detection is possible only by referring to the initial situation, no longer present as a whole, of which the subject has stored a memory or representation that needs to be compared to the present; novelty *per se* does not exist, but only by reference to familiarity. However, in spite of the simplicity and reliability of the above method, there is still as pointed out in the introduction, the pending and crucial problem of the transformation of information gathered during exploration.

The hippocampus and spatial representations

It is well known that, in rats at least, the hippocampal function is primarily concerned with spatial learning and memory conceived as consequences of exploratory activity (O'Keefe and Nadel 1978). Lesions of the hippocampus and its associated structures (fimbria-fornix, septum, entorhinal cortex, subiculum) induce severe and permanent deficits in spatial orientation in a wide variety of situations (Rasmussen *et al.* 1989). Among the most recent studies, spatial deficits have been observed in the Morris navigation task (Morris *et al.* 1986; Kelsey and Landry 1988), in the cross maze (O'Keefe and Conway 1980) and in the radial-arm maze (Olton 1982). All these tasks require the use of a spatial representation in order to be solved.

Electrophysiological studies support the spatial function of the hippocampal formation. Single-unit recordings have revealed that a number of cells in the CA1 and CA3 areas of the hippocampus fire in relation to the animal's location within the environment (O'Keefe and Conway 1978; Olton *et al.* 1978; Kubie and Ranck 1983; McNaughton *et al.* 1983; Muller and Kubie 1987; O'Keefe and Speakman 1987).

However, although behavioural and electrophysiological studies often converge, many questions still remain unanswered. One such question concerns the distribution of spatial information across the hippocampus and, thus, the organizing principle linking the different 'place cells' that encode the various locations of the animal. The few studies that deal with this issue (O'Keefe and Speakman 1987; Eichenbaum and Cohen 1988; Eichenbaum *et al.* 1989) suggest that the representations of the different parts constituting an environment are distributed across the hippocampus. 'One of the great challenges for theories of hippocampal function will be to devise models which explain how neighbouring cells with similar inputs can represent different parts of the environment and how the distributed representation of a place can be decoded by other areas of the brain' (O'Keefe and Speakman 1987, p. 24). O'Keefe (1990, and Chapter 16) has now attempted to solve this problem.

The convergence of the issues raised both in electrophysiological studies and in those that consider the relationships between exploration and spatial knowledge are striking and intellectually stimulating. Both sets of data, again, raise the inescapable problem of how the brain organizes the gathered information, which on the one hand depends on the subject's position, and on the other hand is processed so as to constitute a representation that is independent of these positions.

The hippocampus and exploration

The main argument in favour of the role of hippocampus in exploration is that place cells are active during exploration (O'Keefe and Nadel 1978; O'Keefe 1983; Muller and Kubie 1987; Muller et al. 1987). Ranck (1973) reports the existence of multimodal neurons that habituate rapidly to repeated stimulus presentation but are responsive to novelty, with some cells firing during orienting behaviour. More recently, Muller and Kubie (1989) have shown that when rats are exposed to a new stimulus in an open field, place cells become progressively active while the rat is at a given location in relation to a visual cue. However, according to McNaughton et al. (1989), the spatial selectivity of place cells would not depend on the prior experience of the rat within the environment. No learning period appears to be required for spatially selective firing to occur (Hill 1978). Thus the status of exploration in the emergence of place fields is an issue that remains to be clarified. Moreover, the firing rates of hippocampal place cells have been demonstrated to be related to behavioural variables such as speed, direction, and the turning angle of the rat as it moves through the environment (Wiener et al. 1989). Finally, spatially selective firing of hippocampal cells is totally removed by head and/or body restraint (Forster et al. 1989). On the other hand, some characteristics of dentate granule-cell activity (such as the growth in synaptic strength, excitatory post-synaptic potential, and increase in the population-spike components of the response) are specifically related to the exploration of a new environment (Sharp et al. 1989).

   The role of the hippocampus in exploration is also supported by the activity of theta trains time-locked to orienting and investigative movements elicited by novelty (reviews in O'Keefe and Nadel 1978; Foreman and Stevens 1987). Large-amplitude, theta electro-encephalographic (EEG) activity has been recorded in the hippocampal formation during exploration (Vanderwolf 1971). More importantly, the myostatial movements of the vibrissae co-ordinated with head movements, which frequently occur during investigation of a new environment, are phase-related to theta peaks in the EEG (Komisaruk 1970).

   The effects of lesions of the hippocampal formation on exploratory behaviour are consistent with the electrophysiological data. Hippocampal rats are often hyperactive in the open field but this is not the expression of exploratory activity, as inter- and intra-session habituation is delayed or absent (Foreman 1983; Poucet 1989). Hippocampal lesions also abolish or decrease the orienting responses, which are one of the components of exploratory activity (Raphelson et al. 1985). Although sensory discriminative abilities are left intact, hippocampal rats are also impaired in terms of their reactions to novelty (Markowska and Lukaszewska 1981; Poucet 1989).

All of these findings have considerable implications with regard to the hippocampal function in exploration. The hippocampus is the site of convergence of pre-processed, multimodal, sensory information (via the entorhinal cortex and perforant path) and of movement-related information (via the septum generating theta rhythm, and fimbria-fornix), particularly during investigative activity. The same cells would therefore be able to match place- and movement-related information (Wiener *et al.* 1989). During exploratory behaviour, different types of investigative movements (eye and head scanning movements, rearings, etc.) generate ever-changing sensory stimulation. The integration and registering of these movements and of their sensory 'results' would be the basis of the formation of spatial invariants or spatial maps.

Reversible inactivation of the hippocampus and exploration

Thus, past studies suggest that the hippocampus is directly involved in spatial learning abilities, but the stage of spatial information processing which is specifically hippocampal-driven is yet to be understood. Therefore, with respect to the study of the functions of the hippocampus, it is necessary to design experiments in which the various stages of information processing can be dissociated. Of course, classical lesion techniques do not permit such an approach. However, Barnes (1988) has advocated a promising technique, which consists of reversible inactivation of the hippocampus (or other brain structures) by means of a local injection of short-term, tricaine anaesthetics (e.g. lidocaine or tetracaine). This method has two advantages. First, it circumvents the problem of synaptic rearrangements (sprouting, reafferentation) which occur after brain damage. Secondly, and more interestingly in this case, it allows for the functions of the hippocampus to be neutralized at any time in the course of a given behavioural process. Additionally, it is possible to adopt a within-subject design in which animals may alternatively be treated (i.e. resulting in a dysfunctioning hippocampus) or not treated (i.e. so that the hippocampal function is left intact).

Using the reversible inactivation method, Mizumori *et al.* (1989a) have now shown that septal inactivation induces a decrease in the spontaneous firing of place cells in the stratum granulosum and in the hilar CA3 region for periods of up to 15 min. Although the firing rates of CA1, complex spike cells (place cells) were not changed, severe impairment of spatial working memory was caused by inactivation of the medial septum (Mizumori *et al.* 1989b). Other studies have demonstrated that hippocampal inactivation induces deficits in a delayed alternation task, but not in a reference memory task in which rats are trained to return to the same arm of an apparatus (Barea *et al.* 1988).

Recently, this method was used to study the role of the hippocampus in terms of response-to-change behaviour. Only after the acquisition of spatial information had taken place under normal conditions of hippocampal functioning was the hippocampus inactivated. In the following two experiments, the procedure was based on the same principle as in our previous studies (Poucet *et al.* 1986; Thinus-Blanc *et al.* 1987) except that instead of modifying the spatial arrangement of the objects, the change consisted of removing a single stimulus object during the test trial. Response-to-change behaviour was assessed by measuring the time spent by the animal at the place (hereafter referred to as Z1) where the stimulus was previously located, which was compared to the time spent at a neutral zone (hereafter referred to as Z2) arbitrarily defined in the field.

The animals (Long-Evans rats) were subjected to four, 5-min exploratory sessions of a circular open field in a curtained environment with a single conspicuous pattern on the wall of the field. During session 1, the animal explored the empty field (Fig. 18.1A,C) During sessions 2 and 3, the 'stimulus' (a box containing another rat) was placed under the transparent

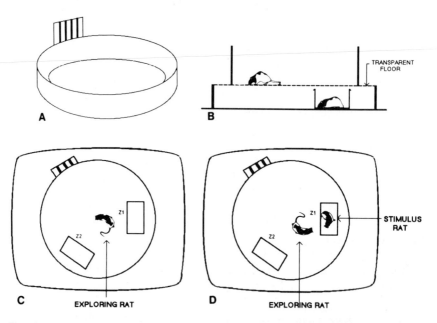

Fig. 18.1. A schematic representation of the apparatus: (A) the empty, circular, open field used during session 1 (reference session) and session 4 (test session); (B) the same open field during session 2 (first session with the stimulus) and 3 (last session with the stimulus)—the stimulus consisted of a box with a rat inside placed under the transparent floor of the arena; (C and D) the video image of the open field during sessions 1 and 4, and sessions 2 and 3, respectively—the time spent by the animals in the two zones Z1 (corresponding to the location of the stimulus) and Z2 (an arbitrarily chosen neutral zone) was recorded.

glass floor of the field (Fig. 18.1B,D). Finally, the test session (session 4) consisted of removing the stimulus. A video camera above the field was connected to a TV screen, which allowed for the observation of the animal without the observer being seen. During each session, the time spent by the animal at the two zones, Z1 and Z2, was recorded. The 5-min sessions were separated by a 3-min interval, with the exception of the test session, which was preceded by a one-hour delay. This longer between-session interval was adopted because pilot study had demonstrated that a delay of at least 60 min was necessary for consolidation, and for the rats to detect the change. Throughout the experiment, olfactory cues were carefully neutralized. Before the experiment, all animals were surgically implanted with guide cannulas in which the injection needle could be inserted. The guide cannula was aimed at the ventral hippocampus (Fig. 18.2), which, at this location, is about 2 mm in medial-lateral extent. An injection of 1.5 µl at this location is completely confined to the hippocampus and blocks all of the hippocampal formation at this level (Sandkuhler *et al.* 1987). Half of the animals were injected with lidocaine while the other half were sham-injected. The injections were made 5 min before the test session.

As shown in Fig. 18.3, the time spent above the neutral zone (Z2) did not vary during the course of the experiment. On the other hand, the stimulus elicited strong investigative reactions, as indicated by the increase of time spent by the animals above the corresponding zone Z1 during

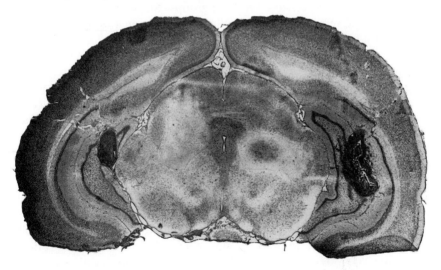

Fig. 18.2. Photograph of a brain section stained with cresyl violet, taken through the plane of the ventral hippocampus of a representative animal. Before removing the brain, 1.5 µl of china ink was injected to mark the location and extent of the diffusion of the drug. The diffusion of the dye is clearly indicated by the dark area within the ventral hippocampus. The track of the guide cannula is also visible.

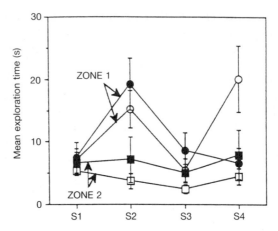

Fig. 18.3. The time course of exploratory activity in the two zones (see Fig. 18.1) Z1 (circles) and Z2 (squares) by normal (sham-injected: open symbols) and experimental (lidocaine-injected: filled symbols) rats during experiment 1. Exploratory activity was measured by time spent (mean ± SE, in seconds) in each zone. During sessions (S) 1 and 4, the circular open field was empty; during sessions 3 and 4 the stimulus was present. The same pattern of exploratory activity was found in experiment 2.

session 2 as compared to session 1. This investigative behaviour decreased during the following session 3 in both groups. Sham-injected rats reacted strongly to the removal of the stimulus during session 4 by spending more time at the place Z1 (where the stimulus was previously located) than at the neutral zone Z2. In contrast, lidocaine-injected rats did not display any sign of having noticed the change (Fig. 18.4). To sum up, reversible inactivation of the hippocampus did prevent the animals from reacting to the spatial change, in spite of a normal phase of exploration. This result parallels the effects of classical hippocampal lesions when they are made after spatial learning has occurred over a larger time scale.

In a second experiment, we attempted to make localization of the change easier to detect by adding some cues to the field. As a matter of fact, in experiment 1, the 'task' was very difficult, because except for the pattern on the wall, there were no cues inside the field. Several previous studies have shown that hippocampal lesions have no harmful influence on the performance scores when the animal is guided by cues that are closely associated to the goal. In contrast, hippocampal lesions have drastic effects when the cues are far from a hidden goal, when its location must be inferred from their configuration. This suggests that the hippocampus is not involved in 'simple associative processing' (such as that involved in sensory guided displacements), but in 'configural associative processing', such as that which underlies orientation relying upon spatial cognitive

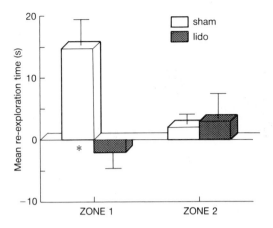

Fig. 18.4. Behaviour in response to the change in experiment 1. The histograms represent the difference between the time (mean ± SE, in seconds) spent investigating the two zones, Z1 and Z2, during session 4 (test session with the stimulus removed), and the corresponding time during session 3 (with the stimulus present under the floor of the apparatus) for the two treatments, 'sham' and 'lido' (lidocaine-injected). * indicates a significant difference between the two sessions ($p < 0.05$).

maps (Sutherland and Rudy 1989). In this case, therefore, cues closely associated to the stimulus in the exploration paradigm could facilitate the localization and search for the disappeared stimulus in lidocaine-injected animals.

The principle of experiment 2 was that of the previous experiment except that two objects were placed under the glass floor. For half of the subjects these objects were located close to the stimulus whereas, for the other half, they were spatially dissociated from the stimulus. During the test session, the box containing the rat was removed but the objects remained at their respective locations in the field. The overall time course of exploratory activity was the same as in experiment 1. After removal of the stimulus, sham-injected rats displayed a consistent, although weak, reaction to the change, both when the objects were close to the stimulus (Fig. 18.5, left-hand side), and when they were dissociated (Fig. 18.5, right-hand side). On the other hand, the lidocaine-injected animals did not react at all to the change and continued to habituate in both conditions. The lack of reactions in the lidocaine-injected rats to the 'associated object' condition may be due to several factors: the strength of the association between the stimulus and the cues may have been too weak, either because of the absence of a strong reinforcer or because the procedure involved only a short period of acquisition time as compared to classical spatial learning procedures where the acquisition time is much longer.

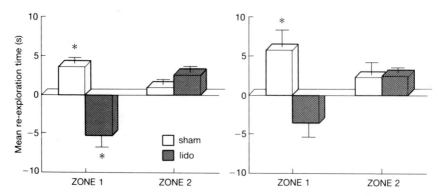

Fig. 18.5. Behaviour in response to the change in experiment 2. The histograms represent the difference between the time spent (mean ± SE, in seconds) investigating the two zones, Z1 and Z2, during session 4 (test session with the stimulus removed), and the corresponding time during session 3 (with the stimulus present under the floor of the apparatus) for 'sham' and lidocaine-injected (lido) rats. * indicates a significant difference between the two sessions ($p < 0.05$). Left-hand side: Condition with the objects placed under the transparent floor close to the stimulus. Right-hand side: Condition with the objects placed under the transparent floor far from the stimulus. In both conditions, the test session (session 4) consisted of removing the stimulus but not the objects, which remained in their respective locations as in sessions 2 and 3.

These two experiments revealed that lidocaine injections into the hippocampus are effective in blocking the response-to-change behaviour displayed by normal animals, although the initial phase of exploration occurred under normal conditions for all the animals. There are a number of explanations for the observed lack of reactions in the injected animals to the change, namely (a) a failure to notice that a change has occurred; (b) an impaired spatial memory of the location of the disappeared stimulus; (c) a more general memory deficit. These different possibilities are discussed elsewhere (see Note 2).

At least, these experiments hint at the usefulness of the technique of reversible inactivation in the search for the neural bases of spatial knowledge. Such a method could be applied, in the near future, in the various approaches aimed at testing new concepts, in which it is possible to intervene at any given time during the experiment, and where the effects can be tested immediately. This possibility of testing the role of a given brain structure at any time is of the greatest importance in the study of a process in which space and time are related dimensions. This allows us to study short- and intermediate-term, spatial memory and perhaps to focus on the particular moment(s) when the hippocampus is likely to play a crucial role in spatial processes.

Conclusions

In this brief overview we have attempted to emphasize the functional, reciprocal relationships linking exploratory activity, spatial knowledge, and the hippocampus. Of course, there are other important psychological theories which, although not mentioned here, support this view. For example, both Piaget (1936) and Gibson (1988) have extensively developed the idea that exploratory activity and play are important factors in the child's development and spatial behaviours. The list of theoretical arguments that supports the reciprocal links between exploration and spatial knowledge could easily be extended. However, it may be suspected that there is a host of interrelated factors, which may lead us to suspect that we are discussing something trivial, but these heterogeneous findings may allow us to generate new hypotheses or ideas.

Throughout this chapter we have referred to the main question raised by the classical conception of spatial representations, namely the transition from an egocentric to an allocentric frame of reference (Paillard 1987). This problem is not exclusively a theoretical one; it is also related to the practical aspects of spatial representations. Strelow (1985), p. 241) has clearly highlighted this point: 'One basic problem with cognitive-map concepts is that the survey-map characteristics they posit in memory have no obvious connection to the traveler's actual perceptual experience of the environment . . . That is, the survey-map is a bird's eye view of the environment, whereas what we experience is a frontal view.' Thus, it appears quite justified to call into question the classical cartographic conception of spatial knowledge because it does not fully account for the subject's real experience. Collett's hypothesis about panoramic snapshots used by honey bees and gerbils to locate a hidden goal appears to hint at a more realistic approach to spatial orientation mechanisms and lends itself to further implementations. As a matter of fact, this hypothesis involves a very simple process of comparison between the current retinal images and the one, unique, stored snapshot (e.g. that taken from the goal) of the layout. The local view that best matches the stored snapshot indicates the location of the goal (Cartwright and Collett 1983; Collett *et al.* 1986). Such a mechanism is extremely rigid and basic, and does not satisfactorily account for more complex spatial behaviours, such as short-cut and detour behaviours.

However, one may ask whether higher cognitive functions would not have their roots in simpler mechanisms. This idea has been recently put forward by P. S. Churchland (1989, p. 451) in the following terms: 'If we can see how the complexity in behaviour that we call cognition evolved from solutions to basic problems in sensorimotor control, this can provide

the framework for determining the nature and dynamics of cognition ...
Higher functions are surely not discontinuous with lower functions; there
are not a sphere unto themselves'. Granted the schematic and perhaps
disputable idea that egocentred activities (such as exploration and comparison between stored and currently perceived snapshots) belong to the
'lower' level, and that the use of complex spatial exocentred representations or maps is a 'higher' function, we outline here a concept that involves
basic elements, such as the snapshots or local views, as well as far more
complex processing.

We assume the existence of at least two levels of spatial processing.
First, visual images of parts of the environment similar to the panoramic
snapshots would be stored. However, instead of the one, unique snapshot
used by the honey bees, many different local views would be interconnected so that they could be recognized as belonging to the same environment. One of the functions of exploration would be to multiply the number
of perspectives (Thinus-Blanc 1988).

The second level is made up of more abstract representations conceived
as schemata or prototypes. The function of these schemata is two-fold. In
addition to their role in orientation processes, they are conceived of as a
system that both guides and organizes the further gathering of new information and extracts spatial invariants. This view is classical in cognitive
psychology (Neisser 1976). Because of their high level of abstraction and
generality, these schemata would obviously be stripped of details relative
to a particular environment to allow the deciphering, detection, and anticipation of the environmental regularities.

During orientation, spatial behaviour is controlled by both perceptual
images and stored local views. For example, short-cut and detour problems
imply an inferential process for the emergence of a new solution, such as
the choice of a path that has never been experienced before. Such an
inferential process relies upon a reorganization of previously acquired
information (Ellen 1987). Thus, the available information, i.e., the stored
and currently perceived local views of the environment, would be processed according to the general rules of transformation generated by the
schemata. O'Keefe (1990, Chapter 16) and Zipser (1986), for instance,
have provided useful models involving various kinds of transformation
rules.

At the brain level, structures such as the associative areas of the neocortex would be involved in the higher-level functions subserved by the
schemata or prototypes. The main argument for this assumption is the
correlative and dramatic increase of the relative importance of the neocortex on the phylogenetical scale, and the development of symbolic processes in higher mammalian species.

The hippocampus would ensure the basic processing and organization of local views. Its role in 'configurational processing' is now well acknowledged, and has been extensively discussed by Wiener *et al.* (1989) and Sutherland and Rudy (1989). The close relationships between place-cell activity and the environmental layout provide some experimental support for these hypotheses (O'Keefe and Speakman 1987; Muller and Kubie 1987). Specifically, the existence of place cells, the activity of which depends not only on the absolute location of the subject but also on the direction in which the subject faces a local view (McNaughton *et al.* 1983), is of particular interest to us. Such findings have led O'Keefe and Speakman (1987) to propose that a spatial representation could be made up of several 'maps' of the environment each corresponding to a different place or view point. These particular 'maps' would have to be partial, egocentric, and visual. Evidence supporting the role of vision in such a process is provided by studies showing that rearranging the configuration of distal (visual) cues induces a modification of the firing patterns of previously identified place cells (O'Keefe and Conway, 1978; Kubie and Ranck 1983; Muller *et al.* 1987, and Chapter 17).

At least two additional processes are required for the hippocampus to integrate the various local views of a given environment: (a) during exploration, a memory trace of the individual local views continuously impinging upon the organism must be kept in order so that invariants can be extracted from the progressive visual transformation resulting from the displacements; (b) during orientation, local views must be compared to each other to determine if they belong to the same environment. Such a process implies that the hippocampus functions as a short-term memory store and as a comparator, two functions which have been proposed by different investigators (Olton *et al.* 1979; Gray 1984).

One issue that remains to be clarified concerns the way spatial information is handled in the hippocampus, i.e. the relationship between the locations of place cells within the hippocampus and their corresponding environmental place fields. Growing evidence suggests that (a) the representation of an environment is distributed across the surface of the hippocampus, with several units firing in relation to the animal's current location; and (b) there is no isomorphic relationship between the location of various firing units within the hippocampus and the parts of the environment they represent (O'Keefe and Speakman 1987; Muller *et al.* 1987). These electrophysiological data support the general concept developed above. If there was a strict topographical encoding of the spatial features as in the visual system, generalizations would become impossible. For example, the various local views of the same landmark configuration would not be classified as belonging to the same environment because of different perceived distances between the landmarks. Overall, the distribution of spatial information and its non-topographical projection onto the hippocampus supports a holographic conception of spatial encoding (Pribram 1969). The advantage of a holographic encoding as opposed to a topographical one is related to the fact that it gives some biological plausibility to the extraction of spatial information from various experiences related to differing view points and reconstructed as a single, unified structure of space. Within the several local views of a single environment, there exist common elements which, however, are ordered in different ways according to the direction in which the animal is facing.

Other simpler means of orienting, involving only specific local views of the environmental can also be effective. For example, according to McNaughton *et al.* (1989) and Sutherland and Rudy (1989), spatial tasks are performed on the basis of conditional associations between internal representations of local views and the body movements that link these representations. This explanatory framework is valuable with regard to spatial tasks where fairly strong associations can be constituted, but, like the snapshot hypothesis, it fails to account for more complex spatial performances relying, for example, on inferential processes. Thus, although our concept leaves many issues unresolved, it offers the advantage that we can acknowledge the coexistence of different systems of orientation that are not mutually exclusive because they involve the same basic elements (local views), which are processed and manipulated in different ways according to the constraints and requirements of the task, to the degree of completion of exploration for a given situation, and to the species that is being considered.

Acknowledgements

Funding for these studies was provided by a grant from the Scientific Affairs Division of the North Atlantic Treaty Organisation (grant NATO n° 0169-87). We also thank A. Christolomme and M. Gavioli for their help in histological processing, and P. Scardigli and H. Lucchessi for their technical assistance.

Notes

1. Thinus-Blanc, C., Durup, M., Lucchessi, H., and Poucet, B. (1990). Further studies on the spatial parameters encoded during exploration by hamsters (in preparation).
2. Save, E., Buhot, M.-C., Foreman, N., Poucet, B., and Thinus-Blanc, C. (1990). Effects of posterior parietal lesions and reversible inactivation of the hippocampus on response to spatial change (in preparation).

References

Barea, E. J., Hickey, M. R., and Smith, D. C. (1988). Hippocampal inactivation effects on spatial memory. *Society for Neuroscience Abstracts*, **14**, 233.

Barnes, C. A. (1988). Spatial learning and memory processes: the search for their neurobiological mechanisms in the rat. *Trends in Neuroscience*, **11**, 163–9.

Berlyne, D. E. (1966). Curiosity and exploration. *Science*, **153**, 25–33.

Buhot, M.-C., Rage, P., and Ségu, L. (1989a). Changes in exploratory behaviour of hamsters following treatment with 8-Hydroxy-2-(di-n-Propylamino)tetralin. *Behavioural Brain Research*, **35**, 163–79.

Buhot, M.-C., Soffié, M., and Poucet, B. (1989b). Scopolamine affects the cognitive processes involved in selective object exploration more than locomotor activity. *Psychobiology*, **17**, 409–17.

Cartwright, B. A. and Collett, T. S. (1983). Landmark learning in bees. *Journal of Comparative Physiology*, **151**, 521–43.

Chapuis, N., Thinus-Blanc, C., and Poucet, B. (1983). Dissociation of mechanisms involved in dogs' oriented displacements. *Quarterly Journal of Experimental Psychology*, **35B**, 213–19.

Chapuis, N., Durup, M., and Thinus-Blanc, C. (1987). The role of exploratory experience in a shortcut task by golden hamsters (*Mesocricetus auratus*). *Animal Learning and Behaviour*, **15**, 174–8.

Churchland, P. S. (1986). *Neurophilosophy. Toward a unified science of the mind-brain* (2nd edn). MIT Press, Cambridge, Mass.

Collett, T. S., Cartwright, B. A., and Smith, B. A. (1986). Landmark learning and visuo-spatial memories in gerbils. *Journal of Comparative Physiology A*, **158**, 835–51.

Eichenbaum, H. and Cohen, N. J. (1988). Representation in the hippocampus: what do hippocampal neurons code? *Trends in Neuroscience*, **11**, 244–8.

Eichenbaum, H., Wiener, S. I., Shapiro, M. L., and Cohen, N. J. (1989). The organization of spatial coding in the hippocampus: a study of neural ensemble activity. *Journal of Neuroscience*, **9**, 2764–75.

Ellen, P. (1987). Cognitive mechanisms in animal problem-solving. In *Cognitive processes and spatial orientation in animal and man* (ed. P. Ellen and C. Thinus-Blanc), pp. 20–35. Martinus Nijhoff, Dordrecht.

Ellen, P., Parko, E. M., Wages, C., Doherty, D., and Herrmann, T. (1982). Spatial problem solving by rats: exploration and cognitive maps. *Learning and Motivation*, **13**, 81–94.

Foreman, N. P. (1983). Head-dipping in rats with superior collicular, frontal cortical and hippocampal lesions. *Physiology and Behavior*, **30**, 711–17.

Foreman, N. P. and Stevens, R. (1987). Relationships between the superior colliculus and hippocampus: neural and behavioral considerations. *Behavioral and Brain Sciences*, **10**, 101–52.

Foster, T. C., Castro, C. A., and McNaughton, B. L. (1989). Spatial selectivity of rat hippocampal neurons is dependent on preparedness for movement. *Science*, **244**, 1580–2.

Gibson, E. J. (1988). Exploratory behavior in the development of perceiving, acting, and acquiring of knowledge. *Annual Review of Psychology*, **39**, 1–41.

Gray, J. A. (1984). The hippocampus as an interface between cognition and emotion. In *Animal cognition* (ed. H. L. Roitblat, T. J. Bever, and H. S. Terrace), pp. 607–26. Erlbaum, Hillsdale, NJ.

Hill, A. J. (1978). First occurrence of hippocampal spatial firing in a new environment. *Experimental Neurology*, **62**, 282–97.

Joubert, A. and Vauclair, J. (1986). Reactions to novel objects in a troop of guinea baboons: approach and manipulation. *Behaviour*, **96**, 92–104.

Kelsey, B. A. and Landry, J. E. (1988). Medial septal lesions disrupt spatial mapping ability in rats. *Behavioral Neuroscience*, **102**, 289–93.

Komisaruk, B. R. (1970). Synchrony between limbic system theta activity and rhythmical behaviors in rats. *Journal of Comparative and Physiological Psychology*, **70**, 284–92.

Kubie, J. L. and Ranck, J. B., Jr. (1983). Sensory-behavioral correlates in individual hippocampus neurons in three situations: space and context. In *Neurobiology of the hippocampus* (ed. W. Seifert), pp. 433–48. Academic Press, London.

Maier, N. R. F. (1929). Reasoning in the white rat. *Comparative Psychology Monographs*, **6**, 1–93.

Markowska, A. and Lukaszewska, I. (1981). Response to stimulus change following observation or exploration by the rat: differential effects of hippocampal damages. *Acta Neurobiologica Experimentalis*, **41**, 325–38.

McNaughton, B. L., Barnes, C. A., and O'Keefe, J. (1983). The contributions of position, direction, and velocity to single unit activity in the hippocampus of freely-moving rats. *Experimental Brain Research*, **52**, 41–9.

McNaughton, B. L., Barnes, C. A., Meltzer, J., and Sutherland, R. J. (1989). Hippocampal granule cells are necessary for normal spatial learning but not for spatially-selective pyramidal cell discharge. *Experimental Brain Research*, **76**, 485–96.

McNaughton, B. L., Leonard, B., and Chen, L. (1989). Cortical–hippocampal interactions and cognitive mapping: a hypothesis based on reintegration of the parietal and inferotemporal pathways for visual processing. *Psychobiology*, **17**, 230–5.

Mizumori, S. J. Y., Barnes, C. A., and McNaughton, B. L. (1989a). Reversible inactivation of the medial septum: selective effects on the spontaneous unit activity of different hippocampal cell types. *Brain Research*, **500**, 99–106.

Mizumori, S. J. Y., McNaughton, B. L., Barnes, C. A., and Fox, K. (1989b). Preserved spatial coding in hippocampal CA1 pyramidal cells during reversible suppression of CA3c output: evidence for pattern completion in hippocampus. *Journal of Neuroscience*, **9**, 3915–28.

Morris, R. G. M., Hagan, J. J., and Rawlins, J. N. P. (1986). Allocentric spatial learning by hippocampectomised rats: a further test of the 'spatial mapping' and 'working memory' theories of hippocampal function. *Quarterly Journal of Experimental Psychology*, **38B**, 365–95.

Muller, R. U. and Kubie, J. L. (1987). The effects of changes in the environment on the spatial firing of hippocampal complex-spike cells. *Journal of Neuroscience*, **7**, 1951–68.

Muller, R. U. and Kubie, J. L. (1989). The firing of hippocampal place cells predicts the future position of freely moving rats. *Journal of Neuroscience*, **9**, 4101–10.

Muller, R. U., Kubie, J. L., and Ranck, J. B., Jr., (1987). Spatial firing patterns of hippocampal complex-spike cells in a fixed environment. *Journal of Neuroscience*, **7**, 1935–50.

Neisser, U. (1976). *Cognition and reality*. W. S. Freeman, San Francisco.

O'Keefe, J. (1983). Spatial memory within and without the hippocampal system. *Neurobiology of the hippocampus* (ed. W. Seifert), pp. 375–403. Academic Press, London.

O'Keefe, J. (1990). A computational theory of the hippocampal cognitive map. *Progress in brain research* (ed. J. Storm-Mathisen, J. Zimmer, and O. P. Ohersen), pp. 301–12. Elsevier, Amsterdam.

O'Keefe, J. and Conway, D. H. (1978). Hippocampal place units in the freely moving rat: why they fire where they fire. *Experimental Brain Research*, **31**, 573–90.

O'Keefe J. and Conway, D. H. (1980). On the trail of the hippocampal engram. *Physiological Psychology*, **8**, 229–38.

O'Keefe, J. and Nadel, L. (1978). *The hippocampus as a cognitive map*. Clarendon, Oxford.

O'Keefe, J. and Speakman, A. (1987). Single unit activity in the rat hippocampus during a spatial memory task. *Experimental Brain Research*, **68**, 1–27.

Olton, D. S. (1982). Spatially organized behaviors of animals: behavioral and neurological studies. In *Spatial abilities. Developmental and physiological foundations* (ed. M. Potegal), pp. 335–60. Academic Press, New York.

Olton, D. S., Branch, M., and Best, P. (1978). Spatial correlates of hippocampal unit activity. *Experimental Neurology*, **58**, 387–409.

Olton, D. S., Becker, J. T., and Handelmann, G. E. (1979). Hippocampus, space and memory. *Behavioral and Brain Sciences*, **2**, 313–65.

Paillard, J. (1987). Cognitive versus sensorimotor encoding of spatial information. *Cognitive processes and spatial orientation in animal and man* (ed. P. Ellen and C. Thinus-Blanc), pp. 97–106. Martinus Nijhoff, Dordrecht.

Piaget, J. (1936). *La naissance de l'intelligence chez l'enfant*. Delachaux et Niestlé, Neuchâtel.

Poucet, B. (1985). Spatial behaviour of cats in cue-controlled environments. *Quarterly Journal of Experimental Psychology*, **37B**, 155–79.

Poucet, B. (1989). Object exploration, habituation and response to a spatial change in rats following septal or medial frontal cortical damage. *Behavioral Neuroscience*, **103**, 1009–16.

Poucet, B., Thinus-Blanc, C., and Chapuis, N. (1983). Route-planning in cats, in relation to the visibility of the goal. *Animal Behaviour*, **31**, 594–9.

Poucet, B., Chapuis, N., Durup, M., and Thinus-Blanc, C. (1986). A study of exploratory behaviour as an index of spatial knowledge in hamsters. *Animal Learning and Behavior*, **14**, 93–100.

Pribram, K. H. (1969). The neurophysiology of remembering. *Scientific American*, **200**, 73–86.

Ranck, J. B., Jr. (1973). Studies on single neurons in dorsal hippocampal formation

and septum in unrestrained rats. Part I. Behavioral correlates and firing reper-
toires. *Experimental Neurology*, **41**, 462–531.

Raphelson, A. C., Isaacson, R. L., and Douglas, R. J. (1985). The effect of
distracting stimuli on the runway performance of limbic-damaged rats. *Psychonomic Science*, **3**, 483–4.

Rasmussen, M., Barnes, C. A., and McNaughton, B. L. (1989). A systematic test
of cognitive mapping, working memory, and temporal discontinuity theories of
hippocampal formation. *Psychobiology*, **17**, 335–48.

Renner, M. J. (1988). Learning during exploration: the role of behavioral
topography during exploration in determining subsequent adaptive behaviour.
International Journal of Comparative Psychology, **2**, 43–56.

Sandkuhler, J., Maisch, B., and Zimmermann, M. (1987). The use of local anes-
thetic microinjections to identify central pathways: a quantitative evaluation of
the time course and extent of the neuronal block. *Experimental Brain Research*,
68, 168–78.

Sharp, P. E., McNaughton, B. L., and Barnes, C. A. (1989). Exploration-
dependent evoked responses in fascia dentata: fundamental observations and
time-course. *Psychobiology*, **17**, 257–69.

Strelow, E. R. (1985). What is needed for a theory of mobility: direct perception
and cognitive maps—Lessons from the blind. *Psychological Review*, **92**, 226–48.

Sutherland, R. J. (1985). The navigating hippocampus: an individual medley of
space, memory and movement. In *Electrical activity of the archicortex* (ed. G.
Buzsaki and C. H. Vanderwolf), pp. 255–79. Akadémiai Kiado, Budapest.

Sutherland, R. J. and Rudy, J. W. (1989). Configural association theory: the role of
the hippocampal formation in learning, memory, and amnesia. *Psychobiology*,
17, 129–44.

Thinus-Blanc, C. (1988). Animal spatial cognition. In *Thought without language*
(ed. L. Weiskrantz), pp. 371–95. Clarendon Press, Oxford.

Thinus-Blanc, C. and Ingle, D. (1985). Spatial behavior in gerbils (*Meriones
unguiculatus*). *Journal of Comparative Psychology*, **99**, 311–15.

Thinus-Blanc, C., Bouzouba, L., Chaix, K., Chapuis, N., Durup, M., and Poucet,
B. (1987). A study of spatial parameters encoded during exploration in hamsters.
Journal of Experimental Psychology: Animal Behavior Processes, **13**, 418–27.

Vanderwolf, C. H. (1971). Limbic–diencephalic mechanisms of voluntary movement. *Psychological Review*, **78**, 83–113.

Wiener, S. I., Paul, C. A., and Eichenbaum, H. (1989). Spatial and behavioral
correlates of hippocampal neuronal activity. *Journal of Neuroscience*, **9**, 2737–
63.

Zipser, D. (1986). Biologically plausible models of place recognition and goal
location. Parallel distributed processing. Exploration in the microstructure of
cognition. Vol. 2. *Psychological and biological models* (ed. J. L. McClelland, D.
E. Rumelhart, and the PDP Research Group), pp. 432–70. MIT Press, Cambridge, Mass.

19

Functions of the primate hippocampus in spatial processing and memory

EDMUND T. ROLLS

The aims of this chapter are to consider which spatial functions are performed by the primate hippocampus, how these are related to its memory functions, and how it performs these functions. In addition to the evidence that is available from anatomical connections, the effects of lesions to the system, and recordings of the activity of single neurons in the system, neuronal network models of hippocampal function will also be introduced, as they have the promise of enabling one to understand what and how the hippocampus computes, and thus the functions being performed. Many of the studies described have been with macaque monkeys in order to provide information as relevant as possible to understanding amnesia in humans. Effects on memory are produced by damage to the hippocampus or to some of its connections, such as the fornix, and these structures are collectively referred to below as the hippocampal system.

Damage to the hippocampal system and spatial function

Damage to the hippocampus or to some of its connections, such as the fornix, produced, in monkeys, deficits in simple left–right discrimination learning in which, for example, food is hidden consistently on the right or left under one of two identical objects, and the monkey must learn whether to displace the left or right object in order to find food (Mahut 1972). Fornix lesions also impair conditional left–right discrimination learning, in which the visual appearance of an object specifies whether a response is to be made to the left or right (Gaffan *et al.* 1984b; Rupniak and Gaffan 1987; [and in humans] Petrides 1985). (An example of such a conditional spatial-response task is that if two objects shown are red, then the object on the left must be chosen to obtain a reward, and if the two objects shown are green, then the object on the right must be chosen to obtain a reward.) Two possible interpretations of these impairments of spatial learning produced by fornix section are as follows.

First, the learning system so disrupted may only be for the acquisition of map-like knowledge about the environment, such as that there is food in a certain place. However, this is not the case, in that lesioned monkeys were impaired in learning to make a response to one side when one picture was shown, and to the other side when a different picture was shown (Rupniak and Gaffan 1987), that is, impaired in conditional spatial-response learning as described above. The spatial environment was held constant, and thus damage to the hippocampal system does not impair only the ability to acquire map-like knowledge of the environment. The experiment does show, on the other hand, that there is an impairment when monkeys must learn to make spatial responses on the basis of non-spatial stimuli.

Second, the hippocampal learning system may only be for the control of spatially directed movements, such as 'go left' and 'go right'. However, this is not the case either, for fornix-sectioned monkeys are impaired in learning on the basis of a spatial cue for which object to choose (e.g. if two objects are on the left, choose object A, but if the two objects are on the right, choose object B; Gaffan and Harrison 1989a). Thus the deficit is not just in learning spatial responses, for in this task the response was not spatial. The spatial aspect of this task was in the position of the stimuli.

These findings suggest that fornix damage can impair learning both about the places of objects and the places of responses. Gaffan and Harrison (1989b) have analysed further what it is that characterizes the spatial-learning deficit of monkeys with damage to the hippocampal system in experiments in which the animal was moved to different positions in a room. Impairments were found when which of two or more objects it had to choose from depended on its position in the room, provided that the same parts of the room were in view from both of its positions so that the relative positions of room cues had to be remembered in order to solve the task (Gaffan and Harrison 1989b; experiment 1). This requirement is referred to as 'whole scene analysis'. If the parts of the room visible from the monkeys' positions were different, then there was no impairment in learning which object to choose (Gaffan and Harrison 1989b; experiment 2). However, if the monkeys had to make a spatial response to one of two identical objects that depended on different environmental cues (whether room-based or local), then those that were fornix-sectioned displayed a learning impairment (Gaffan and Harrison 1989b; experiments 3 and 5). These experiments suggest that fornix-sectioned monkeys can predict which of two different objects is rewarded, based on a conjunction of background items in the environment and the object displaced. Accordingly, they can thus choose one of two (visually) different objects in a scene, provided that the scene has different items visible in it, whether locally or distantly. However, a deficit is produced by fornix section when the monkey has to store the spatial relations of the background items and of identical objects in a scene. Accordingly, the fornix-sectioned monkeys are impaired in learning to select different objects, depending on the spatial relations of items in the scene, or in learning to make spatial responses to identical objects in a scene, as these involve storing the relative positions of places to which to respond (Gaffan and Harrison 1989b).

Another spatial task that is impaired by damage to the hippocampal system in monkeys (Gaffan and Saunders 1985; Parkinson *et al.* 1988) and humans (Smith and Milner 1981) is an object–place memory task. In this task, not only which objects have been seen before but where in space each object was located, must be remembered. The task has been run with macaques by showing a picture in each of four positions on a screen twice (Rolls *et al.* 1989). The first time the monkey saw the picture in a particular position, he had to withold a lick response (in order to avoid saline). The second time a picture appeared in a given position on the screen, the monkey could lick to obtain fruit juice. Each picture was shown in each position twice, once as novel and once as familiar for that position, and many different pictures were used in sequence. Thus, in order to perform the task, the monkey had to remember not only which pictures had been seen before but also the position on the screen in which the picture had been seen. In humans, the object–place task was run by showing the subjects a tray containing a set of objects, and then asking later not only which objects had been seen before but where they were on the tray (Smith and Milner 1981). Such object–place tasks require a whole scene or snapshot-like memory, in which spatial relations in a scene must be remembered. It is not enough just to be able to remember the objects that have been seen before. The deficit in the object–place memory task is thus analogous to the deficit in the spatial tasks described above, in that it is fully apparent when not just objects but objects and their spatial relations to each other must be remembered.

Non-spatial aspects of the function of the hippocampus in primates: its role in memory.

In addition to these spatial deficits produced by damage to the hippocampal system in primates, there are also deficits in non-spatial memory tasks. For example the anterograde amnesia that is associated with damage to the hippocampus in humans is evident as a major deficit in learning to recognize new stimuli, and the deficit in recognition memory encompasses non-spatial items (e.g. objects and people) as well as places (Scoville and Milner 1957; Milner 1972; Squire 1986; Squire and Zola-Morgan 1988). Recognition memory is also impaired in monkeys with damage to the hippocampal system (Gaffan 1974, 1977; Gaffan and Weiskrantz 1980; Owen and Butler 1981; Zola-Morgan *et al.* 1986), although it is possible that severe deficits of recognition memory are only found when there is also damage to the amygdala (Mishkin 1978, 1982; Murray and Mishkin

1984). In a typical recognition-memory task in the monkey, a stimulus is shown to the animal, and when it is shown again later, it can choose it to obtain a reward. If no other stimuli intervene between the first and second present-ations of a given stimulus, then the task is described as a match-to-sample task. If other stimuli intervene between the first (novel) and second (familiar) presentations, then the task is described as a serial or running recognition task. A serial recognition task is often used when analysing the role of the hippocampus in memory, because a memory task with intervening stimuli is more difficult than a delayed match-to-sample task, and may therefore be a more sensitive indicator of an effect on memory (Gaffan 1974, 1977).

It is interesting that the impairment produced by damage to the hippo-campal system in recognition-memory tasks as usually implemented (e.g. choose or respond to objects seen before—that is, delayed match to sample—perhaps with intervening stimuli) is much less clear if delayed, non-match to sample is used (choose the novel stimulus; Gaffan *et al.* 1984a). The impairment is also much less severe if the monkeys are trained initially with the long (and therefore difficult) intervals between stimuli with which they are tested later (Gaffan *et al.* 1984a). The implication of these findings is that the deficit produced by the fornix section is not simply due to an inability to distinguish novel from familiar stimuli, but is due perhaps just as much to a difficulty these lesioned animals have in altering their instrumental response strategies—for example, so that they respond to familiar stimuli when the natural tendency is to respond to novel stimuli, and so that they start responding at long memory intervals when they have been trained previously to respond with short memory intervals (see Gaffan *et al.* 1984a,b). However, although the deficit usually found in recognition-memory tasks may not strictly be due to an inability to distinguish novel from familiar stimuli, there is nevertheless a non-spatial impairment apparent in recognition-memory tasks. Another non-spatial impairment produced by fornix section in monkeys is a deficit in learning the unnatural, instrumental response rule 'Choose the object not previously paired with reward' (sometimes called a win–shift rule; Gaffan *et al.* 1984b). (Fornix section did not impair use of the natural instrumental rule 'Choose the object previously associated with reward', sometimes called the win–stay rule; Gaffan *et al.* 1984b). Thus, in monkeys, hippocampal function is not only involved in some types of spatial learning, but also in some aspect of non-spatial learning, even if this latter may not be pure novelty versus familiarity learning but is instead related in some way to organizing flexibly adaptive, instrumental responses.

There is also the evidence from humans that the hippocampus is in-volved in non-spatial (as well as spatial) memory, for example in paired (word) associate learning, and in episodic memory, such as the memory of events that happened and of people met on previous days.

Relation between spatial and non-spatial aspects of hippocampal function

One way of relating the impairment of spatial processing to other aspects of hippocampal function is to understand that this processing involves a snapshot type of memory, in which one whole scene must be remembered. This memory may then be a special case of episodic memory, which involves an arbitrary association of a set of events that describes a past episode. Further, the non-spatial tasks impaired by damage to the hippocampal system may be impaired because they are tasks in which a memory of a particular episode rather than of a general rule is involved. Thus the learning of tasks with non-general rules, such as choose the object not previously rewarded (i.e. win–shift, lose–stay) may be impaired because, to solve them, the particular pairing in the particular context (of performing with this special rule) must be remembered in order to choose the correct object later. (The natural rule, which will in the natural environment usually lead to reward, is to choose the object previously associated with reward.) Another example is that choosing familiar rather than novel objects in a recognition-memory task may be particularly difficult for monkeys with damage to the hippocampal system because it involves a special rule—choose the familiar object in this task—rather than what may be a more general tendency, that is to choose the novel rather than the familiar object. The latter rule is what normally guides behaviour, as this rule is more likely to lead to reward for objects without an explicit reward association already in the natural environment. Further, recognition memory may be particularly impaired when this involves the memory of particular and arbitrary associations between parts of the image, especially when the same elements may occur in different combinations in other images. Also, the deficit in paired associate learning in humans may be especially evident when this involves arbitrary associations between words; for example, window—lake. I suggest that the reason why the hippocampus is used for the spatial and non-spatial types of memory described above, and the reason that makes these two types of memory so analogous, is that the hippocampus contains one stage, the CA3 stage, which acts as an auto-association memory. (The structure, operation, and properties of auto-association memories are described below.) An auto-association memory implemented by the CA3 neurons would equally enable whole (spatial) scenes or episodic memories to be formed, with a snapshot quality which depends on the arbitrary associations that can be made and on the short temporal 'window' that characterizes the synaptic modifiability in this system (see below, and Rolls 1987, 1989a,b). The way in which the architecture of the hippocampus is specialized to perform these functions in spatial, snapshot, and episodic memory is described next, in order to lead towards a deeper understanding of hippocampal function in these types of learning.

The computational significance of the functional architecture of the hippocampus

The internal connections of the hippocampus and the learning rules implemented at its synapses will be described first to delineate its functional architecture, which provides the basis for a computational theory of the hippocampus.

Schematic diagrams of the connections of the hippocampus are shown in Figs. 19.1 and 2. In primates, major input connections are from the association areas of the cerebral cortex, including the parietal cortex (which processes spatial information), the temporal-lobe visual and auditory areas, and the frontal cortex. Within the hippocampus, there is a three-stage sequence of processing, consisting of the dentate granule cells (which receive from the entorhinal cortex via the perforant path), the CA3 pyramidal cells, and the CA1 pyramidal cells (see below). Outputs return from the hippocampus to the cerebral cortex via the subiculum, entorhinal cortex, and para-hippocampal gyrus.

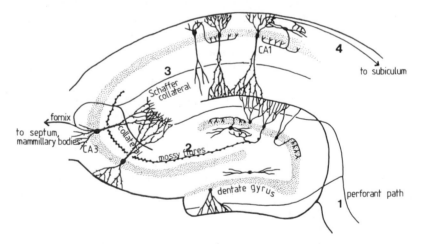

Fig. 19.1. Representation of connections within the hippocampus. Inputs reach the hippocampus through the perforant path (1), which makes synapses with the dendrites of the dentate granule cells and also with the apical dendrites of the CA3 pyramidal cells. The dentate granule cells project via the mossy fibres (2) to the CA3 pyramidal cells. The well-developed, recurrent collateral system of the CA3 cells is indicated. The CA3 pyramidal cells project via the Schaffer collaterals (3) to the CA1 pyramidal cells, which in turn have connections (4) to the subculum.

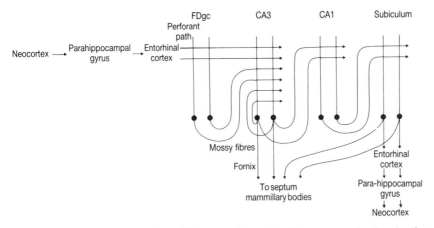

Fig. 19.2. Schematic representation of the connections of the hippocampus, showing also that the cerebral cortex (neocortex) is connected to the hippocampus via the para-hippocampal gyrus and entorhinal cortex, and that the hippocampus projects back to the neocortex via the subiculum, entorhinal cortex, and para-hippocampal gyrus; FDgc—dentate granule cells.

The CA3 pyramidal cells

One major feature of hippocampal neuronal networks is the recurrent collateral system of the CA3 cells, formed by the output axons of the CA3 cells having a branch that returns to make synapses with the dendrites of the other CA3 cells, as shown in Figs. 19.1 and 2. Given that the region of the CA3 cell dendrites on which the recurrent collaterals synapse is long (approximately 12 mm), that the total dendritic length is approximately 16 mm and has approximately 16 000 spines (Amaral, Ishizuka, and Claiborne 1990; Squire, Shimamura, and Amaral 1989), and that each spine receives one synapse, approximately 12 000 synapses per CA3 pyramidal cell could be devoted to recurrent collaterals, which with 304 000 CA3 neurons on each side of the brain in the (Sprague–Dawley) rat (Boss *et al.* 1987; Amaral *et al.* 1990), makes the probability of contact between the CA3 neurons 3.9 per cent. ((The quantitative values given here have been updated a little from those given by Rolls (1989a,b) in the light of new estimates provided by Amaral *et al.* (1990).) It is remarkable that the contact probability is so high, and also that the CA3 recurrent collateral axons travel so widely in all directions that they can potentially come close to almost all other CA3 neurons (D. G. Amaral, personal communication; Amaral and Witter 1989; Squire, Shimamura, and Amaral 1989; Rolls 1989a,b). The connectivity of these CA3 cells is even more remarkable than this, for in addition there is a commissural system in which CA3 neurons on one side of the brain send axons to end primarily on the dendrites of the CA3 neurons of the other side of the brain. The terminals are made on the same

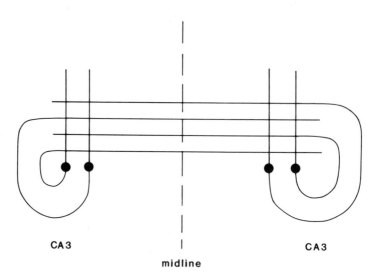

Fig. 19.3. Schematic representation of the connections of the CA3 neurons, showing that they are interconnected across the midline by commissural connections, as well as on each side of the brain via the recurrent collateral axons.

stretch of the CA3 dendrites as the recurrent collaterals, so that the contact probability calculated above must be reduced (with the lower limit being perhaps 2.0 per cent, representing 12 000 synapses shared among 608 000 CA3 neurons). The remarkable effect achieved by this is that the CA3 neurons provide one interconnected network of neurons for both sides of the brain, with a reasonably high probability that any CA3 neuron will be connected to any other CA3 neuron, irrespective of the side of the brain, as illustrated in Fig. 19.3. Although connectivity across the midline is likely to be high in the rat, as implied in Fig. 19.3, the two sides of the hippocampus are probably not fully interconnected in humans, as indicated by the evidence that damage to the right temporal lobe affects spatial tasks (such as conditional, spatial-response learning) more than non-spatial memory tasks, whereas damage to the left temporal lobe affects non-spatial tasks (such as paired-word associate learning) more than spatial tasks (Milner 1982; Kolb and Whishaw 1985).

There is evidence from studies of long-term potentiation (Bliss and Lomo 1973; Kelso et al. 1986; Wigstrom et al. 1986; Andersen 1987) that the synapses in this recurrent collateral system are Hebb modifiable, that is that they become stronger when there is strong conjunctive post-synaptic and pre-synaptic activity (Miles 1988).

INPUT STIMULUS

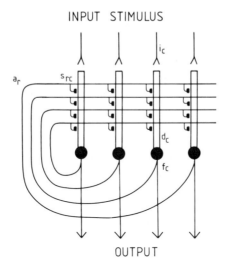

OUTPUT

Fig. 19.4. An auto-association matrix memory. The dendrites, d_c, have recurrent collateral axons, a_r, which make Hebb-modifiable synapses, s_{rc}, with the other neurons in the population. The inputs i_c reach the network through unmodifiable synapses, and produce firing rate f_c.

An auto-association memory implemented by the CA3, recurrent collateral system

This functional anatomy of the CA3 pyramidal cells immediately suggests that this is an auto-association (or autocorrelation) matrix memory. The auto-association arises because the outputs of the CA3 cells are fed back by the recurrent collateral axons to make Hebb-modifiable synapses with the dendrites of the other CA3 neurons. The result of implementation of the Hebb rule in this architecture is that any strongly activated cell or set of cells becomes linked by strengthened synapses with any other conjunctively strongly activated cell or set of cells. During learning, the matrix of synaptic weights that links the cells together (see Fig. 19.4) comes to reflect the correlations between the activities of the CA3 cells. Because the matrix of synaptic weights stores the correlations between the activities of the cells of the memory, this type of memory is called an autocorrelation or auto-association matrix memory. During recall, presentation of even a part of the original pattern of activity of the CA3 cells, which might represent one part of, or key to, the memory, comes to elicit the firing of the whole set of cells that was originally conjunctively activated. This important property is termed completion, and is fundamental to any biological memory system. During recall, if a pattern similar to one learned by the system is presented, then, in so far as some of the neurons active in the key stimulus were also part of a pattern stored previously in the memory, the previously stored pattern is recalled. This property, which is also fundamental to biological memory, is termed generalization. Another property of this type of memory is that it continues to function moderately well if it is partially damaged, or if, for example, not every synapse in the matrix is present, either because of limitations of fan in of individual neurons, or because of limitations of the precision of development. This property is also important for a biological memory system, and is termed graceful degradation or fault tolerance. More extensive descriptions of the properties of auto-association matrix memories are given by Kohonen et al. (1981), Kohonen (1984) and Rolls (1987). The suggestion made here is that the output of the CA3 pyramidal cells is fed back along the horizontally running, recurrent collateral axons that make Hebb-modifiable synapses with other CA3 dendrites so that the pattern of activity in the CA3 pyramidal cells is associated with itself.

For this auto-association to work correctly it is important that a depolarization produced by synaptic input on one part of the dendrite is effective on other parts of the dendrite, such that even distant, active synapses experience the post-synaptic term required for the Hebb rule to be implemented. This condition does appear to be met, as shown by the short electrical length of the dendrites and by the co-operativity which occurs between inputs that synapse on different parts of the dendrite in setting up the post-synaptic depolarization required for long-term potentiation (Andersen 1987; McNaughton 1984). This co-operation between active synapses made at different positions along the post-synaptic membrane, such that active synapses on to a neuron alter their strength only when other synapses are active on the same dendrite and produce post-synaptic activation, enables associations to be formed which are based on temporal conjunctions that occur between any set of conjunctively active afferents. In a sense, the large number of synapses of these CA3 cells devoted to the recurrent collaterals allows correlations of firing across a large information space to be detected. Consistent with this suggestion about the computational role of the CA3 system of the hippocampus, it is known that the probability of contact of the neurons in an auto-association matrix memory must not be very low if it is to operate usefully (see Marr 1971; Gardner-Medwin 1976). The synaptic modifiability implemented in the CA3 recurrent collateral system may use NMDA receptors (N-methyl-D-aspartate), which allow synaptic modifiability only when the post-synaptic membrane is strongly activated. This interesting non-linearity of the learning rule means that only correlations between strongly activated CA3 pyramidal cells are stored, which may help to maximize the storage capacity of the system and to minimize interference.

It is suggested below that the systems-level function of this auto-association memory is to enable events occurring conjunctively in quite different parts of the association areas of the cerebral cortex to be associated together to form a memory that could well be described as episodic. Each episode would be defined by a conjunction of a set of events, and each episodic memory would consist of the association of one set of events (such as where, with whom, and what one ate at lunch on the preceding day). It is suggested that the 'snapshot, whole scene' spatial memory in which the hippocampus is implicated, as shown above, is what the hippocampus can achieve for spatial information processing, by allowing all the parts of a whole scene to be associated together to provide a memory of that scene. The importance of the hippocampus in episodic and in 'whole scene' memory may arise from the fact that in one part of it, the CA3 region, there is one association matrix with a relatively high contact probability which receives information originating in many different areas of the cerebral cortex, and from both sides of the brain. One reason why there may not be more cells in the CA3 region is that it is important that the connectivity be kept relatively high so that any event represented by the firing of a sparse set of CA3 cells can be associated with any other event represented by the firing of a different set of CA3 cells. Because each CA3 pyramidal cell has a limited fan in or number of synapses (perhaps 16 000, see above), the total number of cells in the auto-association memory cannot be increased beyond the limit set by the fan in and the connectivity. The advantages of sparse encoding and a well-interconnected matrix are that a large number of different (episodic) memories can be stored in the CA3 system, and that the advantageous, emergent properties of a matrix memory, such as completion, generalization, and graceful degradation (see Kohonen *et al.* 1977, 1981; Kohonen 1984; Rolls 1987) are produced efficiently. Completion may operate particularly effectively here with a sparse representation, because it is under these conditions that the simple, autocorrelation effect can reconstruct the whole of one pattern without the interference that would arise if too high a proportion of the input neurons was active.

The dentate granule cells and the CA1 pyramidal cells

The theory is developed elsewhere that the dentate granule-cell stage of hippocampal processing which precedes the CA3 stage acts in two ways to produce the sparse yet efficient (i.e. non-redundant) representation in CA3 neurons that is required for the auto-association to perform well (Rolls 1989a,b). The first way is that the perforant path–dentate granule-cell system, with its Hebb-like modifiability, could act as a competitive learning matrix to remove redundancy from the inputs, so producing a more orthogonal and categorized set of outputs. The second way arises because there is a very low (0.005 per cent in the rat) contact probability in the mossy fibre–CA3 connections, which achieves, by pattern separation, relatively orthogonal representations (compared to those on the dentate granule cells, and within the limits set by the relative numbers of dentate granule and CA3 cells—see Rolls 1989a and Amaral *et al.* 1990). This separation is required if the auto-association matrix memory formed by the CA3 cells is to operate with a usefully large capacity and with minimal interference (see Kohonen *et al.* 1977, 1981; Rolls 1987). As the neurons have positive, continuous firing rates, the only way in which relatively orthogonal representations can be formed is by making the number of neurons active for any one input stimulus relatively low (see, for example, Jordan 1986), and this sparse representation is exactly what can be achieved by the low contact probability, pattern separation effect of the mossy fibres (Rolls 1989a,b). By the pattern separation effect is meant that input patterns which are correlated produce output patterns which are less correlated with each other.

The function of the CA1 stage that follows the CA3 cells (see Figs. 19.1 and 2) is also considered to be related to the CA3 auto-association effect, in which several arbitrary patterns of firing occur together on the CA3 neurons and become associated together to form an episodic or 'whole scene' memory. It is essential for this operation that several different, sparse representations are present conjunctively in order to form the association. Moreover, when completion operates in the CA3 auto-association system, all the neurons firing in the original conjunction can be brought into activity by only a part of the original set of conjunctive events. For these reasons, a memory in the CA3 cells consists of several, different, simultaneously active ensembles of activity. It is suggested that the CA1 cells, which receive these groups of simultaneously active ensembles, can detect the conjunctions of firing of the different ensembles that represent the episodic memory and allocate, by competitive learning, a relatively few neurons to represent each episodic memory. The episodic memory would thus consist, in the CA3 region, of ensembles of active cells, each ensemble representing one of the sub-components of the episodic memory (including context), whereas the whole episodic memory would be represented not by its parts but as a single collection of active cells at the CA1 stage. It is suggested below that one role of these economical (in terms of the number of activated fibres) and relatively orthogonal signals in the CA1 cells is to guide information storage or consolidation in the cerebral cortex. To understand how the hippocampus may perform this function for the cortex, it is necessary to turn to a systems-level analysis to show how the computations performed by the hippocampus fit into overall brain function. It may be noted that by forming associations of events derived from different parts of the cerebral cortex (the CA3 stage), and by building new economical (i.e. less redundant) representations of the conjunctions detected (the CA1 stage), the hippocampus provides an output that is suitable for directing the long-term storage of information.

Systems-level analysis of hippocampal function, including neuronal activity in the primate hippocampus

I have just used the functional architecture (internal anatomy and physiology) of the hippocampus to suggest a computational theory of how it operates. In order to understand what these computations are used for, and how they contribute to the information processing being performed by other parts of the brain, I now turn to a systems-level analysis in which I consider the connections of the hippocampus with the rest of the brain, and the activity of single neurons in the hippocampus when it is performing its normal function, as assessed by the effects of selective damage to the hippocampus described above.

Systems-level anatomy

The primate hippocampus receives inputs via the entorhinal cortex (area 28) and the para-hippocampal gyrus from many areas of the cerebral association cortex including the parietal cortex, which is concerned with spatial functions, the visual and auditory temporal association cortical areas, and the frontal cortex (Van Hoesen 1982; Amaral 1987; Rolls 1989a, b). In addition, the entorhinal cortex receives inputs from the amygdala. There are also sub-cortical inputs from, for example, the amygdala and septum. The hippocampus in turn projects back via the subiculum, entorhinal cortex, and para-hippocampal gyrus (area TF–TH), to the cerebral cortical areas from which it receives inputs (Van Hoesen 1982), as well as to sub-cortical areas such as the mammillary bodies (see Figs. 19.1 and 19.2).

Systems-level neurophysiology

Information processing by the primate hippocampus while it is performing the functions for which lesion studies have shown it is needed has been investigated in experiments in which the activity of single hippocampal neurons has been analysed during the performance and learning of these (and related) spatial tasks. Watanabe and Niki (1985) analysed hippocampal, neuronal activity while monkeys performed a delayed spatial-response task. In such a task, a stimulus is shown on, for example, the left; there is then a delay period, and after this the monkey can respond by, for example, touching the left stimulus position. They reported that 6.4 per cent of hippocampal neurons responded differently while the monkey was remembering left as compared to right. The responses of these neurons could reflect preparation for the spatial response to be made, or they could reflect memory of the spatial position in which the stimulus was shown. To provide evidence on which was important, Cahusac *et al.* (1989) analysed hippocampal activity in this task, and in an object–place memory task. In the object–place task, the monkey was shown a sample stimulus in one position on a video screen, there was a delay of 2 s, and then the same or a different stimulus was shown in the same or in a different position. The monkey remembered the sample and its position, and if both matched the delayed stimulus, he licked to obtain fruit juice. Of the 600 neurons analysed in this task, 3.8 per cent responded differently for the different spatial positions, with some of these responding differentially during the sample presentation, some in the delay period, and some in the match period. Thus some hippocampal neurons (those differentially active in the sample or match periods) respond differently to stimuli shown in different positions in space, and some (those differentially active in the delay period) respond differently when the monkey is remembering different positions in space. In addition, some of the neurons responded to a combination of object and place information, in that they responded only to a novel object in a particular place. These neuronal responses were not due to any response being made or prepared by the monkey, for information about which behavioural response was required was not available until the match stimulus was shown. Cahusac *et al.* also found that the majority of the neurons that responded in the object–place memory task did not respond in the delayed spatial response task. Instead, a different population of neurons (5.7 per cent of the total) responded in the delayed spatial response task, with differential left–right responses in the sample, delay, or match periods. Thus this latter population of hippocampal neurons had activity that was related to the preparation for, or initiation of, a spatial response, which in the delayed response task could be encoded as soon as the sample stimulus was seen. These recordings showed there are some neurons in the primate hippocampus with activity that is related to the spatial position of stimuli or to the memory of the spatial position of stimuli (as shown in the object–place memory task); and that there are other neurons in the hippocampus with activity related not to the stimulus or the memory of the stimulus, but instead to the spatial response that the monkey is preparing and remembering (as shown in the delayed spatial response task).

The responses of hippocampal neurons in primates to activity related to the place in which a stimulus is shown was further investigated using a serial, multiple object–place, memory task. The task required a memory for the position on a video monitor in which a given object had appeared previously (Rolls *et al.* 1989). This task was designed to allow a wider area of space to be tested than in the previous study, and was chosen also because memory of where objects had been seen previously in space was known to be disrupted by hippocampal damage (Gaffan and Saunders

1985; Gaffan 1987). In the task, a visual image appeared in one of four or nine positions on a screen. If the stimulus had been seen in that position before, the monkey could lick to obtain fruit juice; but if it had not, the monkey had not to lick in order to avoid the taste of saline. Each image appeared in each position on the screen only twice, once as novel, and once as familiar. The task thus required memory not only of which visual stimuli had been seen before, but of the positions in which they had been seen, and is an object–place memory task. It was found that 9 per cent of neurons recorded in the hippocampus and para-hippocampal gyrus had spatial fields in this and related tasks, in that they responded whenever there was a stimulus in some but not in other positions on the screen. Of the neurons, 2.4 per cent responded to a combination of spatial information and information about the object seen, in that they responded more the first time a particular image was seen in any position. Six of these neurons were found that showed this combination even more clearly, in that they, for example, responded only to some positions, and only provided it was the first time that a particular stimulus had appeared there. Thus, not only is spatial information processed by the primate hippocampus, but also it can be combined, as shown by the responses of single neurons, with information about which stimuli have been seen before (Rolls *et al.* 1989).

The ability of the hippocampus to form such arbitrary associations of information (probably originating from the parietal cortex) about position in space with information originating from the temporal lobe about objects may be important for its role in memory. Moreover, these findings provide neurophysiological support for the computational theory described above, according to which such arbitrary associations should be formed onto single neurons in the hippocampus.

These 'space' neurons (Cahusac *et al.* 1989; Rolls *et al.* 1989) may be compared with 'place' cells recorded in the rat hippocampus (see McNaughton *et al.* 1983; O'Keefe 1984). The place cells described in the rat respond when the animal is in a particular place in the environment as specified by extra-maze cues, whereas the cells described here respond to particular positions in space, or at least when stimuli are shown in particular positions in space (see further Feigenbaum and Rolls 1990).

These studies therefore showed that some hippocampal neurons in primates have spatial fields. In order to investigate how space is represented in the hippocampus, Feigenbaum *et al.* (1987), and Feigenbaum and Rolls (1990), investigated whether the spatial fields use egocentric or some form of allocentric co-ordinates. This was done by finding a neuron with a space field, and then moving the monitor screen and the monkey relative to each other, and to different positions in the laboratory. For 10 per cent of the spatial neurons, the responses remained in the same position relative to the monkey's body axis when the screen was moved or the monkey was rotated or moved to a different position. These neurons thus represented space in egocentric co-ordinates. For 46 per cent of the spatial neurons analysed, the responses remained in the same position on the screen or in the room when the monkey was rotated or moved to a different position. These neurons thus represented space in allocentric co-ordinates. Evidence for two types of allocentric encoding was found. In the first type, the field was defined by its position on the monitor screen, independently of the position of the monitor relative to the monkey's body axis and independently of the position of the monkey and the screen in the laboratory. These neurons were called 'frame of reference' allocentric, in that their fields were defined by the local frame provided by the monitor screen. The majority of the allocentric neurons responded in this way. In the second type of allocentric encoding, the field was defined by its position in the room, and was relatively independent of position relative to the monkey's body axis or to position on the monitor screen. These neurons were called 'absolute' allocentric, in that their fields were defined by position in the room. These findings provide evidence that in addition to neurons with egocentric spatial fields, which have also been found in other parts of the brain (Sakata 1985; Andersen 1987), there are neurons in the primate hippocampal formation that encode space in allocentric co-ordinates.

In another type of task for which the primate hippocampus is needed—conditional spatial-response learning—in which the monkeys had to learn which spatial response to make to different stimuli (that is, to acquire associations between visual stimuli and spatial responses), 14 per cent of hippocampal neurons responded to particular combinations of stimuli and responses (Miyashita et al. 1989). The firing of these neurons could not be accounted for by the motor requirements of the task, nor wholly by its stimulus aspects, as demonstrated by testing their firing in related, visual discrimination tasks. These findings showed that single hippocampal neurons respond to combinations of the visual stimuli and the spatial responses with which they must become associated in conditional response tasks; they are consistent with the computational theory described above, according to which, part of the mechanism of this learning involves associations between visual stimuli and spatial responses learned by single hippocampal neurons. In a following study, it was found that during such conditional spatial-response learning, 22 per cent of this type of neuron in the hippocampus and para-hippocampal gyrus altered their responses so that their activity, which was initially equal to the two new stimuli, became progressively differential to the two stimuli when the monkey learned to make different responses to the two stimuli (Rolls et al. 1990b). These changes occurred, for different neurons, just before, at, or just after the time when the monkey learned the correct response to make to the stimuli. In addition to these neurons, which had differential responses that were sustained for as long as the recordings continued, another population of neurons (45 per cent of this type of neuron analysed) developed differential activity to the two stimuli, yet showed such responses transiently for only a small number of trials at about the time when the monkey learned. These findings are consistent with the hypothesis that some synapses on hippocampal neurons become modified during this type of learning so that some neurons come to respond to particular stimulus–spatial-response associations that are being learned. Further, the finding that many hippocampal neurons started to reflect the new learning, but then stopped responding differentially (the transient neurons), is consistent with the hypothesis that the hippocampal neurons with large, sustained changes in their activity inhibited the transient neurons, which then underwent reverse learning, thus providing a competitive mechanism by which not all neurons are allocated to any one learned association or event. These transient modifications are consistent with the computational theory outlined above and elsewhere (Rolls 1989a, b), for the return of the neuronal activity to non-differential responsiveness is consistent with an implementation of competitive networks using reverse learning when the post-synaptic neuron is inhibited conjunctively with active afferents (see Rolls 1989c).

The activity of hippocampal neurons in non-human primates has also been analysed during the performance of non-spatial tasks for which the hippocampus is needed, such as recognition memory tasks (Rolls *et al.* 1985, 1990a). It has been found that, in the macaque hippocampus, some neurons do respond differently to novel and familiar stimuli in a serial, recognition memory task, with those that did so typically responding more to novel than to familiar visual stimuli. It was notable that only a small proportion (2.3 per cent) of hippocampal neurons responded in this way, but this is not inconsistent with the hypothesis that the hippocampus is involved in episodic memory. It might be of interest in future studies of recognition memory and hippocampal function to investigate whether there are hippocampal neurons that are tuned to respond to only rather few of a set of stimuli being remembered, and whether the representation found is sparse, as would be useful if the CA3 neurons are to store many different stimuli using an auto-association network. Brown (1982) has also found context sensitivity of hippocampal neurons recorded during a delayed, match-to-sample, memory task (which is consistent with a role in episodic memory, in which context is important), but the task also included a conditional-response component that may have contributed to the neuronal responses found.

Systems-level theory

The effects of damage to the hippocampus indicate that the very long-term storage of information is not in the hippocampus, at least in humans, in that the retrograde amnesia produced by damage to the hippocampal system is not always severe, and in that very old memories (e.g. for events which occurred 30 years previously) are not destroyed (Squire 1986; Squire and Zola-Morgan 1988). On the other hand, the hippocampus does appear to be necessary for the storage of certain types of information (character- ized by the description 'declarative', or 'knowing that', as contrasted with 'procedural', or 'knowing how', which is spared in amnesia). Declarative memory includes what can be declared or brought to mind as a proposition or an image. It includes episodic memory, that is memory for particular episodes, and semantic memory, that is memory for facts (Squire and Zola- Morgan 1988; Squire et al. 1989).

These computational and systems-level analyses suggest that the hippo- campus is specialized to detect the best way in which to store information, and then, by the return paths to the cerebral cortex, to direct memory storage there. The hypothesis is that the CA3 auto-association system is ideal for remembering particular episodes, for perhaps uniquely in the brain it provides a single, auto-association matrix that receives from many different areas of the cerebral association cortex. It is thus able to make almost any arbitrary association, including incorporation, by association, of the context in which a set of events occurred. This auto-association type of memory is also what is required for paired-associate learning, in which arbitrary associations must be made between words and impairment of which is almost a defining test of anterograde amnesia. Impairment of this ability to remember episodes by using the CA3 auto-association matrix memory may also underly many of the memory deficits produced by damage to the hippocampal system. For example, conditional spatial response learning (see Miyashita et al. 1989) may be impaired by hippo- campal damage because a monkey or human cannot make use of the memory of the episode of events on each particular trial, for example that a particular stimulus and a particular response were made, and reward was received. Similarly, object–place memory tasks, also impaired by hippo- campal damage, require associations to be made between particular loca- tions and particular objects—again a natural function for an auto- association memory. Further, the difficulty with memory for places pro- duced by hippocampal damage (see Barnes 1988) may be because a place is normally defined by a conjunction of a number of features or environmen- tal cues or stimuli, and this type of conjunction is normally made by the auto-association memory capability of the hippocampus (see further Rolls et al. 1989). Clearly, the hippocampus—with its large number of synapses on each neuron, its potentiation type of learning, and its CA3 auto- association system—is able to detect when there is conjunctive activation of arbitrary sets of its input fibres, and is able, as indicated both theoretically and by recordings made in the behaving monkey, to allocate neurons economically (i.e. with relatively few neurons active) to code for each complex input (by the output or CA1 stage). Such output neurons could then represent an efficient way in which to store information, in that complex memories with little redundancy could have been generated. In this theory the hippocampus sets up a representation using Hebbian learning, which is useful in determining how information can best be stored in the neocortex, and this representation could provide a useful working memory and therefore this theory is not inconsistent with the possibility that the hippocampus provides a working memory. It may be that by understanding the operations performed by the hippocampus at the neuronal network level, it can be seen how it could contribute to several functions that are not necessarily inconsistent.

The question of how the hippocampal output is used by the neocortex (i.e. cerebral cortex) will be considered next. Given that this output returns to the neocortex, a theory of back-projections in the neocortex will be needed. This is developed elsewhere (Rolls 1989a,b). By way of introduction to this, it may be said that which particular hippocampal neurons happen to represent a complex input event is not determined by any teacher or forcing (unconditioned) stimulus. Thus the neocortex must be able to use the signal rather cleverly. One possibility is that any neocortical neuron, with a number of afferents active at the same time as the hippocampal return fibres in its vicinity, modifies its responses so that it comes to respond better to those afferents the next time they occur. This learning by the cortex would involve a Hebb-like mechanism. One function served by what are thus, in effect, back-projections from the hippocampus is some guidance for, or supervision of, neocortical learning. It is a problem of unsupervised learning systems that they can detect local conjunctions efficiently, but that these are not necessarily those of most use to the whole system. It is exactly this problem that it is proposed the hippocampus helps to solve, by detecting useful conjunctions globally (i.e. over the whole of information space), and then directing storage locally at earlier stages of processing so that filters are built locally which provide representations of input stimuli that are useful for later processing. I also suggest (Rolls 1989a,b) that the back-projections are used for recall, for dynamic adjustment of the processing of earlier stages to facilitate the optimal satisfaction of multiple constraints, and for attention.

Conclusion

A computational theory of the hippocampus is proposed: a key feature is the ability to implement an auto-association memory using the CA3 pyramidal cells. The hippocampus would thereby be involved in both spatial and episodic memory as a result of its ability to form arbitrary associations between input stimuli, so that whole spatial scenes or all the events that comprise a single, episodic memory can be associated together. Recordings from single neurons in the primate hippocampus are consistent with the theory that inputs to it, originating from different parts of the cerebral cortex, are brought together there onto single neurons, and that synaptic modifications within the hippocampus implement the associations. Further work is needed to test the detailed predictions of the theory.

Acknowledgements

The author has worked on some of the experiments and neuronal network modelling described here with A. Bennett, P. M. B. Cahusac, D. Cohen, J. D. Feigenbaum, R. P. Kesner, G. Littlewort, Y. Miyashita, H. Niki, R. Payne, and A. Treves, and their collaboration is sincerely acknowledged. Discussions with David G. Amaral of the Salk Institute, La Jolla, were also much appreciated. This research was supported by the Medical Research Council.

References

Amaral, D. G. (1987). Memory: anatomical organization of candidate brain regions. In *Handbook of neurophysiology,* Section 1, *The nervous system*, Vol. V, Part 1, pp. 211–94. American Physiological Society, Washington, DC.

Amaral, D. G. and Witter, M. P, (1989). The three-dimensional organization of the hippocampal formation: a review of anatomical data. *Neuroscience*, **31**, 571–91.

Amaral, D. G., Ishizuka, N., and Claiborne, B. (1990). Neurons, numbers and the hippocampal network. *Progress in Brain Research*, **83**, 1–11.

Andersen, R. A. (1987). Inferior parietal lobule function in spatial perception and visuomotor integration. In *Handbook of physiology*, Section 1, *The nervous system*, Vol. V, *Higher functions of the brain. Part 2,* pp. 483–618. American Physiological Society, Washington, DC.

Barnes, C. A. (1988). Spatial learning and memory processes: the search for their neurobiological mechanisms in the rat. *Trends in Neurosciences*, **11**, 163–9.

Bliss, T. V. P. and Lomo, T. (1973). Long-lasting potentiation of synaptic transmission in the dentate area of the anaesthetized rabbit following stimulation of the perforant path. *Journal of Physiology*, **232**, 331–56.

Boss, B. D., Turlejski, K., Stanfield, B. B., and Cowan, W. M. (1987). On the numbers of neurons in fields CA1 and CA3 of the hippocampus of Sprague–Dawley and Wistar rats. *Brain Research*, **406**, 280–7.

Cahusac, P. M. B., Miyashita, Y., and Rolls, E. T. (1989). Responses of hippocampal formation neurons in the monkey related to delayed spatial response and object-place memory tasks. *Behavioural Brain Research*, **33**, 229–40.

Feigenbaum, J., Cahusac, P. M. B., and Rolls, E. T. (1987). The coding of spatial information by neurons in the primate hippocampal formation. *Society for Neurosciences Abstracts*, **13**, 608.

Feigenbaum, J. D. and Rolls, E. T. (1990). Allocentric and egocentric spatial information processing in the hippocampal formation of the behaving primate. *Psychobiology* (in press).

Gaffan, D. (1974). Recognition impaired and association intact in the memory of monkeys after transection of the fornix. *Journal of Comparative Physiological Psychology*, **86**, 1100–9.

Gaffan, D. (1977). Monkey's recognition memory for complex pictures and the effects of fornix transection. *Quarterly Journal of Experimental Psychology*, **29**, 505–14.

Gaffan, D. (1987). Amnesia, personal memory and the hippocampus: experimental neuropsychological studies in monkeys. In *Cognitive neurochemistry* (ed. S. M. Stahl, S. D. Iversen, and E. C. Goodman), pp. 46–56. Oxford University Press, Oxford.

Gaffan, D. and Harrison, S. (1989a). A comparison of the effects of fornix section and sulcus principalis ablation upon spatial learning by monkeys. *Behavioural Brain Research*, **31**, 207–20.

Gaffan, D. and Harrison, S. (1989b). Place memory and scene memory: effects of fornix transection in the monkey. *Experimental Brain Research*, **74**, 202–12.

Gaffan, D. and Saunders, R. C. (1985). Running recognition of configural stimuli by fornix transected monkeys. *Quarterly Journal of Experimental Psychology*, **37B**, 61–71.

Gaffan, D. and Weiskrantz, L. (1980). Recency effects and lesion effects in delayed non-matching to randomly baited samples by monkeys. *Brain Research*, **196**, 373–86.

Gaffan, D., Gaffan, E. A., and Harrison, S. (1984a). Effects of fornix transection on spontaneous and trained non-matching by monkeys. *Quarterly Journal of Experimental Psychology*, **36B**, 285–303.

Gaffan, D., Saunders, R. C., Gaffan, E. A., Harrison, S., Shields, C., and Owen, M. J. (1984b). Effects of fornix transection upon associative memory in monkeys: role of the hippocampus in learned action. *Quarterly Journal of Experimental Psychology*, **26B**, 173–221.

Gardner-Medwin, A. R. (1976). The recall of events through the learning of associations between their parts. *Proceedings of the Royal Society, London*, **B194**, 375–402.

Jordan, M. I. (1986). An introduction to linear algebra in parallel distributed processing. In *Parallel distributed processing*, Vol. 1, *Foundations* (ed. D. E. Rumelhart and J. L. McClelland), pp. 365–442. MIT Press, Cambridge, Mass.

Kelso, S. R., Ganong, A. H., and Brown, T. H. (1986). Hebbian synapses in the hippocampus. *Proceedings of the National Academy of Science*, **83**, 5326–30.

Kohonen, T. (1984). *Self-organization and associative memory*. Springer-Verlag, Berlin.

Kohonen, T., Lehtio, P., Rovamo, J., Hyvarinen, J., Bry, K., and Vainio, L. (1977). A principle of neural associative memory. *Neuroscience*, **2**, 1065–76.

Kohonen, T., Oja, E., and Lehtio, P. (1981). Storage and processing of information in distributed associative memory systems. In *Parallel models of associative memory* (ed. G. E. Hinton and J. A. Anderson), pp. 105–43. Erlbaum, Hillsdale, NJ.

Kolb, B. and Whishaw, I. Q. (1985). *Fundamentals of human neuropsychology*, (2nd edn). Freeman, New York.

Mahut, H. (1972). A selective spatial deficit in monkeys after transection of the fornix. *Neuropsychologia*, **10**, 65–74.

Marr, D. (1971). Simple memory: a theory for archicortex. *Philosophical Transactions of the Royal Society, London*, **B262**, 23–81.

McNaughton, B. L. (1984). Activity dependent modulation of hippocampal synaptic efficacy: some implications for memory processes. In *Neurobiology of the hippocampus* (ed. W. Seifert), pp. 233–52. Academic Press, London.

McNaughton, B. L., Barnes, C. A., and O'Keefe, J. (1983) The contributions of position, direction, and velocity to single unit activity in the hippocampus of freely-moving rats. *Experimental Brain Research*, **52**, 41–9.

Miles, R. (1988). Plasticity of recurrent excitatory synapses between CA3 hippocampal pyramidal cells. *Society for Neurosciences Abstracts*, **14**, 19.

Milner, B. (1972). Disorders of learning and memory after temporal lobe lesions in man. *Clinical Neurosurgery*, **19**, 421–46.

Milner, B. (1982). Some cognitive effects of frontal lobe lesions in man. *Philosophical Transactions of the Royal Society, London*, **B298**, 211–26.

Mishkin, M. (1978). Memory severely impaired by combined but not separate removel of amygdala and hippocampus. *Nature*, **273**, 297–8.

Mishkin, M. (1982). A memory system in the monkey. *Philosophical Transactions of the Royal Society, London*, **B298**, 85–95.

Miyashita, Y., Rolls, E. T., Cahusac, P. M. B., Niki, H., and Feigenbaum, J. D. (1989). Activity of hippocampal neurons in the monkey related to a conditional spatial response task. *Journal of Neurophysiology*, **61**, 669–78.

Murray, E. A. and Mishkin, M. (1984). Severe tactual as well as visual memory deficits follow combined removal of the amygdala and hippocampus in monkeys. *Journal of Neuroscience*, **4**, 2565–80.

O'Keefe, J. (1984). Spatial memory within and without the hippocampal system. In *Neurobiology of the hippocampus* (ed. W. Seifert), pp. 375–403. Academic Press, London.

Owen, M. J. and Butler, S. R. (1981). Amnesia after transection of the fornix in monkeys: long-term memory impaired, short-term memory intact. *Behavioural Brain Research*, **3**, 115–23.

Parkinson, J. K., Murray, E. A., and Mishkin, M. (1988). A selective mnemonic role for the hippocampus in monkeys: memory for the location of objects. *Journal of Neuroscience*, **8**, 4059–167.

Petrides, M. (1985). Deficits on conditional associative-learning tasks after frontal- and temporal-lobe lesions in man. *Neuropsychologia*, **23**, 601–14.

Rolls, E. T. (1987). Information representation, processing and storage in the brain: analysis at the single neuron level. In *The neural and molecular bases of learning* (ed. J.-P. Changeux and M. Konishi), pp. 503–40. Wiley, Chichester.

Rolls, E. T. (1989a). Functions of neuronal networks in the hippocampus and neocortex in memory. In *Neural models of plasticity: experimental and theoretical approaches* (ed. J. H. Byrne and W. O. Berry), pp. 240–65. Academic Press, San Diego.

Rolls, E. T. (1989b). The representation and storage of information in neuronal networks in the primate cerebral cortex and hippocampus. In *The computing neuron* (ed. R. Durbin, C. Miall, and G. Mitchison), pp. 125–59. Addison-Wesley, Wokingham.

Rolls, E. T. (1989c) Functions of neuronal networks in the hippocampus and cerebral cortex in memory. In *Models of brain function* (ed. R. M. J. Cotterill), pp. 15–33. Cambridge University Press.

Rolls, E. T. (1990). Visual information processing in the primate temporal lobe. In *Models of visual perception: from natural to artificial* (ed. M. Imbert). Oxford University Press.

Rolls, E. T., Miyashita, Y., Cahusac, P. M. B., and Kesner, R. P. (1985). The responses of single neurons in the primate hippocampus related to the performance of memory tasks. *Society for Neuroscience Abstracts*, **11**, 525.

Rolls, E. T., Miyashita, Y., Cahusac, P. M. B., Kesner, R. P., Niki, H., Feigenbaum, J., and Bach, L. (1989). Hippocampal neurons in the monkey with activity related to the place in which a stimulus is shown. *Journal of Neuroscience*, **9**, 1835–45.

Rolls, E. T., Cahusac, P. M. B., Feigenbaum, J. D., and Miyashita, Y. (1990a). Responses of single neurons in the hippocampus of the macaque related to recognition memory. *Experimental Brain Research* (in press).

Rolls, E. T., Cahusac, P. M. B., Miyashita, Y., and Niki, H. (1990b). Modification of the responses of hippocampal neurons in the monkey during the learning of a spatial response task. (In preparation.)

Rupniak, N. M. J. and Gaffan, D. (1987). Monkey hippocampus and learning about spatially directed movements. *Journal of Neuroscience*, **7**, 2331–7.

Sakata, H. (1985) The parietal association cortex: neurophysiology. In *The scientific basis of clinical neurology* (ed. M. Swash and C. Kennard), pp. 225–36. Churchill Livingstone, London.

Scoville, W. B. and Milner, B. (1957). Loss of recent memory after bilateral hippocampal lesions. *Journal of Neurology, Neurosurgery and Psychiatry*, **20**, 11–21.

Smith, M. L. and Milner, B. (1981). The role of the right hippocampus in the recall of spatial location. *Neuropsychologia*, **19**, 781–93.

Squire, L. (1986) Mechanisms of memory. *Science*, **232**, 1612–19.

Squire, L. R., Shimamura, A. P., and Amaral, D. G. (1989). Memory and the hippocampus. In *Neural models of plasticity: theoretical and empirical approaches* (ed. J. Byrne and W. O. Berry), pp. 208–39. Academic Press, New York.

Squire, L. R. and Zola-Morgan, S. (1988). Memory: brain systems and behavior. *Trends in Neurosciences*, **11**, 170–5.

Van Hoesen, G. W. (1982). The parahippocampal gyrus. New observations regarding its cortical connections in the monkey. *Trends in Neurosciences*, **5**, 345–50.

Watanabe, T. and Niki, H. (1985). Hippocampal unit activity and delayed response in the monkey. *Brain Research*, **325**, 241–54.

Wigstrom, H., Gustaffson, B., Huang, Y.-Y., and Abraham, W. C. (1986). Hippo-campal long-term potentiation is induced by pairing single afferent volleys with intracellularly injected depolarizing currents. *Acta Physiologica Scandinavica*, **126,** 317–19.

Wilson, F. A. W., Riches, I. P., and Brown, M. V. (1988). Neuronal activity in the inferomedial temporal cortex compared with that of the hippocampal formation: implications for amnesia of medial temporal lobe origin. In: *Cellular mechanisms of conditioning and behavioral plasticity* (ed. C. D. Woody, D. L. Alkon, and J. L. McGaugh), pp. 313–98. Plenum Press, New York.

Zola-Morgan, S., Squire, L. R., and Amaral, D. G. (1986). Human amnesia and the medial temporal region: enduring memory impairment following a bilateral lesion limited to field CA1 of the hippocampus. *Journal of Neuroscience*, **6,** 2950–7.

PART 5

Models of space representation

20

Interaction of multiple representations of space in the brain

MICHAEL A. ARBIB

Concepts of space

My concern in this presentation is with the space of everyday action. The representation of this quotidian space in the brain is not one absolute space, but rather a patchwork of approximate spaces (partial representations) that link sensation to action. I mean '*partial*' and '*approximate*' in two senses: a representation will be *partial* because it represents only one small sample of space (that within reaching distance, that within sight, the features of an object relevant to grasping it, or more abstract 'allocentric' or cognitive representations), and it will be *approximate* in that it will be based on an incomplete sample of sensory date and may be of limited accuracy and reliability. I will suggest that our behaviour is mediated by the interaction of these partial representations: both through their integration to map ever larger portions of the territory relevant to behaviour, and through their mutual calibration to yield a shared representation more reliable than that obtainable by any one alone with its limited sample of sensory data.

Although, with the use of various co-ordinate systems, Euclidean geometry provides a useful framework for measuring the stimuli to, and the responses of, the subjects whose behaviour we study, there is seldom a *direct* mapping of these co-ordinates into neural activity and connectivity. For the animal, 'space is the measure of movement', and as the animal moves in diffcrent ways, or makes use of different sensory cues in guiding its movement, so will we find a variety of different representations in its brain. For example, we can distinguish between representations of oculomotor space, itself possibly subdivided to meet the needs of other motor systems, and of those that guide locomotion and reaching. The brain's multiple maps gain their coherence not by their subservience to some over-arching, mathematical definition of space but with respect to a repertoire of movement.

A number of formal studies show how different types of sensorimotor experience could yield different forms of abstract mathematical structure for representing space. Room (1967) showed how the experience that a farmer gains in learning how to lay out a field and plough it in regular furrows might eventually lead to systematic observations that could be encapsulated in the axioms of Euclidean geometry. Nicod (1970) has imagined how different creatures with different sensorimotor systems might induce quite different geometrical structures for their worlds. For example, one might contrast the visual and motor repertoire of our farmer with that of a creature confined to running up and down a piano keyboard with the sound of the notes thus struck providing its only sensory input.

Another view of the diversity of space comes from contemplating the trip from my home in Los Angeles to the conference hall in Marseille to take part in this conference. In travelling, I went by car, plane, two trains, a taxi, and a bus. When driving a car I needed a rather detailed representation of space, although one that was accurate in the small rather than the large. In choosing to travel by plane, I needed to select the appropriate flight but needed to know little more than the destination to co-ordinate that with plans for further travel. While on the plane, my space was the Euclidean space inside the cabin, with glances out the window giving me a small sample of the planet, small enough to still be Euclidean. Meanwhile, a hundred feet in front of me, the pilot was living in a non-Euclidean world, for in plotting his trajectory on or near a great circle around the globe, he was living in a Riemannian spherical geometry.

Nonetheless, leaving aside our pilot and a few others whose profession forces them to work on a planetary scale or beyond, we may say that we move in a world where the position and orientation of objects can be described in Euclidean terms. But we do not receive signals corresponding to some co-ordinate system for this Euclidean space. We receive arrays of stimulation based on visual, auditory, tactile, chemical, and other indications of our relationship with the object and other energy sources (sun, wind, and so on) of the world. The task of perception is *not to reconstruct* a Euclidean model of the surroundings. Perception is *action-oriented*, combining current stimuli and stored knowledge to determine a course of action appropriate to the task at hand: brain state and state of effectors determine movement, while sensory stimuli and brain state determine brain state. Our task is to understand where notions of space may enter into our analysis of these transformations. When we draw a map of the city or countryside, or give instructions to a friend, it is paths that define the space as much as the landmarks. Instructions usually are of the form 'follow a path until you see a landmark', but may be augmented by indications of duration, a primitive coupling of space and time. Space is then best defined by this graphical duality of paths/edges and landmarks/nodes (Lieblich and Arbib 1982). But just as a feature on a map is never a true Euclidean point, so an object of the real world has a non-zero extent which allows a whole variety of actions to effect an interaction with it. We must learn how the brain encodes neighbourhoods of space and the actions that link them.

Eye movements: from co-ordinates to distributed codes

Descartes taught us to think of points as being represented by sets of numbers, the (x, y, z) of three-dimensional space, for example, but mathematicians have long since abstracted from this the notion that *any* string of measurements can be seen as a point in the abstract space of all such measurements. However, topologists have taught us that space is not to be seen just as a set of measurement vectors, but as a set enriched with relations that tell us when points are close together (topology) or let us measure the distance between points (metrics and norms). From this Olympian viewpoint, the firing patterns of millions or even billions of neurons can be seen as constituting a space, and various neural models (e.g. of associative memory) are based on the notion that similar situations in the input correspond to similar firing patterns in the neural assembly. This section will present a model that highlights the way in which the vector of neural firing that represents space may not be structured to correspond in a simple way to an (x, y, z)-like, co-ordinate system. The next section will argue that it may be dangerous to view a point-wise representation of space as providing the most useful way to map onto neural activity.

The classic models of eye movements due to David A. Robinson and his colleagues were based on control systems analyses in which particular co-ordinates of the system were mapped onto single, neural-activity variables in the model. Thus, in the model of Van Gisbergen *et al.* (1981) shown in Fig. 20.1, the desired position of the eye in, let us say, the horizontal plane is represented by the firing rate E_d of a specific neuron, and the actual position of the eye is represented by an internal copy given by the firing rate E' of the neuron T, the neural integrator. (The model was developed before it was discovered that there were indeed proprioceptive signals generated by the extra-ocular muscles.) Without going into further details (see, for example, Arbib 1989, Section 6.2 for an exposition), we may note that the functions of the neurons in the model directly encode basic numerical operations on the co-ordinates, so that the neuron B which receives excitation in the amount of E_d and inhibition in the amount of E' carries out the subtraction necessary to generate a signal as to whether or not an error has occurred.

One step beyond such a model is to observe that the position of a target relative to the current direction of gaze is not encoded by a particular number E_d but is, in fact, coded by the position of a peak of activity on the retina, which is in turn transformed back to the position of a peak of activity on the superior colliculus (SC) (Pitts and McCulloch 1947; Arbib 1972). In taking account of this effect, Scudder (1988) has suggested how one might adapt the model of Van Gisbergen *et al.* so that, while the

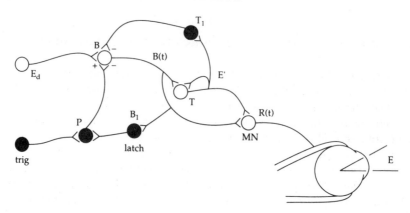

Fig. 20.1. Saccade control diagram: the desired position of the eye is represented by the firing rate E_d of a specific neuron, and the actual position of the eye is presented by an internal copy given by the firing rate E' of the neuron T, the neural integrator.

control system calculations are still carried out in the type of network that they described, the input for that network comes from a population of activity in the SC, with the transformation carried out by topographical weighting from the collicular array to specific, long-lead, burst neurons (LLBN).

However, the control of eye movements does not depend only on visual signals but, as in the case of the vestibulo-ocular reflex (VOR), depends crucially on vestibular signals. It has been observed that the planes in which the semicircular canals lie do not match the planes in which the eye muscles lie, and so there is no easy separation of the vestibular control of eye movements into three separate, co-ordinate planes. One of the people to most imaginatively address the problem has been Pellionisz (e.g. 1984), who has shown that the Moore–Penrose generalized inverse can describe the transformation[1] from the co-ordinates provided by the three planes of the semicircular canals to the co-ordinates provided by the three planes of the extra-ocular muscles (Pellionisz and Graf 1987). However, Anastasio and Robinson (1989) emphasize that between the firing pattern that directly represents the three dimensions of vestibular activity and the firing pattern that represents the three co-ordinates of extra-ocular muscle activity (with each dimension given by the activity of mononeurons controlling a paired set of muscles) there lies the large neural population of the vestibular nucleus. Measurements of this nucleus show that the activity of these neurons is not neatly segregated in terms of the particular co-ordinates so far described. Thus the synaptic weights which connect the various levels do not correspond to a matrix transformation from one co-ordinate system to another, let alone the Moore–Penrose generalized inverse. Although the matrix offers a useful behavioural description of the system *as observed from the outside*, it does not make explicit the detailed neural transformations that mediate this behavioural transformation.

In seeking to understand this phenomenon, Anastasio and Robinson used back propagation[2] to train the 'hidden units' that lie between the sensory activity and the motor activity of the vestibulo-ocular system. As do others, they stress that in training the network this way, they do not claim that back propagation is an accurate representation of the neurophysiological, developmental mechanisms whereby the connections are formed. Rather, it is a computational technique for identifying a set of possible connection patterns which could indeed mediate the given transformation from the input layers to the output layers of the network. They find that such training yields a network with remarkable similarities to the actual scatter of tuning of the neurons in the modelled vestibular nucleus. This represents a distributed code that is very different in character from the direct neural implementation of a simple matrix from one three-dimensional co-ordinate system to another. Once again, the vector of firing patterns in neurons does not map directly to a co-ordinate system that provides an economical representation of our measurements of animal stimulation and behaviour.

Space may be pointless

Having now emphasized that the distributed coding of space in a neural network may differ greatly from the simple Cartesian co-ordinates of Euclidean space, I now want to suggest that in some cases it may even be a mistake to view points as the building blocks of space when we consider neural encoding. In *Process and Reality*, Whitehead (1929) used neighbourhoods as building blocks for describing space. He defined a point by an 'abstractive set' of ever-decreasing neighbourhoods—an infinite Russian doll. Thus, a point is never exactly defined; rather, it can be more and more precisely localized. Perhaps we can see the development of the child in similar terms when it develops its skills for reaching. The infant starts by flailing in the general direction of the visual target. Experience refines the neighbourhood, rather than shifting a target point, to yield more and more accurate reaching towards the target (von Hofsten 1990).

Jeannerod (1981) has shown that, as the hand reaches towards an object, it pre-shapes itself (Fig. 20.2A)—not in such a way as to offer an exact matching of hand co-ordinates with object co-ordinates, but rather so that the hand defines a neighbourhood of the shape of the target which is large enough to encompass the target but small enough to ensure that tactile control of the grasp during the second phase of the movement will not take

M. A. Arbib

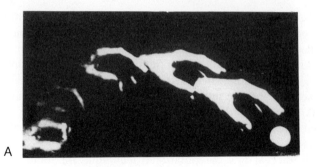

A

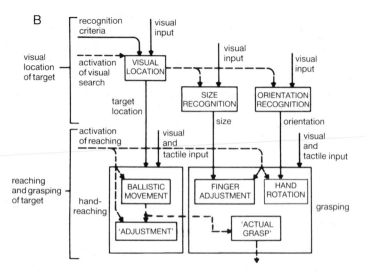

B

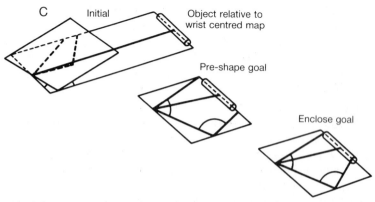

C

Fig. 20.2. (A) Hand reaching (Jeannerod 1981); (B) co-ordinated control programme for hand reaching; (C) opposition space for pre-shaping.

very long (indicated by the observation of a slowing of the movement, in the final portion of the trajectory of Fig. 20.2A). The strategy is thus to define a neighbourhood large enough to encompass the object, and then use tactile feedback to find the exact pattern of neural firing to grasp the object securely. Of course, the initial stages must bring the system into the right ballpark (to use the terminology of Peter Greene 1971) for feedback to be able to carry out its role of fine tuning. In current, dynamic systems parlance, we may say that the initial stage must bring the system into the basin of the appropriate attractor.

A more specific breakdown of the various components (Fig. 20.2B; Arbib 1981) emphasizes the perceptual schemas required to characterize the object and the motor schemas acting in parallel to control the arm and hand movements.[3] In subsequent work, Iberall *et al.* (1986) gave more detailed co-ordinates for the behaviour. Their three, basic, opposition spaces of pad-opposition, palm-opposition and side-opposition provide the elements for a rich vocabulary for the description of a variety of hand movements (including those which can be seen as the conjoint activity of several oppositions as, for example, grasping a screwdriver with both a palm-opposition and a side-opposition). Figure 20.2C shows the in-gredients for a theory of pre-shaping. The visual system must analyse the object to determine an opposition space embedded therein that provides the axis along which the opposing fingers must advance. The goal of the pre-shape must include a safety margin. This goal determines the appropri-ate offset of the wrist from the centre of the object—and so planning the *hand* shape modifies the plan for *arm* movement. In other words, the different spatial representations, in this case for the arm and for the hand, must be appropriately coupled. There is no one absolute space represented in one place in the brain, only a coupling of sensory and motor spaces in such a way as to yield movement to achieve some goal.

Superior colliculus and tectum

In relating the visual system (including the control of eye movements) to reaching and grasping, Paillard and Beaubaton (1975) distinguished the *parallel* contribution of three visual processes.

1. One extracts from the *object space*, specific features that allow the perceptual *identification* of the object and the pre-shaping of the hand on the basis of visual cues (shape and size) in order to grasp the object appropriately.
2. The second derives from the fixation of gaze on the target, the oculo-motor and depth cues that allow the *localization* of the object in a body-centred *reaching space*, and the triggering of a programmed transport of the arm, which brings the hand to a position near the target.

3. The third provides visual cues about directional and positional errors of the on-going movement that allow the feedback correction of the trajectory and the final wrist *adjustment* to match the grip to the orientation of the object. After contact has been established, tactile cues intervene to shape the hand to the object.

What is to be emphasized is the interaction throughout this task of diverse representations of 'reaching space' and 'object space', involving a variety of sensorimotor dialogues (visuomotor, tactuo-motor, propriocepto-motor, and combinations thereof). Moreover, Paillard's (1989) overview of the neural systems involved in these performances demonstrates a central role of the SC both in the control of eye, head, and trunk movements for directing the gaze of the animal to the appropriate place, and in the control of limb movements to allow the animal to move towards and then reach towards the intended, target object. Complementary cortical pathways control the hands and digits for fine reaching, but these systems co-operate, rather than acting independently.

This centrality of the SC provides a graceful transition to studies of the role of the homologous structure, the tectum, in approach, avoidance, and detour behaviour in frog and toad. These behaviours involve the co-ordination of different maps or vector fields. Several chapters in this book emphasize the vital role of the SC of the primate in saccadic eye movements, which cause the animal's eyes to approach a visual target. Here, I want to emphasize the role of the SC in animals for which it is whole-body movements, rather than eye movements, that are primarily implicated. Recent work by Dean *et al.* (1989) has shown that the rat SC has a rich involvement in avoidance behaviour, as well as the better understood involvement in approach behaviour—suggesting that the study of avoidance activity in the SC of the primate merits further study. Different portions of the colliculus are more implicated in avoidance and orienting, and one may characterize the types of movement which stimuli make to yield these different performances. A looming object may yield defence or avoidance, while a fluttering object like a butterfly may yield pursuit. Underlining the general theme of interaction of multiple representations of space in the brain, Dean *et al.* show that these maps do not control behaviour in isolation but through their conjoined activity with contextual representations encoded elsewhere in the brain, including the basal ganglia.

The finding of important activity correlated with avoidance in the rat SC comes as no surprise to those who study the homologous tectum of frog and toad, for here the role of tectal–pretectal interactions in the mediation of both approach and avoidance behaviour has long been a subject of study. Figure 20.3a (Ewert 1987) shows how the toad's response to a worm not only can be modulated by motivational representations in

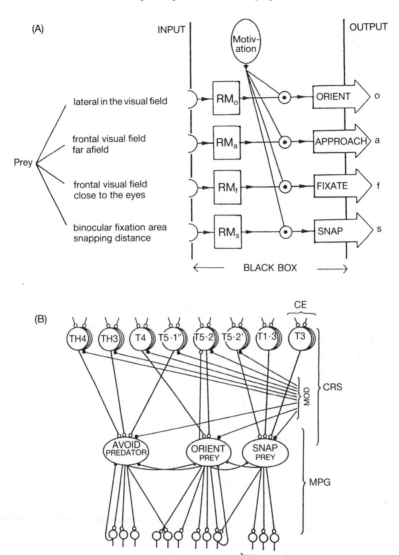

Fig. 20.3. (A) Releasing mechanisms (RMs) for four different components of the toad's acquisition of prey; (B) neural groupings for different releasing mechanisms. Various neuron types from thalamus (TH) and tectum (T) (functioning as command elements, CE) are combined to form command releasing systems (CRS) which, under various modulatory influences (MOD) control the motor pattern generators (MPG) involved in avoiding predators and catching prey (after Ewert 1987).

the brain, but also depends upon the location of the stimulus in the visual field.

Over many years, Ewert and other workers have refined this ethological type of description to provide neural correlates. As Fig. 20.3B (also Ewert 1987) shows, certain combinations of identified neurons in both thalamus–pretectum and tectum seem to be required to trigger different types of behaviour. For example, the conjoined activity of TH4, TH3, and T5.1″ neurons seems necessary for the animal to move to avoid a predator, while the conjoined activity of T5.2, T1.3, and T3 neurons seems involved in the decision to snap.

But how is the movement to be directed appropriately into the animal's environment? The basic coding principle here, of course, is retinotopy. However, retinotopy alone is not enough. If we take the retinotopic position of a stimulus on one eye and continue it out into space we need further information to determine how far away the prey object is and thus determine what angle the toad must turn and what distance it must advance to approach or snap at the prey. Grobstein (1989) has carried this analysis even further. He finds that the result of lesioning one half tectum in the frog is to stop the animal from orienting towards stimuli that are not available in the visual field of the other eye, but still leaves it able to orient correctly to stimuli still visible to the remaining half tectum. However, if the descending ipsilateral pathway of the tectum is severed, the frog does not orient to stimuli on the side which has lost vision. The deficit does *not* correspond to the visual field of the remaining tectum.

It might at first be thought that this is a simple motoric deficit, and that the motor schema for turns to that side of the animal no longer receives any input. However, Grobstein argues that what is lost is rather part of a generalized spatial representation (what he calls an 'activity-gated divergence'). The evidence for this is as follows. The normal frog will snap at an object that is close but hop towards a prey that is somewhat further away. The transition from the snap zone to the hop zone is about two body-lengths from the centre of the animal in the forward direction, but only one body-length in the lateral direction. The animal with the lesion that we have just discussed will orient and snap or hop like an unlesioned frog for stimuli on the normal side. For stimuli on the other side, it will snap or hop without orienting, whether or not the target is straight ahead. The significant observation, however, is that the transition between the snap and hop zones now occurs for all directions of the stimulus at the distance of two body-lengths, appropriate to a target that is straight ahead. Grobstein thus concludes that this quite different aspect of motor planning, the decision whether to hop or snap, is making use of a zero-turn co-ordinate. In other words, it is the representation of space in this orientation dimension, rather than the trigger signal for the orienting movement, that seems to be removed by the lesion described above.

Depth and detours

The various studies mentioned so far all report the behaviour of the animal in response to a single object, and so may encourage us to think falsely of the brain as encoding the properties of the target alone. In general, however, the animal must act within a complex and structured environment, and so a number of features of that world relevant to its action must be encoded simultaneously in the animal's brain. I will illustrate this with a particular study of toad behaviour that yields a model which, though rather far removed from the neurophysiology, is conceptually challenging, and has already been applied in the design of controllers for mobile robots (Arkin 1989).

The basic phenomena have been well explored by Collett (e.g. 1982). A toad is placed in front of a barrier or some combination of barriers, and a worm is placed behind the obstacle. In general, the animal will make a detour appropriately to go around the obstacle to reach the prey. It is clear, then, that the animal must build some type of spatial representation in which the positions of some at least of these objects are displayed relative to the animal. There are now a number of models that address these effects, but here I will focus on one model, the Path Planning model (Arbib and House 1987), which is part of a continuing project on *Rana computatrix*, the 'frog that computes'. Figure 20.4 shows four representations of the world of the toad. Each of these is based on a common geometry for the ground plane in front of the animal. Each motor schema (Fig. 20.4A–C) contributes one summand of the vector field that will direct the action. In Fig. 20.4A a worm is represented by a vector field giving, for each position in the ground plane, the 'attraction' for the animal to move towards the worm, with the attraction being greater the closer is the toad to the worm. By contrast, the vector field for a fence post gives, for each position in the ground plane, the 'repulsion' for the animal to move away from the post. Figure 20.4B shows that a fence post has little effect upon the behaviour of the toad unless the toad is within a body width of the post, in which case it will move slightly to the side to avoid contact. Finally, Fig. 20.4C suggests the propensity of the animal to move forward from its present position. The superposition of the fence posts yields no disposition to move within the vicinity of the fence itself and a strong lateral push to detour from one end of the fence or to the other. When we combine this (Fig. 20.4D) with the field for the worm, we see a vector field that determines the animal's detour behaviour.

In summary, then, the suggestion is that the brain will contain at least two separate representations of the ground plane, one showing the presence of targets, and the other showing the presence of obstacles. These

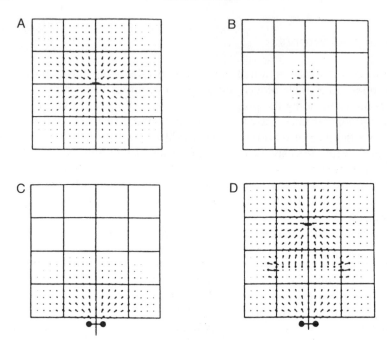

Fig. 20.4. The Path Planning (vector field) model sees objects in the animal's visual world as determining a space of potential motor activities. The potential fields depicted here represent an exploratory attempt at defining a set of primitive fields that will interact in interpreting a more complex scene. Each field provides, for each position in the ground plane, a vector showing the direction and 'strength' of a movement the animal might make were it situated at that position. (A) A single prey object sets up a radially symmetrical, attractant field whose strength decays gradually with distance from the prey. (B) A single, barrier object sets up a repellent field whose effect is more localized to its point of origin than is that of the prey field. The barrier field is not radially symmetrical but has a lateral component that is stronger but decays more rapidly with distance than does its opposing component. (C) The vector field model also contains a representation of the animal itself. This representation is simply the converse of the prey representation, i.e., it is radially symmetrical but diverges from its point of origin. (D) The effect of the interaction of the fields from several objects arranged to form a fence is to provide a strong lateral thrust at the fence ends. The lateral components produced by the interior posts is effectively cancelled by neighbouring posts. The net field produced by the interaction of all of the elements of the configuration can then be thought of as tracing out a set of paths, most of which are diverted around the fence ends (Arbib and House 1987).

must be brought into appropriate register to play down upon those neural networks that actually determine the behaviour of the animal to yield an appropriate detour nonetheless to achieve its prey. Much remains to be done to determine where and how these partial representations are encoded. In particular, must the entire vector field be explicitly represented in the brain at any one time, or is it only the local field required to guide the next phase of action that must be encoded? Moreover, as is suggested by studies of rat hippocampus (e.g. O'Keefe 1984; Olton 1984), whatever 'egocentric' encoding of local space there may be should be related to more global 'allocentric' encoding which represents the animal's overall know-ledge of the position of motivationally important landmarks in its world (Lieblich and Arbib 1982).

Maps may be implicit or explicit

It should also be stressed that the map of the ground plane or any other external spatial structure may be implicit or explicit. For example, in those cases where retinotopy determines the code, we may say that space is explicitly represented. However, this is not always so. A simple example comes from a network for landmark learning studied by Barto and Sutton (1981). The 'animal' is placed in a simple environment (Fig. 20.5A) in

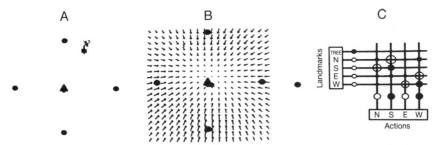

Fig. 20.5. (A) A simple environment in which there are four landmarks and a central goal; (B) the vector field showing the appropriate direction in which to go at each point of the terrain (cf. Fig. 20.4); (C) a neural network whose 16 synaptic weights provide an implicit representation of the vector field of (B).

which there are four landmarks, with the current sensory input to the animal providing signals that represent the strength of 'odours' of each landmark. The training is to enable the animal to learn, without being explicitly programmed, how to proceed from any position in the landscape to reach the goal shown by the tree at the middle of the figure. Here it is not necessary to explain the learning process, but rather to show that in the end the animal has a map of its world, indicated in Fig. 20.5B that pro-vides the appropriate direction in which to go no matter at which point it may be in its terrain. However, as Fig. 20.5C shows, the map of Fig. 20.5B is not explicitly represented by a vast array of neural structures, with each 'column' encoding the vector for the corresponding position, but is simply given by the strength of 16 synaptic weights which, for example, can translate the sensory signal 'strong smell of north' into 'strong activa-tion of the motor command to go south' as follows.

Inputs $x_i(t)$, for $i =$ N, S, E, and W, denote the signals at time t from the North, South, East and West landmarks respectively. Input $x_i(t)$ affects the jth 'motor neuron' via a synaptic weight $w_{ji}(t)$ which encodes a degree of confidence that, when the asterisk is near landmark i, it should proceed in direction j to get nearer the tree. The four neurons control motions in the respective cardinal directions. Connection weights between input and output elements are shown in Fig. 20.5C as circles centred on the intersections of the input pathways with the element 'dendrites'. Positive weights appear as open circles, and negative weights appear as filled circles.[4] Let:

$$s_j(t) = \Sigma_i w_{ji} x_i(t) \qquad (1)$$

so that $s_j(t)$ sums up the degrees of confidence for a move in direction j on the basis of the current signals received from the four landmarks. If $s_j(t)$ is big enough to exceed threshold when noise is added, the robot will run in direction j. If, on the other hand, the value is below 0, there will be no j-movement. In case two elements fire simultaneously, then the appropriate compound move is made, e.g. North-west if N and W fire; no move if N and S fire. The reader may check that for each position in the terrain, the vector whose co-ordinates are:

$$(s_W(t) - s_E(t), \ s_N(t) - s \ S(t))$$

is indeed that given in Fig. 20.5B—but the 400 vectors of Fig. 20.5B depend only on the 16 synaptic weights w_{ji} of Fig. 20.5C, via the formula (1).

We are thus challenged to investigate, should the vector fields of the previous section be 'neurally real', whether they are represented explicitly as in Fig. 20.4 or implicitly in the way that the network of Fig. 20.5C encodes the vector field of Fig. 20.5B.

The scratch reflex

Before returning to a final look at the relationship of retinotopy to the diverse, partial representations within the brain, I want to briefly look at somatotopy. It is ironical that the scratch reflex, a classic underpinning for much of what Sherrington taught us about the basic synaptic structure of the brain, remains little explored after almost a century. The precise neural mechanisms for transforming position on the body into the direction of an appropriate movement to reach and scratch at the target has not been properly worked out. In my group, we have only achieved a preliminary model of a one-dimensional restriction of the scratch reflex in the cat. This work models a simple circuit that provides a flexor drive during the positioning phase and then an alternating flexor and extensor drive during the rhythmic phase of scratching at the scratch site [Fig. 20.6(A)]. The current

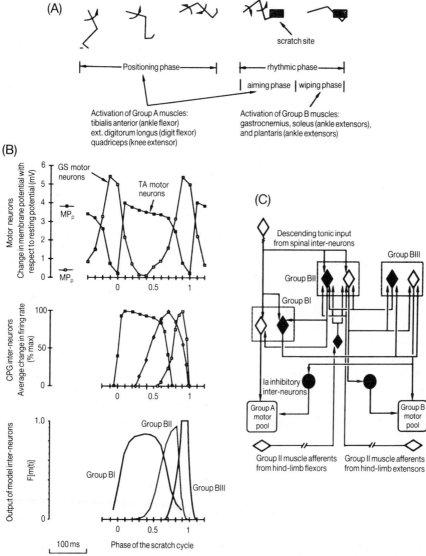

Fig. 20.6. (A) A one-dimensional rendition of the scratch reflex in cat. An initial positioning phase involving flexion is following by repeated cycles of scratching, alternating flexion, and extension in the rhythmic phase. (B) Top: average change in membrane potential of motor neurons in TA (tibialis anterior) and GS (gastrochemius) motor pools (corresponding to the Group A and Group B muscles, respectively, of part (A)) by the end of the positioning phase (denoted by MPp), and during the scratch cycle. Change is with respect to resting potential before the reflex was initiated. Middle: activity in three groups of inter-neurons involved in the control pattern generator (CPG) for the scratch groups BI, BII and BIII located in segments L4 and L5 of the spinal cord, during one cycle of the reflex. Bottom: simulated activity of the three groups of inter-neurons yielded by the model. (C) Schematic of the neuronal system postulated to control the positioning and rhythmic portions of the scratch reflex. Open neurons are excitatory; filled are inhibitory.

model is based on the data of Berkinblit *et al.* (1978), which shows that there are three groups of inter-neurons whose firing activity can be correlated with the activity of the flexor and extensor, motor pools [Fig. 20.6(B)], with group I driving the flexor pools and group III driving the extensor pools. Our job was to find a connection scheme and set of parameters that can connect the five pools to yield a model that simulates the given time pattern of behaviour.

The connections in the model are shown in Fig. 20.6(C) (Shadmehr 1989). The excitatory neurons of group BI drive the flexor motor pool (group A), the excitatory neurons of group BIII drive the extensor motor pool (group B), while BII neurons mediate the coupling. Activity in BI and BII is driven by the tonic, excitatory, 'irritation' input, while BIII is driven by activity in BII. BII is given a longer time constant than BI, so that turning on the tonic activity yields a period in which only BI is active, thus driving the flexion activity of the positioning phase. Thereafter, we have the cyclic control of the rhythmic phase: BII activity eventually inhibits BI activity and excites BIII activity; BIII activity yields extension, inhibits flexion, and closes down BII activity; released from BII inhibition, BI closes down BIII activity, produces flexion, and the cycle repeats itself.

With appropriate tuning this network can, as shown at the foot of Fig. 20.6(B), yield a pattern of firing in the modelled neurons that accords remarkably well with the time pattern of firing activity in the real spinal cord of the cat. It should be noted that our model simulates each neuronal pool by a single, leaky, integrator neuron[5] so that there are interesting issues in understanding the distribution of activity across a motoneuron pool that are not touched upon by the present model. As the duration of the positioning phase can be changed as a function of the membrane time-constants of the group 2 pool, it is particularly pressing to understand how the pool time-constant relates to the parameters of neurons within the pool.

It is our postulate that it is the transformation of position of the body into time-constants of the network that yields the appropriate positioning phase for the scratch reflex as a function of one-dimensional position of the irritation site. Here we have in some sense closed the circle back to the first model considered in this chapter, that of the control of saccadic eye movements (Fig. 20.1). Once again we see how action can be controlled by a network that, essentially, transforms spatial position into time-constants of some performance.

The subtlety of such reflexes has been further demonstrated by the finding of Fukson *et al.* (1980) that the wiping reflex in the spinal frog depends on the body schema. As shown in Fig. 20.7, the trajectory used by the tip of the hind limb to reach for the fore-limb shoulder and move along the limb to remove an irritant patch changes dramatically and appropriately when the position of the frog's body and limbs changes. Thus, we must

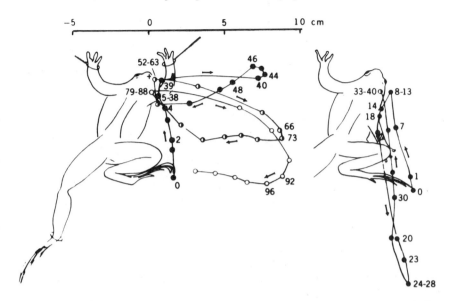

Fig. 20.7. In the frog wiping reflex, the trajectory of the wiping limb varies systematically with the position of the irritant site in three-dimensional space—which varies with the positioning of the frog's limb and body as well as the locus of the irritant on the skin. This is true even in the spinal frog: 'the spinal frog takes into account the scheme of its body during the wiping reflex'. With the wiping trajectory appropriately modified for an irritant of the forelimb when the limb is in different positions as shown in the figure. Numbers indicate successive points observed along the trajectory in a single wiping episode. (Fukson *et al.* 1980).

compound the classic question about the translation of body position to wiping to scratching trajectory into the even more subtle question of how the somatotopic code is modulated by representation of the current state of the body. To model this phenomenon is one of the current targets in my own laboratory.

Retinotopy and multiplicity

Classically, retinotopy corresponds to the co-ordinates laid out on a single retina, but we have already seen that in determining motor behaviour we need further information, such as that for depth, which can only be afforded by integrating this retinotopy with other cues. Stereopsis is based on using cues gained by triangulation from the two eyes, but accommodation and optic flow can also provide powerful depth cues. As a further example of the integration of multiple, partial representations, we consider the Cue Interaction model (House 1989) which shows [Fig. 20.8(A)] how representations based on accommodation and stereopsis might themselves

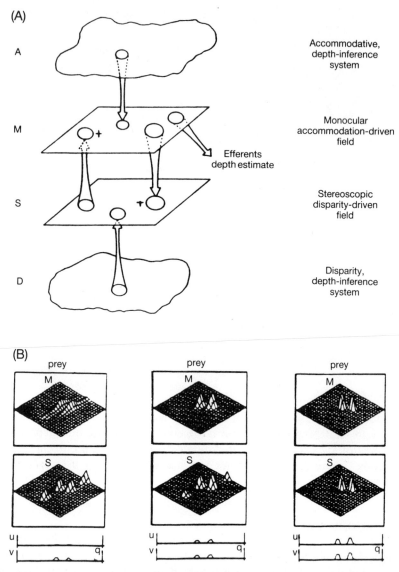

Fig. 20.8. (A) The Cue Interaction model couples two depth systems as explained in the text. The fields M and S are coupled by mutual, excitatory interconnections between each local region (oval) of one field on to the corresponding local region of the other field. By means of these interconnections, points of high excitation in one field provide additional excitation to corresponding points in the other field. Competition among depth estimates within each field ensures that points excited in only one field will have little chance of sustaining this excitation when there are other points receiving stimulation in both fields. (B) The time course of the Cue Interaction model is shown from its immediate response to input to a satisfactory depth segmentation. In each case, the upper, two-dimensional grid shows the level of excitation of the accommodation field, and the lower the disparity field. The line graphs under the grids indicate the intensity and localization on the retinal-angle axis of excitation in the inhibitory pools (House 1989).

be integrated. The model couples two depth systems. The binocular system takes input from layer D and represents an inference system that provides binocular cues from disparity matching and sends it to layer S, a spatially organized field that uses the Dev (1975) algorithm to suppress false targets in a map of space to yield a unique choice of target in each visual direction. The monocular system takes input from layer A, which represents an inference system that provides a monocular depth cues from lens accommodation, and processes it in layer M which, apart from its source of input, is just like S.

The first panel of Fig. 20.8(B) shows two representations of two prey. In the upper representation, accommodation cues yield uncertainty as to the location of the prey so that we have only two targets but with a smeared representation. In the lower representation, stereo cues yield precise localization by triangulation but, initially, also yield ghost targets by pairing the wrong stimuli on the two eyes. Dev's mechanism seeks to find the depth represented by maximal activity in each direction, but with excitatory connections between neurons representing points neighbouring in both depth and direction. The Dev mechanism can sharpen up each estimate in the first panel of Fig. 20.8(B), but has the danger that it might give preference to the ghost target rather than the real target in the stereo representation, or that it might mislocalize the peak of the broad 'hillside' for each target in the monocular representation. To remedy this, the Cue Interaction model [Fig. 20.8(A)] uses an excitatory coupling between corresponding points in the two representations to increase the chance that each system picks the same depth location in each visual direction. Thus, as the attempt to find the peak of maximal activity in each direction progresses, the ghost targets receive no support from the accommodation map and so lose out to the real targets, while the precise localization of these real targets by stereo provides the excitation to make the true peaks of the monocular representation survive while the side lobes are inhibited.

Work on optic flow (reviewed in Arbib 1989; Section 7.2) uses the input not from two eyes but from a succession of eyes, namely one eye making observations over a period of time. Such information can be used to determine whether or not a collision will occur with a target and to give some estimate of the time until collision or adjacency. But, again, we would have the depth cues from stereo and accommodation integrated with the depth cues from optic flow if the animal is most effectively to make use of its visual input. To illustrate this use of coherence of multiple, partial representations, Poggio *et al.* (1988) simulated a low-level vision system on a Connection Machine. Four different cues—colour, texture, motion and stereo—are represented in separate quasi-neural networks (the Markov random fields of Geman and Geman 1984), and each could alone proceed towards a segmentation of the visual field into regions that are candidates for interpretation as different surfaces. However, both to speed the process and to make it more reliable, Poggio *et al.* couple the four segmentation processes with a brightness-based, edge-detection system. The confidence that a change in brightness signals a real edge in the visual world is enhanced if it accords with an edge in the other representations, and vice versa. Thus, the four systems for colour, texture, motion, and stereo, coupled through the edge-detection system, can rapidly converge to a highly reliable segmentation of the world into distinct surfaces.

Integrating knowledge with space

Once those low-level processes have begun to give reasonably reliable information about the structure of the world, the problem remains of interpreting it. Here we go beyond the world of quasi-retinotopy to the more abstract representation of knowledge. Figure 20.9 gives a view of the machine vision system of Riseman and Hanson (1987), which builds on some of my ideas on schema theory (Arbib 1981). At the left, we see data about segmentation and measurements of the regions thus found. These constitute the so-called intermediate representation of the image, which

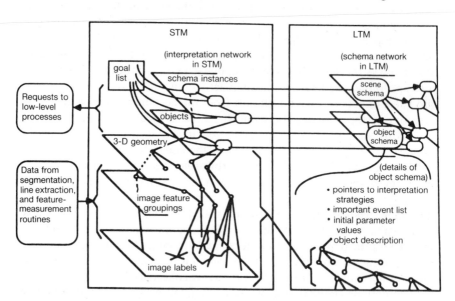

Fig. 20.9. Overview of the VISIONS system. Interpretation strategies are stored in schemas which are linked in a schema network in long-term memory (LTM). Under the guidance of these schemas, the intermediate representation is modified and interpreted by a network of schema instances which label regions of the image and link them to a three-dimensional geometry in short-term memory (STM).

provides the input to what is called short-term memory (STM), which provides a dynamic interpretation of the current visual input by appeal to long-term memory (LTM). In this model, LTM is a network of perceptual schemas for the recognition of objects and their relationships on the basis of visual cues. These schemas provide not only knowledge of how to recognize certain objects but also knowledge of whole–part relationships and of contextual co-occurrence of object. As interpretation proceeds, STM can request further low-level processing to refine the intermediate representation in the light of ongoing attempts to make sense of what objects are really present in the world. STM generates instances of the LTM schemas, links them to regions of the image, and adjusts confidence values back and forth until the instances with high confidence values constitute a coherent interpretation of the image.

In relating this purely computational account to neurophysiology, recall that there are cells in monkey infero-temporal cortex that respond to a complex pattern like 'hand' or 'face', irrespective of spatial location. I thus suggest that their activity encodes schema instances without specifying where the corresponding object is located in space. On the other hand, the parietal cortex seems to hold a spatial representation without knowing what the objects are. De Yoe and van Essen (1988) have suggested how a variety of low-level visual systems may provide the features to drive both the 'what' system of the infero-temporal cortex and the 'where' system of the parietal cortex. To this we must add the necessary 'dynamic links' required to complete the process of perception. The recognition of where an object is must be linked to the representation of what an object is.

This linkage of partial representations must occur up and down the hierarchy. For example, in a stroboscopic presentation of coloured letters, the subject can reliably report what letters and colours have been presented but only reports the colour of specific letters at chance level when the presentation is a very brief one. In other words, there is time for separate representations of colour and letter to be formed, but not time for linkages between them to be put in place. Von der Malsburg (1988) has offered one model for how such linkages might be formed by fast changes of synapses based on temporal or other correlations. Here my point is simply to assert once again the way in which a multiplicity of different representations, whether they be partial representations on a retinotopic basis, or abstract representations of knowledge about types of object in the world, or the specific types of planning involved in generating appropriate motor activity for locomotion and reaching, must be linked into an integrated whole. There is no one place in the brain where one integrated representation of space plays the sole executive role in linking perception and action.

Notes

1. Pellionisz's understanding of such transformations has developed as part of what is called the tensor model of the cerebellum. Elsewhere, Arbib and Amari (1985) explained why it is a mistake to suggest that the cerebellum implements a metric tensor and also showed that the way in which tensor terminology is used by Pellionisz does not accord well with the proper application of the mathematical framework of tensor analysis. They then suggest how tensor analysis might be used to advance brain theory.

2. The Perceptron training scheme of Rosenblatt (1962) gave a way of training a formalized neural network to yield (if possible) the desired output patterns in response to a given set of input patterns by adjusting the synaptic weights of the output neurons of a network on the basis of errors in the outputs of the neurons. Since the set of possible input–output transformations is extended if neurons internal to the network are also subject to synaptic modification, the back-propagation scheme (e.g. Rumelhart *et al*. 1986) extends this method to provide a rule for propagating the error back from output units to neurons within the network (the so-called hidden units) so that their connections may also be adjusted. The rule requires neurons to have output values varying continuously from 0 to 1 rather than being binary. (Further exposition is given in Sections 4.4 and 8.2 of Arbib 1989.)

3. Arbib (1975) introduced schemas as the building blocks for the brain's representation of knowledge. Schema theory provides a knowledge representation protocol which is in some ways related to the frames and scripts of artificial intelligence, but is distinguished by its special attention to perceptual structures and distributed motor control (Arbib 1981). Iberall and Arbib (1990) and Arbib (1990) probe the issue of the 'neural reality' of such schemas as those presented in this section.

4. Barto and Sutton (1981) show how the net can 'learn' appropriate values for the weights. At each step, the weights are adjusted in such a way as to improve the performance of the network. The z input signals proximity to the central goal. With no associated weights of its own, z is the 'teacher' used to adjust the weights linking sensory inputs to motor outputs. We need not consider z further in our present discussion.

5. The leaky integrator model uses the 'firing rate' (e.g. the number of spikes traversing the axon in the most recent 20 ms) as a continuously varying measure of the cell's output, while the internal state of the neuron is described by a single variable, the membrane potential. The firing rate $M(t)$ is approximated by a sigmoid function σ of the membrane potential

$m(t)$, $M(t) = \sigma(m(t))$). The time evolution of the cells' membrane potential is given by the differential equation $\tau\,\dot{m}(t) = -m(t) + \Sigma_{iwi}\,X_i(t) + h$, where $X_i(t)$ is the firing rate at the ith input. Here, τ is the time constant of the neuron, while the w_i are synaptic weights.

References

Anastasio, T. J. and Robinson, D. A. (1989). Distributed parallel processing in the vestibulo-oculomotor system. *Neural Computation*, **1**, 230–41.

Arbib, M. A. (1972). *The metaphorical brain: an introduction to cybernetics as artificial intelligence and brain theory*. Wiley–Interscience, New York.

Arbib, M. A. (1975). Artificial intelligence and brain theory: unities and diversities. *Annals of Biomedical Engineering*, **3**, 238–74.

Arbib, M. A. (1981). Perceptual structures and distributed motor control. In *Handbook of physiology—The nervous system II. motor control* (ed. V. B. Brooks), pp. 1449–80. American Physiological Society, Bethesda, MD.

Arbib, M. A. (1989). *The metaphorical brain 2: Neural networks and beyond*. Wiley–Interscience, New York.

Arbib, M. A.(1990). Programs, schemas, and neural networks for control of hand movements: beyond the RS framework. In *Attention and performance XIII. Motor representation and control* (ed. M. Jeannerod), pp. 111–38. Erlbaum, Hillsdale, NJ.

Arbib, M. A. and Amari, S. (1985). Sensori-motor transformations in the brain (with a critique of the tensor theory of cerebellum). *Journal of Theoretical Biology*, **112**, 123–55.

Arbib, M. A. and House, D. H. (1987). Depth and detours: an essay on visually-guided behaviour. In *Vision, brain, and cooperative computation* (ed. M. A. Arbib and A. R. Hanson), pp. 129–63. Bradford Books/MIT Press, Cambridge, MA.

Arkin, R. C. (1989). Neuroscience in motion: the application of schema theory to mobile robotics. In *Visuomotor coordination: amphibians, comparisons, models, and robots* (ed. J.-P. Ewert and M. A. Arbib), pp. 649–71, Plenum, New York.

Barto, A. G. and Sutton, R. S. (1981). Landmark learning: An illustration of associative search, *Biological Cybernetics*, **42**, 1–8.

Berkinblit, M. B., Deliagina, T. G., Feldman, A. G., Gelfand, I. M., and Orlovsky, G. N. (1978). Generation of scratching. I. Activity of spinal interneurons during scratching. *Journal of Neurophysiology*, **41**, 1040–57.

Collett, T. (1982). Do toads plan routes? A study of the detour behaviour of *Bufo viridis*. *Journal of Comparative Physiology*, **146**, 261–71.

Dean, P., Redgrave, P., and Westby, G. W. M. (1989). Event or emergency? Two response systems in the mammalian superior colliculus. *Trends in Neuroscience*, **12**, 138–47.

Dev, P. (1975). Perception of depth surfaces in random-dot stereograms: a neural model. *International Journal of Man–Machine Studies*, **7**, 511–28.

De Yoe, E. A. and Van Essen, D. C. (1988). Concurrent processing streams in monkey visual cortex, *Trends in Neuroscience*, **11**, 219–26.

Ewert, J.-P. (1987). Neuroethology of releasing mechanisms. *Behavioral and Brain Sciences*, **10**, 337–405.

Fukson, O. I., Berkinblit, M. B., and Feldman, A. G. (1980). The spinal frog takes into account the scheme of its body during the wiping reflex. *Science*, **209**, 1261–3.

Geman, S. and Geman, D. (1984). Stochastic relaxation, Gibbs distributions, and the Bayesian restoration of images. *IEEE Transactions of Pattern Analysis and Machine Intelligence*, **6**, 721–41.

Greene, P. H. (1971). Introduction. In *Models of the structural functional organization of certain biological systems* (ed. I. M. Gel'fand, V. S. Gurfinkel, S. V. Fomin, and M. L. Tsetlin, trans. by C. R. Beard), pp. xi–xxxi. MIT Press, Cambridge, Mass.

Grobstein, P. (1989). Organization in the sensorimotor interface: A case study with increased resolution. In *Visuomotor coordination: amphibians, comparisons, models, and robots* (ed. J.-P. Ewert and M. A. Arbib), pp. 537–68. Plenum, New York.

House, D. (1989). *Depth perception in frogs and toads: a study in neural computing. Lecture Notes in Biomathematics 80*. Springer-Verlag, Berlin.

Iberall, T. and Arbib, M. A. (1990). Schemas for the control of hand movements: an essay on cortical localization. In *Vision and action: the control of grasping* (ed. M. A. Goodale), pp. 204–42. Ablex, Norwood, NJ.

Iberall, T., Bingham, G., and Arbib, M. A. (1986). Opposition space as a structuring concept for the analysis of skilled hand movements. *Experimental Brain Research Series*, **15**, 158–73.

Jeannerod, M. (1981). Le controle de l'oeil sur le geste. *La Recherche*, **12**, 376–8.

Lieblich, I. and Arbib, M. A. (1982). Multiple representations of space underlying behaviour. *Behavioral and Brain Sciences*, **5**, 627–59.

Nicod, J. (1970). *Geometry and induction* (trans. J. Bell and M. Woods). University of California Press.

O'Keefe, J. (1984). Spatial memory within and without the hippocampal system. In *Neurobiology of the hippocampus* (ed. W. Seifert), pp. 375–403. Academic Press, New York.

Olton, D. S. (1984). Memory functions and the hippocampus. In *Neurobiology of the hippocampus* (ed. W. Seifert), pp. 335–73. Academic Press, New York.

Paillard, J. (1990). Basic neurophysiological structure of eye–hand coordination. In *Development of eye–hand coordination across the lifespan* (ed. C. Bard, M. Fleury, and L. Hay) pp. 26–74. University of South Carolina Press.

Paillard, J. and Beaubaton, D. (1978). De la coordination visuo-motrice à l'organisation de la saisie manuelle. In *Du contrôle moteur à l'organisation du geste* (ed. H. Hecaen and M. Jeannerod), pp. 225–60. Masson, Paris.

Pellionisz, A. (1984). Coordination: a vector–matrix description of transformations of overcomplete CNS coordinates and tensorial solution using the Moore-Penrose generalized inverse. *Journal of Theoretical Biology*, **110**, 353–75.

Pellionisz, A. and Graf, W. (1987). Tensor network model of the 'three-neuron vestibulo-ocular reflex-arc' in cat, *Journal of Theoretical Neurobiology*, **5**, 127–51.

Pitts, W. H. and McCulloch, W. S. (1947). How we know universals, the perception of auditory and visual forms. *Bulletin of Mathematical Biophysics*, **9**, 127–47.

Poggio, T., Gamble, E. B., and Little, J. J. (1988). Parallel integration of visual modules. *Science*, **242**, 436–40.

Riseman, E. M. and Hanson, A. R. (1987). A methodology for the development of general knowledge-based vision systems. In *Vision, brain and cooperative computation* (ed. M. A. Arbib and A. R. Hanson), pp. 285–328. Bradford Books/ MIT Press, Cambridge, MA.

Room, T. G. (1967). *A background (natural, synthetic and algebraic) to geometry.* Cambridge University Press.

Rosenblatt, F. (1962). *Principles of Neurodynamics.* Spartan, Washington, DC.

Rumelhart, D. E., Hinton, G. E., and Williams, R. J. (1986). Learning internal representations by error propagation. In *Parallel distributed processing: explorations in the microstructure of cognition*, Vol. 1 (ed. D. Rumelhart and J. McClelland), pp. 318–62. MIT Press/Bradford Books, Cambridge, MA.

Scudder, C. A. (1988). A new local feedback model of the saccadic burst generator, *Journal of Neurophysiology*, **59**, 1455–75.

Shadmehr, R. (1989). A neural model for generation of some behaviours in the fictive scratch reflex. *Neural Computation*, **1**, 242–52.

van Gisbergen, J. A. M., Robinson, D. A., and Gielen, S. (1981). A quantitative analysis of generation of saccadic eye movements by burst neurons. *Journal of Neurophysiology*, **45**, 417–42.

von der Malsburg, C. (1988). Pattern recognition by labelled graph matching. *Neural Networks*, **1**, 141–8.

von Hofsten, C. (1990). Early development of grasping an object in space-time. In *Vision and action: the control of grasping* (ed. M. A. Goodale), pp. 65–79, Ablex, Norwood, NJ.

Whitehead, A. N. (1929). *Process and reality.* Macmillan, London.

21

Neurocomputing concepts in motor control
PIETRO MORASSO and VITTORIO SANGUINETI

Introduction

The nature of the computational processes that underly initiation, generation, and termination of co-ordinated movements is still largely unknown.
Earlier computational metaphors, such as the motor programme concept,
have clearly demonstrated insurmountable difficulties in dealing with
excess degrees of freedom, context sensitivity, and so on.

Neurocomputing concepts are currently being advocated for overcoming
limitations in conventional computing methods in a large variety of applications. This has renewed interest in the old cybernetic idea that computation, communication, and control are just three facets of the same thing,
and has given new strength to the conjecture that biological systems, as
typical *cybernetic machines*, are valuable paradigms for the investigation of
neurocomputing.

Neural networks, as physical systems of multiple, interacting elements,
are dynamic systems of large size that process information in an analogic
way. Moreover, the computational process is intrinsically parallel and distributed, because the basic operation is the transformation of global patterns simultaneously. Programming, as an ordered sequence of explicit
instructions, is substituted by strategies of parameter adjustment, i.e.
learning. Although a very large variety of neurocomputing models exists,
we think that they can be reduced, from our perspective of motor control,
to three main computational paradigms:

- association,
- relaxation,
- self-organization,

that are characterized by basic functional features. Association is the
ability of a system to implement mapping between input and output representations; relaxation characterizes the behaviour of a dynamic system in
the neighbourhood of equilibrium configurations; self-organization may
emerge from non-linear dynamic systems operating far from equilibrium.
We believe that all these computational paradigms have a role in the
human, motor-control system, although in rather different ways.

In particular, it is evident that associative networks, such as multi-layer perceptrons, look at skills as 'black boxes': input and output representations must be clearly defined and an error vector must be available to the motor system for adapting the input–output transformation parameters, i.e. the connection weights of the neurons.

As regards relaxation networks, such as Hopfield networks (Hopfield 1982, 1984), we must acknowledge that these are devices for optimization. There is no question, of course, that movements are optimal in some sense, but the fact that people have such different 'motor styles' means that no single, universal criterion exists. Moreover, we must never forget that, as was clearly remarked by N. Bernstein (1967), movement is not causally determined by *active* efferent patterns only but is shaped by the *passive* influences of the environment as well. In general, we can look at motor optimization in two different ways: (a) as the direct search for active motor patterns that optimize some performance factor; or (b) as the indirect effect of an internal simulation of the interaction between the environment and the motor system. The direct approach to relaxation is essentially the same as association, i.e. it is focused on performance. The indirect approach, on the contrary, is focused on the physical phenomena that underly movements, whatever the task or skill that we are considering. In the following we shall restrict our analysis to the latter sense.

Self-organizing feature maps, as proposed by Kohonen (1988), are powerful devices for discovering regularities in a flow of data. Basic, local mechanisms of competition/co-operation between units in a Kohonen map allow the units to be tuned in such a way that the input vector space is optimally tessellated (from the information point of view). Although Kohonen networks have been studied mainly in perception, we believe that they can also be proved to be useful in motor control. In general, one could think of Kohonen maps as *intelligent tables*, and it is well known that the *tabular* concept has long inspired students of motor control.

We think that the different neurocomputing paradigms, outlined above, are powerful enough to capture the subtle and immense complexities of motor skills or schemas. The 'bottom line', apart from the large number of reflex and perceptuo-motor integration mechanisms, is the formation of *synergies* of motor commands that can support basic actions, such as reaching, hitting, catching, etc. By synergy, we informally mean a generation/distribution mechanism, structured in time and space, that transforms a concise motion plan into an array of time functions, one for each muscle. During everyday life, basic actions of this kind are performed in a limitless number of combinations and variations. Even the simplest movement involves virtually all the muscles and the degrees of freedom of the human body. Therefore, to talk of excess degrees of freedom (as it is done by many students of motor control) is somehow misleading, because it implies that 'excess' is the exception to a 'standard' (a non-redundant, robot-like manipulator) that, in reality, does not exist. On the contrary, the basic neural mechanism for synergy formation must be rather insensitive to the exact number of degrees of freedom and muscles, or to the specific constraints that they must satisfy. Furthermore, it is very unlikely that this mechanism ignores the mechanical properties of muscles; rather, it seems reasonable that evolution has taken advantage of their computational characteristics and has exploited them in the design of the mechanism.

Association does not seem an appropriate computational paradigm for this purpose. It requires a precise identification of input, output, and desired operation that is unreasonable for bottom-line motor abilities; and training is absolutely necessary for achieving performance. For this purpose, as will be argued in the rest of the chapter, relaxation networks are more appropriate: these networks are driven by *attractors*, which, in the case of the motor system, correspond to postures of minimum potential energy, and we postulate that the generation of motor synergies is equivalent to the simulation of an internal model of the visco-elastic system. This model does not need to be learned from scratch because it does not depend on the specific task but mainly reflects the physics of the musculo-skeletal system: it can be 'wired-in' from birth and its parameters can be tuned during practice.

Associative networks, on the other hand, are strongly dependent on the specific nature of a motor schema. Although this makes them unsuitable as a general-purpose mechanism of synergy formation, associative networks are ideal for perfecting a skill, by focusing attention on a selected set of input–output variables and a specific performance criterion, as in sports or other highly practised movements. Relaxation networks are indeed a rather unfocused computational paradigm, which can only offer general-purpose services but is too bulky and possibly too slow for top performance. Therefore, it is natural to think of a complementary relationship between relaxation and associative networks in the sense that the former can be conceived of as a background process that can 'boot strap' the latter in the initial phase of learning a specific skill: moreover, a relaxation network can possibly be *suspended* during the execution of skilled patterns and may eventually be *resumed* during less focused operations.

Self-organizing networks, on the other hand, can provide the *compositional element*, i.e. the tables or catalogues of basic actions from which action sequences can be composed, and this is necessary for both the associative and relaxation modes hypothesized above. For example, we have studied the possible role of Kohonen networks in modelling the production of handwriting, i.e., the generation of strokes and the chaining of stroke sequences into allographs and of allographs into words (Morasso 1989).

Summing up, we can conceive of a nested structure that consists of three layers:

- synergy generation;
- skill adaptation;
- skill composition.

In this chapter, we shall focus on the innermost layer and, in particular, we shall analyse in detail a relaxation model that was presented preliminarily by Morasso *et al.* (1989).

Motor relaxation as a passive-motion paradigm

The idea that relaxation can be a fundamental mechanism of motor planning and control comes from the study of the spring-like properties of muscles. Their role in controlling posture and movement was clearly demonstrated for the first time by Feldman (1966), who observed that in a simple joint the angular position is identified by the intersection of the length–tension curves of agonist and antagonist muscles, i.e. it is a result of *passive* mechanical properties and not of *active* feedback control. Subsequently, experiments with single-joint and multiple-joint movements were performed which confirmed the original idea (Bizzi *et al.* 1976; Kelso 1977, Polit and Bizzi 1979, among others). From this came the *equilibrium* trajectory hypothesis (Bizzi *et al.* 1984; Hogan 1984; Mussa Ivaldi *et al.* 1985), according to which limb movements are achieved by gradually shifting the hand equilibrium position encoded by neuromuscular activities. The next logical step was to formulate a computational mechanism of the formation of equilibrium trajectories. This was done by Mussa Ivaldi *et al.* (1988), who proposed a *passive-motion paradigm* (PMP), i.e. the concept that plans of movement (which include synergies of muscular activities as well as expected muscle contractions, joint rotations, and limb trajectories) can be obtained by the *simulation of an internal model* of the musculo-skeletal system, subjected to virtual disturbances that correspond to the intended movements.

The simulation may produce an overt movement or simply a mental image of it. Furthermore, the power of the concept is that it overcomes the degrees-of-freedom problem that challenges any model of motor control. Motor redundancy (as regards both joints and muscles) is indeed *hidden* by the fact that the passive elastic properties of muscles and ligaments embed the musculo-skeletal system into a potential energy function that has remarkable properties: it uniquely determines posture when neural commands are kept constant, and shapes movement when real disturbances are applied or neural commands are generated in such a way as to represent 'virtual' disturbances. In summary, the basic computational concept is that the mechanical properties of muscles are not just a pure, peripheral topic but have a strong organizational influence at the central, motor-planning level.

The PMP can be naturally implemented by a relaxation network (M-net) which seeks equilibrium states of some computational energy function analogous to the mechanical potential energy of the musculo-skeletal system. This is obtained by a *somatotopic network* of neural assemblies in which we allocate units representing the skeletal segments, the muscles, and the ligaments. Such units are not as fine-grained as neurons but are mid-grained like cortical columns or similar cell assemblies in other parts of the brain; they must deal with vectorial quantities (as regards both input and output) and perform simple but not trivial mechanical calculations. However, these calculations need not be very precise because the same redundancy that challenges the architecture of the motor controller guarantees, at the same time, a certain robustness against 'noise' in the computational process when distributed to a large number of units.

An additional concept, which will be further developed in the following, is that PMP implies an alternation of *passive* and *active phases* during the generation of a motor plan. The internal model that is advocated by the PMP is an analogic device for transforming an intention of movement, expressed as a virtual disturbance applied to the internal model, into a pattern of motions of all the joints and muscles; to this, however, we must add one more logical step, i.e. the derivation of the activation patterns that would have produced the same result as the virtual disturbance. This is the active part of the motor plan and we have two alternatives: one is to perform it concurrently with the passive simulation; the other is to alternate the two phases, by allowing a sequence of equilibrium states along a trajectory and by updating the motor commands intermittently, near their equilibrium configurations. We opted for the second alternative in our model, because a concurrent passive/active network is very complex and highly prone to instability.

Analogy between motor relaxation and Hopfield networks

We defined informally in the previous section the concept of motor M-nets as a distributed implementation of PMP. We wish to discuss here the analogy with Hopfield networks, which are prototypical relaxation sytems. For this purpose, and for clarity of presentation, we will now summarize the structure of Hopfield networks. Discrete Hopfield networks (Hopfield 1982) are arrays of artificial neurons or units interconnected through a matrix of weights T (Fig. 21.1, top). Each unit has an output V, a bias B, an external input I, and an array of connection weights T_{ji} which represent the 'synaptic' influence on unit i from all the other units. The output is computed by means of an activation function which operates on the net input:

$$net_i = \Sigma_j T_{ji} V_j + I_i$$
$$V_i = g(net_i - B_i)$$

where $g(.)$ is the unit-step function. Hopfield demonstrated that for such a network it is possible to define a potential energy function if the connection matrix T is symmetrical and its principal diagonal is null (i.e. there are no self-connections). In these conditions, the network admits equilibrium configurations and its dynamics can be characterized as a convergent flow from the initial configuration towards the nearest equilibrium configuration.

Continuous networks of the same nature have also been studied (Hopfield 1984), in particular, as networks of electronic amplifiers, resistors and capacitors with a stronger analogy to the electrical characteristics of neurons (Fig. 21.1, top). Each unit is made up with an amplifier that has two complementary outputs in order to represent separately the excitatory and inhibitory influence of neurons; the connection weights are now made up by resistors R_{ij} ($T_{ij} = 1/R_{ij}$) that transform output voltages V_i into input currents. These currents, for each unit, are added to an external input current, yielding a net membrane input current net_i. At the synaptic site this current determines a membrane potential U_i when interacting with the membrane resistance R and capacitance C according to the simple equation $C\dot{U}_i + U_i/R = net_i$. Finally, the membrane potential is mapped into the output potential through a non-linear sigmoidal function $V = g(U)$, which represents the approximately sigmoidal relation between membrane potential and the firing rate of neurons. Also, for the continuous Hopfield networks, symmetry of connections is a sufficient condition for assuring a convergent flow of network dynamics to equilibrium configurations.

Let us now consider these networks as continuous, dynamic systems. Standard system equations in state form $\dot{x} = f(x,z)$ (where x is the state vector, z is the input vector, and $f(.)$ is an array of non-linear systems functions) can be represented by the block diagram of Fig. 21.1 (middle), which can be considered as the scheme of an analogue computer, based on integrators and non-linear feedback. Hopfield networks can be interpreted as dynamic systems by considering that the natural choice of the state vector is the set of capacitive voltages U_i. Figure 21.1 (middle) shows the corresponding block diagram that separates the linear and non-linear parts of the system functions and clearly shows the symmetrical element that guarantees convergent flow.

Motor relaxation networks should make up a distributed, computational model that generates the equilibrium trajectories of a musculo-skeletal

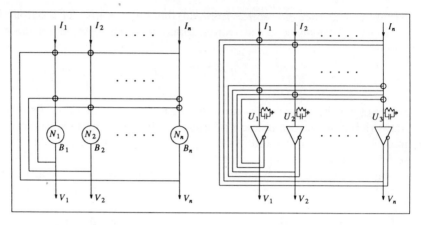

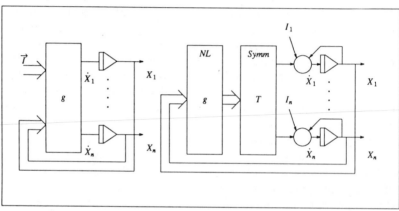

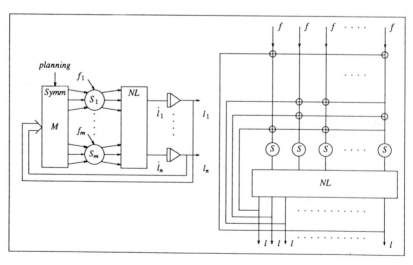

structure, i.e. a *mechanical circuit* of skeletal bodies and visco-elastic elements. Considered as a dynamic system, its state vector is the set of lengths of all the elastic components, i.e. the energy-storage elements. Here we need a few words of comment as regards the elastic elements: in our model we explicitly represent not only muscles but also ligaments. The reason for including them does not come just from a requirement of representational fidelity but from a computational necessity. A generic requirement of a distributed, somatotopic network is that it performs *local* computations. In a complex, articulated structure like the skeleton, the joints are kinematic constraints that are difficult to express in general because the number of degrees-of-freedom changes during actions and exact calculations would require the 'global' analysis of entire kinematic chains. By using ligaments in the computational model, it is possible to transform exact kinematic constraints into soft, elastic constraints, i.e. *local* computations, whatever the interaction between the skeleton and the environment; in other words, the model uses an expanded set of degrees of freedom (six for each S-unit) that are functionally reduced by the action of the ligaments and muscles (L-units and M-units).

Figure 21.1 (bottom) shows a block diagram of an m-net interpreted as a dynamic system. The output stage has an array of n integrators that corresponds to the elastic elements of the system. Informally speaking, the input to this stage is provided by a non-linear transformation of the outputs of another array of units that represents the different skeletal segments (S-units): each S-unit is identified by a cloud of points located on the skeletal segment, which are insertion points of muscles and ligaments or other forces, and its function is to transform a set of incoming force vectors into the velocity vectors $\dot{\mathbf{p}}$ of the corresponding insertion points. Finally, the input to the S-units comes from a generalized, interconnection matrix M, which represents muscles and ligaments. Different from the standard Hopfield net, this matrix implements a non-linear mapping, because the muscles are not ideal springs, but it retains the essential requirement of symmetry, intrinsic to the underlying physical system. Moreover, this generalized interconnection matrix is not constant, but is actively changed during the actual motor-planning process. The figure also shows the same

---

Fig. 21.1. Top box: Hopfield relaxation networks. Left: discrete network; right: continuous network. Small circles identify connection elements (constant weights). Triangular symbols correspond to amplifiers with sigmoidal transfer function and double output: direct and inverted (small circle). Middle box. Dynamic systems and relaxation. Left: structure of a generic, dynamic system (**X**: state vector; **I**: input vector, $g(.)$: system function). Right: structure of a continuous Hopfield network as a dynamical system (the system function consists of a non linear sigmoidal part $g(.)$ and a linear transformation with a symmetric matrix T). Triangle–rectangle symbols correspond to integrators. Bottom box. Motor relaxation networks. Left: M-net as a dynamical system (**I**: state vector of muscle lengths; **f**: input vector of virtual force disturbances). Right: M-net as a generalized Hopfield network.

model drawn as a generalized Hopfield network, which emphasizes the logically layered nature of the network: a layer of skeletal units, one of muscle and ligament units, one of cross-connections, and one of external inputs.

Structure of motor relaxation networks

As outlined in the previous section, there are three types of units in an m-net:

- skeletal segment units (S-units);
- muscle units (M-units);
- ligament units (L-units).

M-units and S-units behave as impedances, i.e. they receive positional information and react by feeding back force information. S-units, on the contrary, behave as admittances, i.e. they receive force information and react by modifying positional parameters. Figure 21.2 (top) sketches the correspondence between these units and the actual musculo-skeletal components.

S-units

S-units model the different skeletal body segments, represented as rigid bodies to which complex sets of forces are applied. Let us define the input variables, output variables, state variables, parameters, and activation function.

- Input variables: $(\vec{f}_1, \vec{f}_2, \ldots)$.
  These are the various types of force vectors applied to the S-unit. We distinguish two types of forces: *internal forces* (applied by M-units, L-units, and gravity) and *external forces* (used to express motor goals or environmental constraints).
- State variable: (homogeneous matrix H).
  It identifies the position/orientation of a Cartesian frame, fixed in the skeletal segment, with respect to a reference frame in the environment.
- Parameters: $(\vec{r}_1, \vec{r}_2, \ldots)$.
  These are the insertion points, i.e., the points where the various force vectors are applied and are referred to the local frame. H performs the transformation from these parameters (which are constant) to the output variables (which change during movement). An additional parameter is the mass of the skeletal segment.

- Output variables: $(\vec{p}_1, \vec{p}_2, \ldots)$
  These are the current position vectors of the insertion points expressed in a reference frame common to all the S-units.
- Activation function: it computes the output variables according to the following algorithm:
  —Computation of the resultant force and torque vectors
  $$\vec{F} = \Sigma_i \vec{f}_i$$
  $$\vec{N} = \Sigma_i (\vec{p}_i - \vec{c}) \times \vec{f}_i$$
  —Computation of vectors of velocity of rotation and translation
  $$\vec{v} = \eta \cdot g(\vec{F})$$
  $$\vec{\omega} = \eta' \cdot g(\vec{N})$$
  —Homogeneous matrix update
  $$H(t + dt) = \Delta H_1(\vec{v} \cdot dt) \cdot \Delta H_2(\vec{\omega} \cdot dt) \cdot H(t)$$
  —Computation of the output variables
  $$\vec{p}_i = H \cdot \vec{r}_i$$

In these equations $\vec{c}$ is the centre of gravity of the unit; $g(.)$ is the sigmoidal function which has the purpose of saturating the speed of relaxation movements (these movements are also controlled by η and η', i.e. apparent computational viscosities); ΔH_1 and ΔH_2 are the matrix operators that identify an infinitesimal translation $\vec{v}_i \cdot dt$ and an infinitesimal rotation $\vec{\omega} \cdot dt$, respectively.[1] In summary, an S-unit rotates and translates as a function of the resultant force and torque vectors, according to a viscous behaviour, and in so doing determines the velocity vectors of the cloud of insertion points. For convenience, instead of computing these vectors explicitly, we compute their integral, i.e. the updated position vectors. At equilibrium, the resultant vectors will be null.

M-units

M-units model single and multi-joint muscles as elastic cables passing through pulleys and fixed at their extremities onto two different bones. As a consequence, these cables are divided into a number of tracts and, if we ignore friction, the tension can be assumed to be constant in all the tracts of the same muscle. Only some tracts change their length during movement (they are dubbed *active* because only their tension influences the equilibrium of S-units), but also the other tracts are relevant because the force of a muscle depends on its total length.

From the computational point of view, an M-unit has two modes of operation: *active* and *passive*. In the passive mode, it behaves as a common spring, i.e. it receives from nearby S-units the co-ordinates of its insertion points and feeds them back with the developed force, computed from the

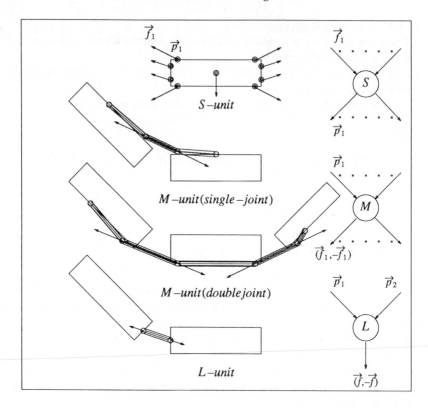

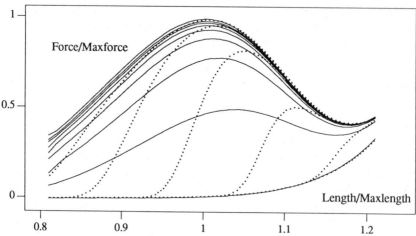

Fig. 21.2. Top box: Components of a motor relaxation network: S-unit; M-unit; L-unit. The small circles identify the insertion points of either muscles or ligaments and the arrows correspond to the pairs of force vectors of each active tract. Bottom box: Normalized length–tension curves of muscles for the α-model (continuous line) and the λ-model (dotted line).

length-tension curves, for the current level of muscle command. In the active mode, which is entered when the network is close to equilibrium, the level of muscle command is changed according to a strategy that will be explained below.

As regards the length–tension curves, it is obviously not necessary to duplicate in the network all the complex mechano-electro-chemical dynamics of the muscles and their distributed structure. M-units are indeed models of the central somatotopic representation of the elastic properties of muscles, which must also take into account their characteristic non-linearity, i.e. the fact that, for a given level of muscular command, there is an optimal length, not far from mid range, which gives maximum force output (Gordon *et al.* 1966; Stevens *et al.* 1980; Inman *et al.* 1981).

The specific length-tension curves used by M-units were derived from a detailed model proposed by Hatze (1981) by considering the steady-state relations of a typical motor unit, representative of the whole muscle. (In Appendix 1 there is a concise summary of the model.) We ignore, as regards the behaviour of M-units, the transients due to electrochemical activation dynamics, to mechanical dynamics (non-linear viscous pheno-mena that do not affect equilibrium), and to recruitment dynamics, be-cause recruitment patterns are probably organized in more peripheral stages of motor control, in accordance with implementation constraints such as the Henneman principle.

The length–tension curves of an M-unit are families of curves indexed by the firing rate V, which is the only control variable,

$$f = f(l, V; \Pi)$$
$$\Pi : \hat{f}, \hat{l}, \sigma$$

parametrized by the maximum isometric force $\hat{f}$, the length $\hat{l}$ at which this is achieved (the *optimal length*) and by a coefficient (σ) which measures the *spread* of the length–tension curves, in a similar way to the standard deviation for a Gaussian function. The first parameter is proportional to the number of motor units in the muscle and the second to the number of sarcomeres in a muscle fibre. Their product is proportional to the total number of sarcomeres in the muscle, i.e. its power. Figure 21.2 (bottom) shows a family of functions valid for the medial head of the triceps ($\hat{f}$:805 N; $\hat{l}$: 8.6 cm; σ: 0.433.)

In summary, in the passive mode an M-unit is defined as follows:

- Input variables: $(\vec{p}_1, \vec{p}_2, \ldots)$.
  These are the insertion points of the muscle; the indication of the active tracts is stored in the unit.
- Parameters: $(\hat{f}, \hat{l}, \sigma)$.
- Output variables: $((\vec{f}_{t1}, -\vec{f}_{t1}), (\vec{f}_{t2}, -\vec{f}_{t2}), \ldots)$.

These are the pairs of force vectors in each active tract. Mono-articular muscles only have one pair. The two vectors of each pair add up to zero and are applied to the two S-units that are connected by that muscle tract.

• Activation function: it uses the length–tension curves for the current length and level of neural command V, after having computed the total muscle length l from the input variables. From this it forms the pairs of force vectors.

The active mode is discussed afterwards.

L-units

L-units are used primarily in order to model joints. Joints are kinematic constraints among adjacent linkages that allow restricted motions within joint limits. L-units model both types of constraints in a soft way, as appropriate ensembles of (high-stiffness) springs. For example, in the case of enarthrosis (ball-and-socket joint), the kinematic constraint can be represented by a single spring with zero rest-length; in the case of ginglymus (hinge joint) we need a pair of springs whose terminals approximately identify the rotation axis; in the case of a saddle joint we need two pairs of springs.

Joint limits can be represented by means of additional springs. For example, two more springs are sufficient for the hinge-type joint in order to constrain the rotations within a specified angular range. For more complex joints, such as the spherical joint, it is well known that the exact and explicit formulation of a joint limit function is very complex (Korein 1985); L-units allow us to approximate these functions implicitly and to generate, at the same time, forces that tend to keep the joints far from them. L-units can also be used to represent multi-joint ligaments, such as the retinacular ligament in the fingers, which is essential for the ordered succession of inter-phalangeal joint rotations (Tubiana 1981).

L-units are basically equivalent to M-units operating in the passive phase. The difference is in the activation function, which is monotonic and is linearized for simplicity. Obviously, L-units do not express kinematic constraints in an exact way. The approximation error depends on the relation between muscle stiffness and ligament stiffness in a very complex way. If ligament stiffness is too small, network relaxation may yield strongly 'dislodged' joints; if it is too large, the overall network may become unstable. In practice, it is sufficient that joint stiffness is about one order of magnitude bigger than the largest muscle stiffness.

In summary, an L-unit is defined as follows:

- Input variables: $(\vec{p}_1, \vec{p}_2, \ldots)$.
  These are the insertion points of the ligaments; the indication of the active tracts is stored in the unit.
- Parameters: (l_0, k).
  The first parameter is the rest-length and the second is the stiffness.
- Output variables: $((\vec{f}_{t1}, -\vec{f}_{t1}), (\vec{f}_{t2}, -\vec{f}_{t2}), \ldots)$.
  These are the pairs of force vectors in each active tract. Mono-articular ligaments only have one pair. The two vectors of each pair add up to zero and are applied to the S-units that are connected by that ligament tract.
- Activation function: it uses the length–tension curve $f = k(l - l_0)$ after having computed the total length l from the input variables. From this it forms the pairs of force vectors.

External inputs

External inputs are additional force vectors applied to S-units in order to take into account motor goals or environmental constraints. Together, these forces are the inputs to an M-net, as a global dynamic system. In the next section, we discuss a larger computational architecture in which external forces come from the interaction between an M-net, considered as a synergy, formation mechanism, and other nets that take into account planning and peripheral feedback. At the moment, let us point out that the PMP can be implemented by means of *attracting* forces that pull selected *end-effectors* toward desired targets. For example, the hand can be attracted to a target object in a reaching task or the swinging foot, during locomotion, can be attracted to a target footstep while, at the same time, the trunk is pulled forward in the direction of locomotion.

Alternation of passive and active phases

During the passive phase, an M-net evolves toward an equilibrium state compatible with a given set of external forces and motor-command variables. Only when equilibrium is reached, the motor commands can safely be updated without risking instability of the network. These changes displace the equilibrium of the network, which is re-gained in another relaxation phase.

In other words, the global dynamic is characterized by an alternation of passive relaxation phases followed by quick adjustments of the motor commands, i.e. a sort of computational nystagmus that induces a basic rhythmicity in the motor activity. Hints of intrinsic motor rhythms are obviously known in many motor activities and this is not the place to discuss them in detail, but let us simply suggest that many experimental data might outline a 'ball-park' figure of 100 ms for the alternation cycle.

During the active phase, the activity levels stored in the m-units can be updated according to four main strategies:

- Passivity (the motor command is left unchanged).
- Compliance (the motor command is changed in such a way to help the motion).
- Resistance (the motor command is changed in order to resist the motion).
- Co-activation (the motor commands are changed in order to increase/ decrease the stiffness level of a posture).

Compliance is the appropriate strategy for implementing the PMP because, if the motion was caused by an attractor, it generates muscle activations that tend to cancel out its effect, i.e. to 'substitute' or 'unload' it. *Resistance*, on the other hand, is appropriate when the cause of a movement is gravity or a contact force and we wish to resist it (e.g. during the stance phase of walking). *Passivity* can allow a smooth transition from compliance to resistance and vice versa. *Co-activation* is the technique for changing the global stability of posture and can be very useful in specific aspects of a skill.

The planning problems that underly strategy selection are outside the scope of this chapter. Let us simply present an implementation algorithm which is compatible with the computational approach presented so far:

- Let Δf_p denote, for a given M-unit, the variation of muscle force due to the last passive phase of relaxation.
- Let us choose the force variation during the active phase as follows: $\Delta f_a = k \cdot \Delta f_p$.
- Let us compute, from the length–tension curves, the corresponding variation of the neural command ΔV.

In this algorithm, k is an appropriate gain factor, whose sign and magnitude must be chosen according to the strategy: negative in the compliance case and positive in the resistance case. In the compliance case, for example, this algorithm automatically produces reciprocal activation patterns for agonist/antagonist groups of muscles.

Neuromotor commands (α-model versus λ-model)

The main purpose of an M-net is to generate a coherent pattern of motor commands, i.e. a synergy, and this is performed by each M-unit, during the active phases, updating values that keep constant during each passive phase. But what is the neural signal V that is kept constant during passive relaxation, updated during the active phase, and then transmitted to periphery? We considered two alternatives:

- One alternative is to identify this signal directly with the average firing rate of the α-motoneurons—what can be called an α-model.
- The second alternative, discussed by Feldman (1986), is to recognize the fact that central commands do not reach the muscular fibres, but must interact with a local neural circuitry in the spinal cord that delivers the final α signal as a function of both the central command V and the actual muscle length l:

$$\alpha = \alpha(V, l).$$

From the analysis of electromyographic patterns, Feldman proposed that in fact what counts is the difference between l and V because the length–tension curves recorded for a constant 'motor intention' tend to be parallel. These curves (that he named invariant characteristics: IC) are obviously different from iso-electric characteristics (the length–tension curves for constant α) because stretching a muscle along an IC gives an increasing and not a constant α, the increase being determined by the stretch reflex.

In this framework, the central command can be interpreted as a *length* (λ), which represents the threshold of the stretch reflex: for values of l below λ, α vanishes and for larger values grows until saturation. This is what Feldman called a λ-model. In our implementation, we used a sigmoidal function S:[2]

$$\alpha / \alpha_{max} = S(l - \lambda)$$

in which we adjusted the range of λ and the function coefficients in such a way that at $\lambda = \lambda_{min}$, the IC coincides with the highest iso-electric curve, and $\lambda = \lambda_{max}$ is not outside the physiological range of l. It turns out that the physiological range of $\lambda / \hat{l}$ is [0.40, 1.22] while $\hat{l} / l$ varies in the interval [0.80, 122]. The ICs of a typical muscle are depicted in Fig. 21.2(bottom) superimposed on the iso-electric curves. From these curves, it is possible to see that ICs tend to have a higher slope than iso-electric curves, i.e. the muscles appear to be 'stiffer' if we use the λ-model.

Both the α-model and the λ-model can be implemented in the framework of an M-net with similar results because both assume spring-like properties for the muscles. The λ-model, however, can allow to obtain more significant results as regards the motor commands. Feldman indeed showed that this mechanism can allow to reproduce the tri-phasic structure of electromyograms found in some simple single-joint movements, and we could reproduced these results in a simple M-net; in more complex M-nets we opted for the α-model because is simpler and the simulation is quicker.

The synergy formation architecture

In the previous sections we outlined the computational characteristics of M-nets, conceived as rhythmically pulsating, pattern generators that are based on a degree of analogy with the musculo-skeletal system. In this section, we briefly consider the additional modules that are necessary in order to have a coherent mechanism of synergy formation. In particular, let us focus on three main factors:

- specification of motor plans;
- adaptation to environmental constraints;
- adaptation to movement errors.

Figure 21.3 (top) shows a sketch of the synergy formation architecture, which has two main parts: an M-net and a P-net (a planning network). As regards the former, we can single out two streams of output signals: a stream of motor commands (either λ-signals or α-signals) and a stream of what we may call *kinematic expectations*. The latter can be considered as a side-effect of the relaxation process, because from the ensemble of units it is possible to extract, by means of appropriate *filters*, the expected time-course of all kinds of kinematic variables, at the muscle, joint, or trajectory level. This is the computational basis for setting up a mechanism of *corollary discharge* (CD) that compares the expected and the actual time-course of a selected set of kinematic variables and relays the detected mis-matches to the re-planning, P-net module.

The main role of the P-net is to communicate to the M-net an appropriate set of external forces (transmitted to S-unit) and contraction strategies (transmitted to M-units). This action can be triggered by different sources: a general motor intention, the CD mechanism, or specific afferences, e.g. tactile, that signal the transition between different phases of a complex task.

If we now consider, among the functions of a P-net, the generation of external forces for trajectory formation, it is remarkable that this function can be filled by means of another relaxation network, similar to the M-net, that operates as an *attractor* to a selected S-unit of the M-net, i.e. an end-effector. Figure 21.3 (bottom) shows a possible solution (a fragment of the P-net), that we used in our simulation experiments; the idea is to model each attractor as a three-units network:

- One S-unit represents the *target* and it simply consists of a single insertion point which is 'grounded' (i.e. its co-ordinates are kept fixed during the life of the attractor). Let us denote with $\vec{p}_T$ this point.
- The other S-unit represents the desired position of the end-effector (the

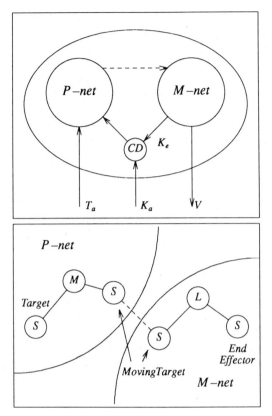

Fig. 21.3. Top box: Synergy formation architecture, composed of a *planning network*, a *motor relaxation network*, and a mechanism of *corollary discharge* (K_a: kinematic afference; K_e: kinematic expectations; T_a: tactile afferences; V: neural motor pattern). Bottom box: Example of interface between P-net and M-net (a target S-unit generates a moving target through a pseudomuscle; the content of the moving-target S-unit is transferred from the P-net to the M-net at each equilibrium state and attracts the designated end-effector through a pseudo-ligament).

moving target) and during the simulation it must move on the desired trajectory with the appropriate velocity profile. Let us denote this point with $\vec{p}_E$.

● The M-unit is the real engine of the attractor because it must generate a force that smoothly accelerates the moving S-unit in the initial phase of the trajectory and then slows it down. This can be achieved if length–tension curve of the unit is simply bell-shaped: $f_M = bell(p_T - p_E)$, with a function support equal to the initial distance between the target and the end-effector.

In these conditions, as the moving S-unit drives the insertion point p_E with a velocity vector proportional to f_M, then the trajectory formed by the attractor will necessarily be straight and with a bell-shaped velocity profile. Furthermore, as the duration of the motion is given by the integral of the velocity profile, then it is possible to synchronize different attractors by scaling the amplitude of the bell functions. In particular, the simplest synchronization strategy is to use an isochrony principle and this can be achieved by adapting the amplitude of the bell function inversely with respect to the support.

The M-net and the different attractor networks can evolve in an independent manner and the rendezvous can occur at each equilibrium state of the M-net. The interface between the attractor and the M-net can be provided by an additional pair of units:

- A copy of the moving target, i.e. a buffer S-unit, which is started off (at each rendezvous) with the current position of the moving S-unit of the corresponding attractor network and is grounded there;
- A linkage L-unit, connected to the end-effector of the M-net, which actually transmits the external force to the M-net.

A powerful characteristic of this approach to trajectory formation is *compositionality*, i.e. multiple networks of this kind can operate concurrently in order to express multiple goals inherent in the same task. Compositionality, however, requires some form of synchronization among attractors, which we wish to obtain in an analogic way, without an explicit clock. The rhythmic behaviour of an M-net itself provides a sort of timebase that can be exploited by the attractors.

Simulation results

Many simulation experiments were performed with an M-net simulator that runs on an HP-9000 work-station under Unix. In particular, let us consider a simulation involving movements of the index finger. The skeletal system consists of four bones (metacarpus and three phalanges) and three joints: metacarpo-phalangeal (MP), proximal inter-phalangeal (PIP), and distal inter-phalangeal (DIP). As regards flexion/extension movements, the main participating muscles are two flexors (superficialis and profundus), the extensor digitorum communis, and the interossei (volares and dorsales). The flexors and the extensor, which are extrinsic muscles of the finger because their origins are outside the hand, influence all the joints in the same way. The interossei, on the contrary, are *oblique* intrinsic muscles that tend to have opposite effects on the MP and DIP joints (MP flexion and PIP extension). To this, we must add the action of the oblique retinacular ligament[3] that replicates the action of the interosseus one joint forward (it favours flexion of the PIP and extension of the DIP joint).

This is a kinematically simple system with a complex co-ordination problem that requires an accurate synergy of all the muscles, integrated with the action of purely passive elements such as the retinacular ligament. In the PIP joint, for example, flexion is favoured by the flexor and the oblique retinacular while it is opposed by the extensor and the interosseus.

Let us consider the physiology of flexion: flexion normally begins at the PIP joint and is then followed by the MP and only later by the DIP joint. This is functionally necessary, because an anticipation of the DIP flexion would greatly disturb grasping, but it is somewhat paradoxical because the more strongly activated muscle (the flexor profundus) would naturally cause the DIP flexion to occur first. The appropriate phasing is assured by the passive properties of both oblique structures. In essence, the causal chain is the following:

- EMG activity of the flexor causes an increase of the tension of the retinacular ligament, which opposes DIP flexion and favours PIP flexion.
- The initiation of the PIP flexion causes a stretch of the interosseus and then an increase of its tension, which favours MP flexion.
- At the same time, PIP flexion unloads the retinacular ligament, which then decreases its tension and does not inhibit the flexion of the DIP joint any more.

In our experiments, we developed a network that consists of four S-units, ten L-units, and three M-units (the network is reported in Appendix 2, according to the formalism of the simulation package).

The S-units identify the three phalanges and the metacarpus. For each of them we defined a reference frame, centred in the proximal joint and oriented in such a way that X points to the subsequent joint and Y is directed as the rotation axis.

Each one of the three joints was modelled by means of three L-units: a pair of collateral ligaments, with high stiffness and zero rest-length, that define the rotation axis, and a volar ligament, with smaller stiffness and non-zero rest-length, which avoids the occurrence of hyperextension. The tenth ligament models, with a soft spring, the retinacular oblique ligament that cross-connects the two inter-phalangeal joints. The three M-units represent the flexor profundus, the extensor digitorum communis, and an interosseus. The first two muscles span all the three joints, following a palmar or dorsal pathway, respectively. The interosseus is a double-joint muscle and has an opposite effect on the two articulations (flexion of the MP joint and extension of the PIP joint).

The parameters of the different units were partly derived from the experimental data reported by Tubiana (1981) and partly from internal constraints of consistency. With this network we performed a number of simulation experiments, like the flexion shown in Fig. 21.4, which is driven

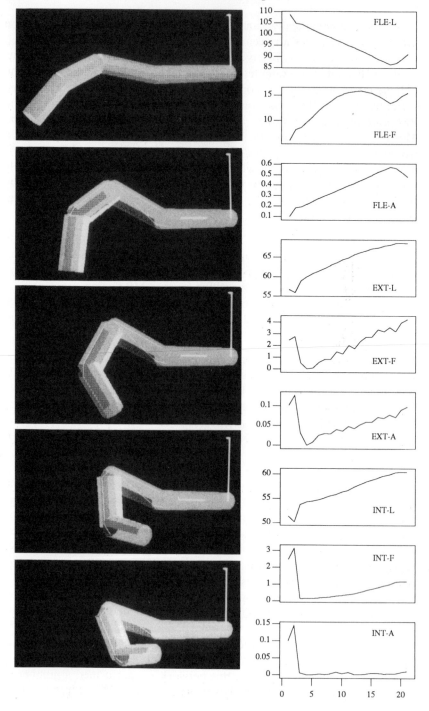

Fig. 21.4. M-net of a finger. Left: photograms of the simulation of a flexion movement. Right: graphs of the profiles of muscle length (L), force (F), and α-activity (A) for the three M-units of the network: flexor (FLE), extensor (EXT), and interosseus (INT). Ordinates for the L-curves are in mm, for the F-curves are in N, and for the A-curves are in normalized activation units (1 is the maximum α activity; abscissas are arbitrary time units.

by a single attractor connected to the fingertip. The right part of the figure, in particular, shows, for each of the three muscles, the time-course of its length, force, and α-activity, i.e. both the motor synergy and the kinematic expectations. This simulation demonstrates that the model can reproduce the appropriate order of joint rotations and the muscle activation patterns (strong activity of the flexor and passive behaviour of the other muscles).

The results are dependent on the fine tuning of all the model parameters and we could indeed reproduce known anomalies, such as the so-called swan-neck deformity, which consists mainly in an hyperextension of the PIP joint and is due to a weakened oblique retinacular. Other support for the model comes from preliminary experiments during which we collected flexion/extension movements of the index finger by means of an opto-electronic device; we then simulated an M-net driven by an attractor mimicking the fingertip of the original movement and we compared the joint rotation in the two cases. The results are encouraging.

In summary, the motor control of a finger is a good example of the fact that the central nervous system must necessarily take into account the interplay of active and passive factors subserving synergy formation.

Discussion

In the framework of the application of neurocomputing concepts to the study of motor control, this chapter has described methods of synergy formation that rely on the force fields and the potential energy function supported by the elastic properties of the musculo-skeletal systems. In this volume and in an associated paper (Arbib 1989), Arbib discusses higher level, visuomotor co-ordination, particularly as regards path planning and schemas for hand control, which is inspired by similar concepts, although at a more abstract level.

Other recent studies are mainly concerned with single kinematic chains (Bullock and Grossberg 1988; Kawato *et al.* 1988; Kuperstein 1988; Eckmiller *et al.* 1989, Massone and Bizzi, 1989). In contrast, the approach presented in this chapter attempts to give a conceptual framework for addressing the general synergy formation problem, which is the basis for the composition and the adaptation of skilled human activity.

Acknowledgements

This work was supported by the Esprit Projects FIRST and ROBIS, by a National Program on Robotics of the Italian Research Council, and by a National Program on Bioengineering of the Italian Ministry of University and Research.

Appendix 1: model of the length–tension curves

The model, which is based on the known mechano-electro-chemical characteristics of sarcomeres, consists of two components: a series elastic element (SE) and a contractile element (CE), serially connected. The force is the same in both elements ($f^{se} = f^{ce} = f$) while the muscle length l is the sum of their lengths ($l = l^{se} + l^{ce}$). The control signal is the repetition rate $v(t)$ of a train of action potentials. The length–tension curves are families of functions

$$f = f(l, V; \Pi)$$

indexed by a set of parameters Π defined in the following. Their shapes come from a combination of the exponential behaviour of the SE and the gaussian behaviour of the CE; The latter expresses the fundamental characteristic of the sliding-filament mechanism of muscle contraction. As a consequence, it is possible to single out an optimum length $\hat{l}$ at which a given muscle attains peak isometric force $\hat{f}$ for a maximum value of the motor command ($v = v_{max}$).

For simplicity, the curves are normalized, considering dimensionless ratios:

- $f/\hat{f}$ the upper limit is 1, the lower limit is close to 0.
- $V = v/v_{max}$ it varies in (0, 1)
- $\xi = l^{ce}/\hat{l}^{ce}$ it varies in (0.58, 1.80).
- $l/\hat{l}$ it varies in (0.80, 1.22).
- $\delta = (l^{se} - l_0^{se})/(\hat{l}^{se} - l_0^{se})$ it varies in (0, 1).

The rest-length of the muscle l_0, achieved when $V = 0$, is close to $\hat{l}$ ($l_0/\hat{l} = 0.954$). This length is accounted for the 60 per cent by the SE and for the 40 per cent by the CE. The same proportion approximately holds for $\xi = 1$ and $V = 1$.

The length–tension curve of the SE is exponential:

$$f^{se}/\hat{f} = (e^{h\delta} - 1)/(e^h - 1)$$

The force exerted by the CE depends on the number of cross-links among sliding filaments and this number is influenced by three factors:

- electro-chemical (active state function q);
- geometric (degree of inter-filamentary overlap ψ);
- sliding speed factor (w).

These factors are combined in a multiplicative way:

$$f^{ce}/\hat{f} = q \cdot \psi \cdot w - \theta_0$$

and are counteracted by an internal resistance θ_0. We can ignore the w factor because we are only interested with steady-state behaviour. As regards ψ, it is possible to assume a Gaussian dependence upon ξ, centred around the optimum length ($\xi = 1$) which identifies, by definition, a 100 per cent overlap between the actin and myosin filaments:

$$\psi(\xi) = e^{-((\xi-1)/\sigma)^2}$$

The spread coefficient σ is dependent on the organization of the specific muscle: number of motor units, number of fibres in each of them, geometrical arrangement of fibres. It varies in the [0.3, 0.5] range.

As regards the active state function q, it can be defined as the percentage of myosin sites ready to form cross-links, i.e. sites which captured Ca anions. This percentage is influenced by the cascade of three phenomena:

- the arrival of a train of action potentials $\alpha(t)$;
- the formation of an intra-cellular, graded potential $\beta(t)$;
- the diffusion of Ca anions, according to a concentration γ which is also influenced by the geometric changes occurring during muscle contraction ($\gamma = \gamma(t, \xi)$).

The transformations from α to β and from β to γ can both be approximated by second-order, damped systems which smooth the incoming spike-train. However, it is more convenient to look at the trend in the signals determined by the instantaneous firing rate v of α. It turns out that, at steady state, the trend function of γ can be approximated by

$$\gamma(\xi, v) = \varepsilon \cdot v(t) \cdot \rho(\xi)$$

where ε is a rate-to-concentration conversion factor and ρ expresses the geometry-dependence of ion diffusion upon the contraction ξ:

$$\rho(\xi) = (\xi_d - 1)/(\xi_d/\xi - 1).$$

The transformation from ion concentration to active state function can be approximated with a sigmoid function

$$q(\xi, \gamma) = (q_0 + (k \cdot \gamma(\xi))^2)/(1 + (k \cdot \gamma(\xi))^2)$$

where k is a constant and q_0 is the background, active-state value.

Finally, the internal resistance θ_0 can be approximated exponentially in the following way:

$$\theta_0 = q_0/(1 - q_0)\cdot(2 - e^{c(\xi-1)})$$

In summary, the normalized length–tension curves $f/\hat{f} = f(l/\hat{l}, V)$ can be computed by numerically solving the implicit set of equations written above in which we used the following set of constants (from Hatze 1981):

Series element
  h 1.531
Primary conversion
  ε $1.373\ 10^{-4}$ moles/Hz
Diffusion
  ξ_d 2.90
Active state
  q_0 0.005
  k 66200
Internal resistance
  c 6.97

and a set of parameters, variable for different muscles: $\hat{f}, \hat{l}, \sigma$.

Hatze shows how these parameters can be estimated for the three heads of triceps brachii and provides the following values (units are N, cm, and pure number, respectively):

medial head   805.4   8.6   0.433
lateral head   482.4   14.1   0.293
long head   486.0   8.9   0.284

Appendix 2: M-net of the index finger

```
S-units
metacarp:X(1,0,0),Y(0,1,0),Z(0,0,1),R(0,0,0),MASS(_),CG(42,0,0)
phalanx1:X(1,0,0),Y(0,1,0),Z(0,0,1),R(84,0,0),MASS(_),CG(24,0,0)
phalanx2:X(1,0,0),Y(0,1,0),Z(0,0,1),R(132,0,0),MASS(_),CG(15,0,0)
phalanx3:X(1,0,0),Y(0,1,0),Z(0,0,1),R(162,0,0),MASS(_),CG(15,0,0)
L-units
mpj_l:STIFF(30),RESTL(0),LEN(0)
     metacarp(84,5,0)->phalanx1(0,5,0)
mpj_r:STIFF(30),RESTL(0),LEN(0)
     metacarp(84,-5,0)->phalanx1(0,-5,0)
mpj_vol:STIFF(5),RESTL(12.02),LEN(9.16)
     metacarp(79.42,0,-5)->phalanx1(4.58,0,-5)
```

```
pipj_l:STIFF(30),RESTL(0),LEN(0)
      phalanx1(48,5,0)->phalanx2(0,5,0)
pipj_r:STIFF(30),RESTL(0),LEN(0)
      phalanx1(48,-5,0)->phalanx2(0,-5,0)
pipj_vol:STIFF(20),RESTL(16.51),LEN(15.7)
      phalanx1(40.15,0,-5)->phalanx2(7.85,0,-5)
dipj_l:STIFF(30),RESTL(0),LEN(0)
      phalanx2(30,5,0)->phalanx3(0,5,0)
dipj_r:STIFF(30),RESTL(0),LEN(0)
      phalanx2(30,-5,0)->phalanx3(0,-5,0)
dipj_vol:STIFF(12),RESTL(9.62),LEN(8.39)
      phalanx2(25.80,0,-5)->phalanx3(4.20,0,-5)
retinac:STIFF(1.5),RESTL(35),LEN(35)
      phalanx1(40.15,0,-5)->phalanx2(7.85,0,-5)
      phalanx2(29.24,0,5)->phalanx3(0.76,0,5)
M-units
   ext:FMAX(9.45),LMAX(62.88),SPD(.433),LEN(56.76)
      metacarp(83.18,0,5)->phalanx1(1.82,0,5)
      phalanx1(47.565,0,5)->phalanx2(.435,0,5)
      phalanx2(29.24,0,5)->phalanx3(0.76,0,5)
   inter:FMAX(5),LMAX(51.05),SPD(.433),LEN(51.38)
      metacarp(79.42,0,-5)->phalanx1(4.58,0,-5)
      phalanx1(47.565,0,5)->phalanx2(.435,0,5)
   flex:FMAX(16.8),LMAX(93.05),SPD(.433),LEN(108.62)
      metacarp(79.42,0,-5)->phalanx1(4.58,0,-5)
      phalanx1(40.15,0,-5)->phalanx2(7.85,0,-5)
      phalanx2(25.80,0,-5)->phalanx3(4.20,0,-5)
```

X, Y, Z are the unit vectors of the co-ordinate axes of each S-unit, R (mm) is the position vector of the origin, and CG is the centre of gravity. For each M-unit, STIFF (N/mm) is the stiffness, RESTL (mm) is the restlength, and LEN is the current length. For each M-unit, FMAX (N) is the peak isometric force at the optimal length LMAX (mm), LEN is the actual length, and SPD(dimensionless) is the spread coefficient.

The active tracts of L-units and M-units are identified by means of their insertion points. The three joints (MP, PIP, DIP) are represented by a pair of stiff L-units, which identify the rotation axis, and a softer L-unit, which limits the extension range. *Retinac* is the double-joint oblique retinacular ligament, *ext* is the triple-joint extensor digitorum communis, *flex* is the triple-joint flexor profundus, and *inter* is the double-joint interosseus.

Notes

1. Given the infinitesimal translation $\vec{dr} = [dx,dy,dz]'$, the homogeneous matrix is: $\Delta H_1 = [I \mid dr]$ where I is the identity metrix.
   Given the infinitesimal rotation $\vec{d\phi} = [d\phi_x, d\phi_y, d\phi_z]' = d\alpha[a_x, a_y, a_z]'$, around the axis $[a_x, a_y, a_z]$, the homogeneous matrix is:

   $\Delta H_2 = [C_1 \mid C_2 \mid C_3 \mid Z]$, where
   $C_1 = [1, d\phi_z, -d\phi_y, 0]'$, $C_2 = [-d\phi_z, 1, d\phi_x, 0]'$, $C_3 = [d\phi_y, -d\phi_x, 1, 0]'$,
   $Z = [0, 0, 0, 1]'$.

2. Setting $x = (l - \lambda)/(l_{min} - \lambda_{min})$, the function $S = S(x)$ is defined as follows:

   $S = x^2(3 - 2x)$ for $0 \leqslant x \leqslant 1$;
   $S = 1$ for $x > 1$.

3. This ligament is considered to be a 'degenerate' muscle, i.e. a muscle that has lost its active contracting mechanism because its basic role, during flexion/extension, is essentially linked to its passive properties. The same is true for the interossei, as it can be seen from the low level of their EMG activity during flexion/extension, which contrasts with the fact that their integrity is essential for the functioning of the movement, as is demonstrated by known motion deformities where there are lesions. On the other hand, the interossei also contribute to finger adduction/abduction and for this the passive properties are not enough.

References

Arbib, M. A. (1989). Visuo-motor coordination: neural models and perceptual robotics. In *Visuomotor coordination* (ed. J. P. Ewert and M. A. Arbib), pp. 121–71. Plenum, New York.

Bernstein, N. (1967). *The coordination and regulation of movement*. Pergamon, London.

Bizzi, E., Polit, A., and Morasso, P. (1976). Mechanisms underlying achievement of final head position. *Journal of Neurophysiology*, **39**, 435–44.

Bizzi, E., Accornero, N., Chapple, W., and Hogan, N. (1984). Posture control and trajectory formation during arm movements. *Journal of Neuroscience*, **4**, 2738–44.

Bullock, D. and Grossberg, S. (1989). VITE and FLETE: Neural modules for trajectory formation and postural control. In *Volitional action* (ed. W. A. Hershberger), pp. 253–97. North-Holland/Elsevier, Amsterdam.

Eckmiller, R., Beckmann, J., Werntges, H., and Lades, M. (1989). *Neural kinematics net for a redundant robot arm.* Proceedings of the International Conference on Neural Networks, **II**, 333–9. Washington, DC.

Feldman, A. G. (1966). Functional tuning of the nervous system with control of movement or maintenance of a steady posture. *Biophysics*, **11**, 565–78.

Feldman, A. G. (1986). Once more on the equilibrium-point hypothesis (Lambda Model) for motor control. *Journal Motor Behaviour*, **18**, 17–54.

Gordon, A. M., Huxley, A. F., and Julian, F. J. (1966). The variation in isometric tension with sarcomere length in vertebrate muscle fibres. *Journal of Physiology*, **184**, 170–92.

Hatze, H. (1981). Myocybernetic control models of skeletal muscle, characteristics and applications. Thesis. University of South Africa, Pretoria.

Hogan, N. (1984). An organizing principle for a class of voluntary movements. *Journal of Neuroscience*, **4**, 2745–54.

Hopfield, J. J. (1982). Neural networks and physical systems with emergent collective computational abilities. *Proceedings of the National Academy of Science, USA*, **79**, 2554–8.

Hopfield, J. J. (1984). Neurons with graded response have collective computational properties like those of two state neurons. *Proceedings of the National Academy of Sciences, USA*, **81**, 3088–92.

Inman, V. T., Ralston, H. J., and Todd, F. (1981). *Human walking*. Williams & Wilkins, Baltimore.

Kawato, M., Uno, Y., Isobe, M., and Suzuki, R. (1988). Hierarchical neural network model for voluntary movement with application to robotics. *IEEE Control Systems Magazine*, **8**, 8–16.

Kelso, J. A. S. (1977). Motor control mechanisms underlying human movement reproduction. *Journal of Experimental Psychology*, **3**, 529–43.

Kohonen, T. (1988). *Self-organization and associative memory*. Springer-Verlag, Berlin.

Korein, J. U. (1985). *A geometric investigation of reach*. MIT Press, Cambridge, Mass.

Kuperstein, M. (1988). Neural model of adaptive hand-eye coordination for single postures. *Science*, **239**, 1308–11.

Massone, L. and Bizzi, E. (1989). A neural network model for limb trajectory formation. *Biological Cybernetics*, **61**, 417–25.

Morasso, P. (1989). *Neural modelling of handwriting*. Proceedings of the International Joint Conference on Neural Networks. IEEE, Washington DC.

Morasso, P., Mussa Ivaldi, F. A., Vercelli, G., and Zaccaria, R. (1989). *Connectionism in perspective* (ed. R. Pfeifer, Z. Schreter, F. Fogelman-Soulie, and L. Steels), pp. 413–20. Elsevier Amsterdam.

Mussa Ivaldi, F. A., Hogan, N., and Bizzi, E. (1985). Neural, mechanical, and geometric factors subserving arm postures in humans. *Journal of Neuroscience*, **5**, 2732–43.

Mussa Ivaldi, F. A., Morasso, P., and Zaccaria, R. (1988). Kinematic networks— A distributed model for representing and regularizing motor redundancy. *Biological Cybernetics*, **60**, 1–16.

Polit, A. and Bizzi, E. (1979). Characteristics of motor programs underlying arm movements in monkeys. *Journal of Neurophysiology*, **42**, 183–90.

Stevens, J. C., Dickinson, V., and Jones, N. B. (1980). Mechanical properties of human skeletal muscle from in vitro studies of biopsies. *Medical and Biological Engineering and Computing*, **18**, 1–9.

Tubiana, R. (1981). *The hand*, Vol. I. W. B. Saunders, Philadelphia.

22

Sensorimotor space representation: a neuromimetic model

JEAN-CLAUDE GILHODES, YVES COITON, and JEAN-LUC VELAY

Introduction

Superior vertebrates, particularly humans, exhibit a great range of motor behaviours, among which spatially oriented activities are fundamental. Activities directed in space require at least the presence of a sensory signal coming from the immediate environment. In principle, this signal should suffice to trigger a correct motor response, assuming that there exists a pre-cabled link between this input and a given motor response. This simple mechanism involves only a primary level of spatial perception and does not necessitate an internal model of space. A great number of primitive animals probably act on the basis of primary mechanisms of this type. Their motor behaviour is fairly restricted, however, and in addition there is no possibility of adaptation to environmental changes. In fact, in the majority of superior organisms, the *sensorimotor relationship* is not completely fixed but can be modified in the course of life, if necessary. Furthermore, the relationship is not given at birth but has to be learned early in life. Highly evolved nervous systems must therefore build and store an internal sensorimotor representation in which motor responses are interconnected with sensory signals. Moreover, the most advanced organisms are equipped with several sensory receptors. Schematically the sensory modalities can be divided into two categories: the *exteroceptive* type, which informs about the outside, and the *proprioceptive* type, which informs about the body positions. Consequently, the existence of processes integrating the various sensory signals and giving rise to a representation of both *extra-personal* and *body-space* has to be considered. A fundamental problem in motor control consists, therefore, of establishing how separate sensory signals are co-ordinated and integrated to produce a coherent, unified, sensorimotor map on which directed movements can be planned.

Internal representations are probably based on the various maps which are known to exist in the central nervous system. Cerebral maps often reproduce the peripheral organization and they can be partly inborn. This is so, for instance, in the case of the somatotopic projections on primary sensory cortical areas, or of the retinal map in the striate cortex. There is also evidence, however, that many cortical areas are able to produce maps that are not innate but acquired through sensory information processing. The sensory projections to these areas are then assumed to be mediated through adaptative connections. The associative areas, which integrate various sensory signals, probably belong to the latter, central, mapping category. Furthermore, there also exist motor maps representing characteristics of the movement such as its direction (Georgopoulos *et al.* 1982; Schwartz *et al.* 1988).

Whatever the biological substrate involved, one of the main characteristics of sensorimotor maps is that they have to be organized during a learning period requiring the activity of the organism itself. The crucial role played by the active motor behaviour in sensorimotor co-ordination has been clearly demonstrated (Held and Hein 1963; Hein *et al.* 1970).

Space representation can therefore be said to result from active motor behaviour generating sensory re-afferents in what Paillard (1986) has called 'sensorimotor dialogues'. The gradual elaboration of sensorimotor representation on the basis of autonomous motor activity implies that nervous structures possess some self-organizational capacities, which probably depend on the one hand on the neural network architecture and on the other hand on the biochemical processes controlling synaptic junctional efficiency.

In order to comply with neurobiological data in simulating these aspects of sensorimotor behaviour, we have elaborated a model, using neuromimetic formulation and techniques. This neuromimetic model, in which we have combined behavioural and neurobiological considerations, was designed to provide answers to the following questions: how is multisensory integration achieved, and how might the sensorimotor relationship then be built up on the basis of active and autonomous motor behaviour?

Description of the model

Our model consists of a set of motor and sensory elements, comprising sensors and effectors, connected to a neuromimetic network (Fig. 22.1). The neuromimetic network determines the position of a mobile organ from orders given to effectors, and it receives information about this position from the sensors, which can be either linked or not to the effector system. It is proposed here to describe the architecture and the functional principles of this model. It was designed in such a way that changes of configuration can be used to test various hypotheses concerning, for example, the effects of changes in the sensory mode.

The neuromimetic network is organized in two layers: a sensory and a motor layer.

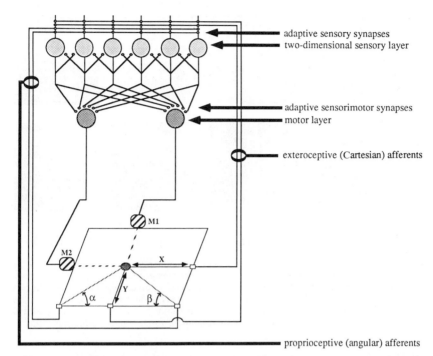

right-side labels:
adaptive sensory synapses
two-dimensional sensory layer

adaptive sensorimotor synapses
motor layer

exteroceptive (Cartesian) afferents

proprioceptive (angular) afferents

Fig. 22.1. Diagram of the model. A network formed by a sensory and a motor layer determine the position of a mobile in the working space, by means of a set of motors (M1, M2). Cartesian and angular sensors feed the bi-dimensional sensory layer with proprioceptive and exteroceptive feedbacks, respectively.

Sensory layer

The sensory or associative layer is composed of a set of formal neurons arranged in a matrix. Recurrent collaterals link these cells in a excitatory manner in the case of neighbouring cells and in an inhibitory manner in that of remote cells. This architecture is based on the cortical architecture. Afferent information from each sensor is distributed to the entire layer, so that each afferent input is linked to each neuron by a synaptic junction that modulates the influence of this activity. The synaptic efficiency that characterizes this influence is variable, depending on the afferent and cellular activity—i.e. the pre- and post-synaptic activity. This law controlling synaptic plasticity is similar to Hebb's (1949) rule.

The properties of this sensory layer have been described by Kohonen (1982, 1984), who showed that by means of a self-organized process (fed by afferent information) this structure is capable of producing a topological map. Thus topological relationships contained in the afferent patterns progressively appear in the sensory layer as activity foci, i.e. spatially

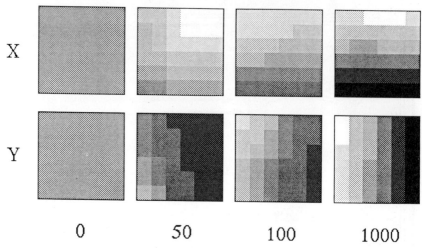

X

Y

0   50   100   1000

Fig. 22.2. Various steps during the development of synaptic efficiency. Each map shows the weights of synaptic junctions connecting two Cartesian sensors (X, Y) to each cell of a 6 × 6 Kohonen's topological network. Weight scale is arranged in ascending order from white to black. Four steps, obtained after 0, 50, 100, 1000 iterations of random position-reaching, are presented. The initial state (0) shows homogeneous distribution of the weights, as opposed to the final state (1000) showing orthogonal weight gradient for X and Y afferent junctions.

neighbouring events are coded by anatomically neighbouring cells. This topology progressively emerges during a learning period, when each sensory pattern characterizing a position in the working space successively induces an activity focus. The synaptic efficacy then changes at the level of this activity focus. We will demonstrate this self-organization property by giving a simple example of this type of network, where the afferents carry information relating to the position of a point in a plane. The information is given in terms of Cartesian co-ordinates. Figure 22.2 shows the changes in the synaptic weight configuration that represents the network memory, from an initial to a final state. During the learning period, points are randomly drawn in a plane. The initial state is arbitrarily characterized by a random distribution of the synaptic coefficient centred around a mean value. The final state is characterized by a gradient of synaptic coefficients organized on both axes of the two-dimensional Cartesian space. After the learning period we can verify that two neighbouring points in the working space give rise to two neighbouring activity foci in the layer, i.e. *the working space has been mapped on to the network*.

Motor layer

The motor layer consists of a set of cells, each controlling an effector component. The connection between the two layers, that is, the sensorimotor connection, is organized in such manner that each element in the sensory layer is connected to every cell in the motor layer. The junctions so resulting are also adaptive. The law controlling the changes in synaptic plasticity at the level of sensorimotor connection is different from that used at the level of the sensory afferents. We have defined and used a law of linear error correction of the type proposed by Widrow and Hoff (1960). The desired activity of the motor cells is not given here by a supervisor but is replaced by the effective motor output, which strengthens the neurobiological plausibility of this model. This plasticity law inclines to make the synaptic efficiency tend towards the post-synaptic level of cellular activity in the motor layer, in order to memorize the relationship between sensory and motor activities.

Peripheral sensory and motor organs

The sensory periphery of the network consists of sensors that can vary in form and in number. In our simulation we have used sensors that symbolize diverse sensorial modalities such as the exteroceptive or proprioceptive ones. In the same way, effectors can be simulated, acting on various degrees of freedom, such as translation or rotation. Afferent and efferent information is represented as activation levels.

Algorithmic procedure

The mathematical formulation and algorithms used can be found in Coiton (1987) and Coiton *et al.* (1991). We will summarize here the algorithmic procedure used in the learning-period simulation. This learning period consists of a randomly chosen series of motor activities. At the beginning all the synaptic weights were randomly defined.

Each cycle leading to a position of the mobile is composed of four steps. First, the random activity of motor cells determines the position. Secondly, the resulting information produced by one or several sensory modalities is sent to the sensory layer. This information then induces an activity focus, the location of which is centred on the sensory cell showing the best match between synaptic weights and afferent information, i.e., the cell in the layer where the weighted sum of the inputs is maximal. At the level of these cells, the synaptic coefficients are then updated. Synaptic changes occur both in afferent junctions and sensory motor junctions; they tend to enhance the correlation between the coefficient and the afferent information in the former, and between the coefficient and the motor activity in the latter.

Both plasticity laws involve a sensibility factor that progressively decreases during the learning period and becomes null at the end.

Results

In order to study the behaviour and the properties of this model, we have performed numerical simulations of various versions of it. Here we shall present some of the results that seem to us to be the most informative. For the sake of clarity, we will describe the results obtained with a version of the model controlling the position of a mobile with two degrees of freedom. This allows us to present the properties of the model in a simple form, especially the transformation of the synaptic-weight configuration and of that of the cellular receptive fields.

We will then, in brief, describe the results obtained with a version of the model controlling the position of an artificial arm in a three-dimensional space, on the basis of two types of afferent information: exteroceptive and proprioceptive.

In the case of the two-dimensional version we will describe the characteristics of sensory and motor representations of space as they are established by learning, along with the sensory and motor modes used. On this basis we will show that it is possible to command movement towards a target (reaching movement).

The nature of space representation in the sensory layer

First, we obtained results showing the network's capacity to establish space representation by associating two modalities on the basis of active movements. The simulated system is consistent with that described in Fig. 22.1. The network is composed of a sensory layer with 36 formal neurons arranged in a 6×6 matrix. Two motor cells, each controlling an effector, determine the position of a mobile in a plane working space. Once the mobile has reached the position, the afferent information characterizing this position is sent to the sensory layer in two forms: in the form of Cartesian co-ordinates, abcissa and ordinate (x,y), and/or in the form of angular values (α,β). Starting from an undifferentiated initial state, learning is accomplished by imposing a uniformly random activity on the motor cells, in such a way that the working space is homogeneously explored during this period. The synaptic plasticity sensibility, or adaptation gain, decreases during the learning period and is null at the end.

If we use only one of these two modalities, we observe the map emergence in the sensory layer (in agreement with Kohonen's results). As described above, this representation of working space is expressed in a synaptic coefficient gradient, which constitutes the network memory (as illustrated in Fig. 22.2). This particular configuration of synaptic efficiency is reflected in the activity of sensory layer cells: a cell is only active when the current

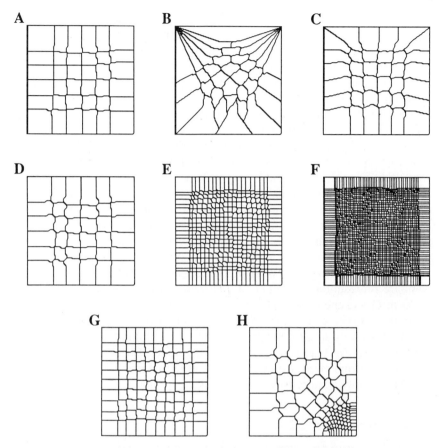

Fig. 22.3. Various sensory maps, represented in the form of receptive fields, can be obtained after the learning period. (A–C) The first three maps show, on a 6 × 6 sensory layer, the various spatial representations induced by Cartesian (A), or angular (B), or both Cartesian and angular (C) sensory afferents. (D–F) The incidence upon spatial resolution of increasing the number of cells. From left to right are shown the receptive fields determined by Cartesian afferents on a sensory layer composed of 36 (6 × 6), 400 (20 × 20), and 2025 (45 × 45) cells, respectively. (G and H) The dependence of the size of the receptive fields upon the way the working space is explored. In (G) exploration was perfectly uniform whereas in (H) the lower right part of the working space was more often explored (0.75 probability).

position belongs to a sub-set of the working space that constitutes its receptive field as determined with Cartesian or angular, unimodal afferents. We would note at this stage that the working-space representation depends on the sensory mode (Fig. 22.3A,B).

Simulations performed using two types of afferent information simultaneously also produce a space mapping, which is the intermediate between the two unimodal maps (Fig. 22.3C). This result shows how a network, by means of a self-organizing process, can produce a topological representation of a working space by associating two modalities.

Apart from sensory information modes, other factors can intervene in determining the nature of the distribution of the receptive fields. The most evident of these factors is the number of cells that compose the sensory associative layer. With the same sensory equipment, the size of the receptive fields will therefore decrease if we increase the number of cells in the layer. Comparisons between the representations of working space obtained on the basis of Cartesian information, with sensory layers composed of 36 (6×6), 400 (20×20) or 2025 (45×45) cells, can be made by consulting Fig. 22.3D,E, and F respectively.

Another important factor lies in the way in which the working space is explored during the learning period. The above results were obtained after a random, uniform exploration of the space, that is, one where every position had the same probability of being adopted. Simulation was also performed with an uneven probability of the mobile being present in various points in space. With Figs. 22.3 G and H, it is possible to compare representations obtained with two types of exploration: the one uniform G and the other favouring one part of the space H. In this case, we observed smaller receptive fields and a proportionally greater number of cells corresponding to this privileged zone of exploration. In neurobiological terms, this biased representation is reminiscent of that observed in somatic or retinal maps, for example. We note that in this case the exploration bias is duly acquired by the network.

Motor representation

The setting up of the sensory map in the model is accompanied by the simultaneous emergence of a motor organization. The former is embedded in the weights of the adaptive junctions connecting sensory afferents and sensory cells. The latter is reflected in the weights of the synapses connecting sensory and motor cells.

The plasticity law that we have developed intervenes when a junction is active at a given moment in time, that is, when the corresponding sensory cells are activated. The states of sensorimotor junction represented in Fig. 22.4 correspond to the version of the model where the two motor cells determine the position of the mobile from angular effector information. Each map represents the coefficient gradient of the sensory–motor junction obtained for the two motor cells after a learning period.

Position control

The main point of interest from the point of view of the existence of a common representation, associating two sensory modalities, lies in the

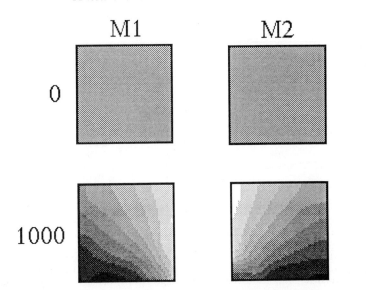

Fig. 22.4. Representation of sensorimotor organization. M1 and M2 denote the two cells of the motor layer. In this example, the sensory layer is composed of 2025 sensory cells, all connected to each motor cell. The weights of the 2025 synaptic junctions are shown before the first learning step (0), when all the weights were uniformly distributed, and after 10 000 movements.

possibility of commanding topocinetic movement. One of the modalities is used to designate the goal, and the other serves to convey the current position of the effector organ. Movements of this kind have been simulated with the model, with a goal designated by Cartesian-type afferents (in this case mimicking the exteroceptive modality), whereas the current position was coded by angular-type afferents. The designation of target involves decorrelating the two sensory modalities, which results in determining the activity of one cell in the sensory layer that represents the best match between current and target position. This cell causes the mobile to move. This cycle is repeated until the target is reached, that is, until the two types of afferent information are again correlated. Figure 22.5 shows changes in the mobile position in two situations. In A the goal is designated and remains unchanged, and in B the goal is designated and then changed while the mobile has already started to move towards the initial goal. The final goal is reached in both cases.

Neuromimetic and robotic model of sensorimotor control

We have developed a version of the model in the form of a neuromimetic network controlling the movement of an artificial arm in a three-dimensional space. This arm comprises goniometers coding the different

A

B

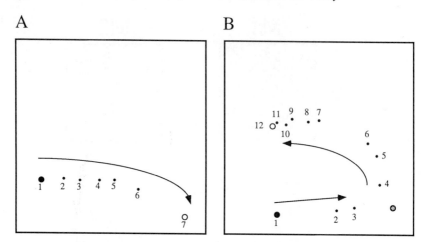

Fig. 22.5. Example of directed movements carried out by the mobile after the learning period. Filled circles show initial position; open circles show both final position and goal. Dots denote successive positions reached by the mobile. In (B) the first goal (grey circle on the bottom right) is replaced during the movement by a new goal (open circle). The trajectory of the mobile changes accordingly.

articulation angles, which play a proprioceptive role. Furthermore, exteroception is provided by three photoreceptors fixed in three orthogonal planes. A light source fixed at the end of the artificial arm stimulates the exteroceptive sensor, thus indicating the current position of the extremity of the arm during the learning period. Any given position of the arm is therefore coded in two ways: the angular values can be said to be intrinsic co-ordinates, as they express the arm configuration in body space, and the exteroceptive signals can be said to be extrinsic co-ordinates in that they inform about the arm-tip position in extra-personal space. The fact that both types of spatial co-ordinates converge on the same cells makes it possible to build up a unified representation of space, integrating extra-personal and body space. The simulations performed with this robotic model confirm the results presented above. Sensory and motor representations gradually emerge in the network and it is possible, after learning, to command movement towards a given target in the working space. The target position is designated by the light source that has been removed from the artificial arm. The network then drives the arm extremity towards the light source.

It is noteworthy that the robot movement mimics a *visual open-loop* pointing movement. Indeed, once the learning has been completed, the exteroceptive information is used solely to define target location, and in no case to convey the position of the arm. In fact, the position of the target in physical space is transformed into the corresponding posture in body-space. This arm configuration defines the equilibrium point to be reached. Neuromimetic models of reaching have been developed that are based on similar networks (Ritter *et al* 1989); however, as only one type of sensory signal is needed, target and arm have to be coded in the same co-ordinates and only closed-loop movements have been simulated.

Another point worth mentioning is that if learning is carried out with passive arm movements, the sensory layer will be structured in exactly the same manner as previously, i.e. the intersensory relationship will be correctly learned under passive conditions. However, despite a perfectly localized target, the network will be unable to command the arm because the synapses linking sensory and motor layers have not been organized during the learning phase. The sensorimotor relationships are not elaborated under passive conditions.

Conclusion

The model described here was developed mainly with a view to proposing possible mechanisms for the genesis of multi-modal space representation in the central nervous system and for the corresponding sensorimotor co-ordination, both of which together result in motor behaviour in external space. One of our concerns in elaborating this model was its neurobiological plausibility: first we took the existence of maps in the central nervous system to be characterized by cellular specializations and assumed these specializations to be acquired during ontogenesis—i.e. due to active motor behaviour inducing synaptic modifications. Here we must stress the fact that this model is not concerned with the numerous neural structures involved in sensory information processing, or in motor-command organization. It can be said to be simply an attempt to formalize behavioural phenomena on the basis of neurobiological considerations. In this context the results of our numerical simulations show how a bimodal space representation and a motor map can emerge in a network of this kind. As far as space representation is concerned, the model shows that it is possible to integrate into the same mapping both exteroceptive and proprioceptive information, leading to a unified representation. It also shows the simultaneous emergence of a motor organization, in close parallel with the sensory map building. On the basis of experimental data from animals and humans, these internal representations are built up during an active learning period involving a self-organization process in the network.

This model thus provides the beginning of an answer to the two questions formulated in the introduction concerning the unified, bimodal representation of space and sensory–motor relationship that can be acquired by autonomous and active learning. Moreover, the use of two types of afferent information—exteroceptive and proprioceptive—means that the system can perform pointing behaviour, i.e., it is able to reach a goal designated in terms of the exteroceptive modality. In this connection, an analogy can be noted between the model behaviour and experimental data obtained on animals' superior colliculus (Roucoux *et al.* 1980; Sparks and Mays 1980). In this structure, electrical stimulation induced gaze displacement toward a position defined only by the stimulus location, whatever the initial gaze orientation. The shape of the space representation obtained after various simulations is determined by two main factors: on the one hand, the characteristics of the afferent information (cf. Fig. 22.3A,B, and C) and on the other hand, the nature of the working space exploration (cf. Fig. 22.3G and H). The same network architecture and the same laws of internal plasticity therefore give rise to very different topological maps, depending on the type and number of the sensory modalities involved and on the exploration behaviour. In the case of the latter we have shown that the working-space part that is privileged during the learning period induces privileged representation in the emergent map. The model's biased exploration behaviour may be due to anatomical and functional characteristics of the effector system leading to uncomfortable or non-optimized positions. It follows that the nature of the peripheral equipment, both sensory and motor, associated with a particular learning story determines the functional structure of the network. This conclusion has a corollary: the same network organization can be involved in various sensorimotor systems, such as those that drive arm, hand, or eye movements. In this case, we can assume that the required co-ordinations between different sensorimotor systems can be organized on the basis of a partial sharing of the sensory information among these systems.

Obviously numerous aspects of natural sensorimotor systems have not been taken into account in this model: they define both its limitations and its potential for future development. It can be reported at this stage that, after the learning period, arm movements were obtained in a pointing task. These movements served no purpose other than reaching a target designated in exteroceptive terms. It is impossible, however, without considerably improving the model, to obtain particular types of movement such as those involved in drawing or hand-writing. By producing a model endowed with basic dynamic characteristics, we have taken the first step towards mimicking more sophisticated skills of this kind. It is well known that natural sensory and motor systems have both static and dynamic properties: muscle-spindle discharges code position and velocity simultaneously (Matthews 1972) and there exist both phasic and tonic motor units. Taking these characteristics into account would probably lead to a fruitful extension of the model.

References

Coiton, Y. (1987). Organisation sensorimotrice: modélisation d'une logique neuro-mimétique. *D.E.A. de Neurosciences*. Université de Provence, Marseille.

Coiton, Y., Gilhodes, J. C., Velay, J. L., and Roll, J. P. (1991) Neural network modelling of the intersensory coordination involved in directed movements. *Biological Cybernetics* (submitted).

Georgopoulos, A. P., Kalaska, J. F., Caminiti, R., and Massey, J. T. (1982). On the relations between the direction of two dimensional arm movements and cell discharge in primate motor cortex. *Journal of Neuroscience*, **2**, 1527–37.

Hebb, D. O. (1949). *The organization of behavior*. Wiley, New York.

Hein, A., Held, R., and Gower, E. (1970). Development and segmentation of visually controlled movement by selective exposure during rearing. *Journal of Comparative Physiology and Psychology*, **73**, 181–7.

Held, R. and Hein, A. (1963). Movement produced stimulation in the development of visually guided behaviour. *Journal of Comparative Physiology and Psychology*, **56**, 872–6.

Kohonen, T. (1982). Self-organized formation of topologically correct feature maps. *Biological Cybernetics*, **43**, 59–69.

Kohonen, T. (1984). *Self-organization and associative memory* (ed. K. S. Fu). Springer-Verlag, Berlin.

Matthews, P. B. C. (1972). *Mammalian muscle receptors and their central actions* (ed. H. Davson, A. D. M. Greenfield, R. Whittam, and G. S. Brindley). Edward Arnold, London.

Paillard, J. (1986). Cognitive versus sensorimotor encoding of spatial information. In *Cognitive processes and spatial orientation in animal and man* (ed. P. Elien and C. Thinus-Blanc), pp. 1–35. Martinus Nijhoff, Dordrecht.

Ritter, H. J., Martinez, T. M., and Schulten, K. J. (1989). Topology conserving maps for learning visuomotor-coordination. *Neural Networks*, **2**, 159–68.

Roucoux, A., Guitton, D., and Crommelinck, M. (1980). Stimulation of the superior colliculus in the alert cat. *Experimental Brain Research*, **39**, 75–85.

Schwartz, A. B., Kettner, R. E., and Georgopoulos, A. P. (1988). Primate motor cortex and free arm movements to visual targets in three dimensional space. I Relation between single cell discharge and direction of movement. *Journal of Neuroscience*, **8**, 2913–27.

Sparks, D. L. and Mays, L. E. (1980). Role of the monkey superior colliculus in the spatial localization of saccade targets. In *Spatially oriented behavior* (ed. A. Hein and M. Jeannerod), pp. 63–85. Springer-Verlag, Berlin.

Widrow, G. and Hoff, M. E. (1960). *Adaptative switching circuits*. Western electronic show and convention record. *IRE, New York*, **4**, 96–104.

23

A model for the co-operation between cerebral cortex and cerebellar cortex in movement learning

Y. BURNOD and M. DUFOSSÉ

Introduction

According to modern control theory, learning requires not only an adaptable system but also the possibility of changing the information-processing rules. Nervous systems seem to learn by modifying the flows of signals transmitted between internal structures. In general, sensorimotor learning occurs in successive steps. Each step has a given role and a time-constant that depends upon the learning properties of the nervous structures involved. A scheme of interactions between the main nervous structures has been proposed by Ito (1984). This hypothetical scheme for motor learning models the cortico-spinal and the cortico-rubral systems and takes the adaptive properties of the cerebellum into account.

The cerebral cortex can rapidly learn the appropriate motor commands for reaching a goal by supplying the spinal servo-mechanisims. When a task is performed repeatedly, the cerebellum gradually intervenes, finely adjusting and automatizing the motor response. The cerebellum can thus help the cerebral cortex during goal-directed tasks (Holmes 1939) as well as in the mental control of more cognitive tasks (Leiner *et al.* 1989).

Our aim was to model the dialogue that takes place between the cerebral and cerebellar cortices during the first steps in sensorimotor learning.

The neural network model described here is based upon known architectural and functional properties of the cerebral and cerebellar cortices. In each cortical structure, it is possible to define a basic unit (Shepherd 1969), a kind of 'crystal' consisting of several neuronal types, which recurs throughout the structure. This crystal is the micro-column of the cerebral cortex and the micro-zone of the cerebellar cortex. The morpho-functional structures, together with their plastic rules, are taken here as the basic units of our neural network model. This model suggests how cellular mechanisms in these two structures may be responsible for two different types of adaptive process, and how their mutual interactions can produce automatic and refined motor sequences.

Cerebral cortex model

The cerebral cortex has six layers: the fourth layer (or granular layer), which receives the external thalamic input, is intermediate between two sub-sets of pyramidal neurons, the one in the supra-granular layer (layers 2 and 3), and the other in the infra-granular layer (5 and 6), which form the two principal output pathways, inside and external to the cortex, respectively.

The pyramidal cells are arranged in vertical columns, perpendicular to the surface, with strong interconnections, sharing afferents with the same sensory or motor significance (Mountcastle 1978; Hubel *et al.* 1978). These connections are accompanied by excitatory and inhibitory pathways, formed by at least five main types of inter-neurons, which can couple or uncouple not only interconnected columns but also the layers within each column, depending upon the patterns of activity involved. This cellular texture shapes the specific operations that each column effects upon its inputs.

It is possible to synthesize known physiological properties of the cortical column in a table that gives the two main outputs of the column (intra- and extra-cortical) along with the two main inputs (cortical and thalamic) and the previous state of the column (Burnod 1989). The model has the following four main properties: (a) the relationship between two columns can be either excitatory or inhibitory, depending upon the level of activity; (b) the activity can spread through the cortical network even without any significant outputs occurring outside the cortex; (c) an amplifying effect is produced when cortical and thalamic inputs are co-active; (d) the relative importance of these two inputs varies from one cortical area to another.

This system is basically an adaptive mechanism producing two types of responses to external events: either a specific cortical action when the inputs are co-active,or an intra-cortical 'call' to other columns. The call can remain in force until one of the columns called produces an extra-cortical action which results in an extra-cortical input to the calling column. The action of each cortical column thus constitutes an equilibrium position or a kind of goal. A call results in an exploration—a search through the possible actions that the cortex can command in order to reach the goal.

Memorization rules make it possible to store the appropriate patterns of activity in the connections between columns. Excitatory connections are strengthened when a called module produces an action outside the cortex that reactivates the calling module (the goal) by an extra-cortical feedback loop (external, causal link). This learning property causes a new functional network to be assembled.

These call trees have a 'top-down' and a 'bottom-up' activation. First, in the top-down direction, calls emanate from possible actions and produce an anticipatory activation of a set of cortical modules which represents possible actions (or sub-goals) that could reduce the distance from the goal. The call spreads until it is in keeping with the environmental con- ditions. Actions are then triggered both in parallel and in sequence, result- ing in the attainment of sub-goals and the goal (bottom-up direction). Numerical simulations during character recognition and speech recognition have shown the efficiency of this kind of neural network processing (Alexandre *et al.* 1989).

Cerebellar cortex model

The basic unit of the cerebellum is the micro-zone, which is longitudinally organized by climbing inputs topographically organized from a specific part of the inferior olive (Oscarsson 1969) and outputs topographically organ- ized on the cerebellar nuclei. Together with their nuclear projecting zones, they form the so-called cortico-nuclear micro-complex (Ito 1984). Another input is provided by the mossy fibre system, which is characterized by its considerable divergence onto wide regions on the cerebellar cortex. The set of mossy fibre inputs constitutes a general context about the present sensorimotor actions, that is, a large set of signals providing information about the states of activity in the various nervous structures, from com- mand structures to more sensory structures. It can be assumed that these micro-zones work in parallel in a relatively independent manner.

Each micro-zone can be viewed as a three-layer neural network (Albus 1971) similar to the perception originally described by Rosenblatt (1958): an input layer formed by cells which originate from the mossy fibres, an intermediate layer of granular cells, and an output layer of Purkinje cells that project to cerebellar output nuclei. During the adaptive phase, this output layer uses an error signal, originating from the inferior olive and conveyed by the climbing fibres. The long-term effect of this error signal is a decrease in the synaptic efficiency between parallel fibres, axons of granular cells, and the output Purkinje cells, whenever the parallel fibre activity is correlated with the error signal (Marr 1969; Albus 1971; Fujita 1982; Ito 1984). The physiological properties of this long-term depression have been described in detail (Ito *et al.* 1982; Ito 1989).

An important feature of the cerebellar design is the great number (10^{11}) of granular cells in the intermediate layer, which is of the same order of magnitude as the total number of cells in the nervous system. The role of this architecture might be to provide an extended set of new combinations of inputs which are very useful for bypassing the mathematical limitations of the classical, two-layer perception for learning abitrary input/output function. Without these combinations wired at the glomerulus level, many functions cannot be learned (see the classical example of the XOR problem given by Minsky and Papert 1969). In the very basic learning that we model, we focus on the plasticity at the level of the output layer. Plasticity at other levels is not necessary but could correspond to more elaborate functions (Chauvet 1986).

Motor learning: cybernetic approach

In the analysis of motor control, cybernetic models have been proposed in order to explain the respective roles of cerebral and cerebellar cortices and have been correlated with experimental data (Ito 1984, 1990).

It is generally assumed that the cerebral cortex first learns an inverse dynamics model of the skeleto-muscular apparatus in order to translate a desired trajectory into the appropriate commands, corrections being effected through a feedback loop. Later, the cerebellar cortex builds a feed-forward control which replaces this closed-loop cerebral process. Two successive phases must be distinguished in this cerebellar take-over.

1. First, the external feedback loope with which the movement can be corrected is replaced by a dynamics model of the skeleto-muscular apparatus which makes it possible to predict and anticipate such corrections. The functioning of this internal model imitates the functioning of the real skeleto-muscular apparatus. The internal model may be built up thanks to the adaptive mechanisms of the cerebellum; this mechanism has been formalized and simulated by Kawato *et al.* (1987).

At the end of this learning phase, in addition to the inverse dynamics model already learned by the cerebral cortex to command the movement, the cerebellum has learned the dynamics model which allows anticipatory corrections because it simulates the movement and, at each step of the command, predicts its mechanical effects.

2. Secondly, with practice, the performance of the command system performed by the cerebral cortex can be taken over by the cerebellum in a feed-forward mode. In this case, the feed-forward system can learn an inverse dyamics model of the skeleto-muscular apparatus, as the whole system is designed to make an actually performed trajectory equal to a desired trajectory. Numerical stimulation has shown that this second phase produces a smooth, efficient trajectory (Kawato *et al.* 1987). This is probably learned by the lateral cerebellum, which can progressively implement the inverse dynamics model previously learned by the cerebrum. The result will be a completely automatic control of the movement, which will free the computational capacity of the cerebral cortex for other tasks.

It is interesting to note that these two phases are not necessarily separate but may overlap considerably. The distinction is more in terms of the relative importance in their behavioural effects, such as refining or automatizing a movement. In the first case, a representation of the effects of a command (direct dynamics) is learned. In the second case, a representation of the command itself (inverse dynamics) is learned.

We propose to develop this cybernetic approach by devising a neural network model taking into account the basic neuronal features of both types of cortex and their interactions.

Motor learning: neural network approach

In a neural network approach, operations performed by the various neural structures are learned in parallel by basic units and their local interactions. The whole processing involves the three components shown in Fig. 23.1: local activation rules and learning rules applicable to the units, and cooperation rules defining the architecture of the network between units.

The activation rules make the transformations between the input and output signals of the basic units. The learning rules describe how the parameters of these transformations, the 'connective coefficients', are tuned depending upon the statistical correlation between inputs and outputs. It should be noted that the cerebral and cerebellar cortices have two different cellular textures, involving very different cell types and local interactions. Consequently, these activation and learning rules have to be defined separately for each cortex. The co-ordination rules model the anatomical connections between the two cortices and define the architecture of the network.

Within the basic units—micro-column and micro-zone—activities are defined by two major parameters. First, they depend upon the main cellular types involved: the upper and lower pyramidal cells ('up' and 'lp') of the cerebral cortex and the thalamic input ('th'); the Purkinje ('pur') and granular cells ('par'); mossy and climbing ('ol') fibre inputs of the cerebellar cortex. Secondly, they also depend upon the position of the unit in the cortical tissue. It is possible to give an address to each unit and to name it (K, X in Fig. 23.1) by giving its main input and output. To simplify, a micro-column is named by giving its thalamic input and its motor output. A micro-zone has a general address, which is defined in terms of its Purkinje cell output, whereas the mossy fibre input has a more local address within this micro-zone.

The activation and learning rules correlate the input and output activities named by a cell type and its address, and this relation depends upon connective coefficients between two addresses (Ki and X).

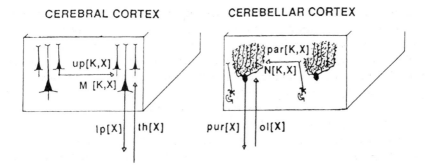

CEREBRAL CORTEX   CEREBELLAR CORTEX

activation rules

cerebral cortex $\text{lp}[X] = \sum M(KI,X).\text{up}[KI] + \text{th}[X]$

cerebellar cortex $\triangle \text{pur}[X] = \sum N(KI,X).\text{par}[KI] + \text{ol}[X]$

learning rules

cerebral cortex

$$\triangle M_{+}[K\,,\,X\,] = P[\ \text{lp}[X](t\text{-}1) > T\ /\ \text{up}[\ K\,,\,X\,](t) > T\ ]$$

$$\triangle M_{-}[K\,,\,X\,] = P[\ \text{lp}[X](t\text{-}1) = 0\ /\ \text{up}[\ K\,,\,X\,](t) > T\ ]$$

cerebellar cortex

$$\triangle N[K\,,\,X\,] = \text{ol}[X].\text{par}[K]$$

coordination rules

$$\text{par}[K] = \text{lp}[K]$$

$$\text{th}[X] = \triangle \text{pur}[X]$$

$$\text{ol}[X] = \text{Fcom}[X] - \text{Fext}[X]$$

Fig. 23.1. Activation, learning and co-ordination rules. Top: two basic units (K and X) are schematized in the cerebral (left) and cerebellar (right) cortex. Below: the corresponding equations for activation, learning and co-ordination rules are given. Note that the symbol = does not denote mathematical equality but merely the transformation from the left to the right part of each equation (see text for abbreviations and details).

The activation rules for both cortices show some similarities: the principal cell integrates major external inputs (thalamic and olivary) with a large set of internal inputs (cortico-cortical and parallel fibre, respectively).

The learning rules are more differentiated. In the cerebral cortex, two learning rules (ΔM+ and ΔM−) depend upon the probability (P) of strong successive co-activation (or inverse activation) occurring between related units; whereas the learning rule in the cerebellar cortex (ΔN) is more like a delta rule (Widrow and Hopf 1960), depending upon a correlation between parallel input activity and an error signal conveyed by the climbing fibre.

The learning rules in the cerebral cortex make it possible for a sub-set of goal-directed actions to be learned. The influence of each unit forming a possible sub-goal will selectively increase toward other units which can themselves command actions whenever those actions increase their own activity through an external loop; whereas the delta rule in the cerebellum can be used to continuously adjust the input/output operations in order to decrease an error signal.

The co-operation between the cortices results from reciprocal actions between the two structures, which are topographically organized. The local address of the mossy fibre input is in contact with a micro-column address in a large sub-set of cortical areas, and each micro-zone has specific connections with micro-columns in the motor cortex through thalamic inputs. The link between the two cortices is also provided by the external loop. It has been suggested that climbing fibres provide an error signal that generally expresses a comparison between a desired command ('Fcom') given by the motor cortex and its actual effect ('Fext'), depending upon the peripheral context.

The learning of the dynamics model

A voluntary movement comprises several components (Paillard 1982). It generally consists of a combination of muscle actions that make it possible to change the relative positions of body segments, in order to reach a goal. In addition, these displacements are accompanied by a set of postural adjustments. Due to the spring properties of muscles (Houk and Rymer 1981), the forces involved in the movement perturb the position of postural segments and may cause a loss of stability and balance (Massion and Dufossé 1988). Learning the co-ordination between posture and movement is therefore essential for efficient motor performance to be possible.

The learning of the whole command is performed in parallel by both cortices and can be analysed in terms of a dialogue between cerebral and cerebellar cortices, as described in Fig. 23.2. During this dialogue, each structure is guiding the processing and learning is taking place in the other structure. Here a distinction is made between the two phases described above.

During the first phase (Fig. 23.2–1), the various muscular actions which are necessary to reach a goal are learned in the cerebral cortex from the changes in the connective coefficients between micro-columns, because the

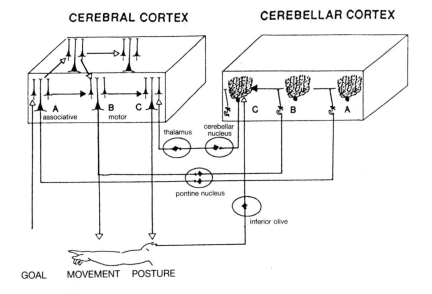

1) Learning of goal/directed movement

$P[\ lp[B]>T\ /\ up[A]>T\ ]\neq 0$

$\Delta M+\ (A-B)\ \nearrow$

2) Perturbation:dynamic compensation

$ol[C] = Fcom[C] - Fext[C] \neq 0$

$\Delta\ pur[C] \neq 0$

3) Learning of postural adjustment

$th[C] \neq 0$

$P[lp[C]>T\ /\ up[A]>T] \neq 0$

$\Delta M+\ (A,C)\ \nearrow$

4) Learning of feed-forward postural adjustment

$par[A] = lp[A]$

$par[A].lp[C] \neq 0$

$\Delta N+\ (A,C)\ \nearrow$

$ol[C] = Fcom[C] - Fext[C] = 0$

$\Delta\ pur[C] = a.par[A] + b.par[C]$

5) Tuning of the command

$lp[C] = \Sigma\ up[\ Ki\ ,\ C] + a.lp[A] + b.lp[B]$

$\Sigma\ up[\ Ki\ ,\ C] \neq 0$

Fig. 23.2. Cerebro-cerebellar co-operation for learning the dynamics model of the skeleto-muscular apparatus. An error signal originating from the periphery is sent to the inferior olive and conveyed to a cerebellar microzone. In the diagram, A, B, and C address cerebral micro-columns (left) and corresponding mossy-fibre inputs to a cerebellar micro-zone (right). Five steps in the dialogue are specified below (see text for abbreviations and details).

learning rules in this tissue are well suited for selecting the appropriate patterns of local actions that produce the expected result.

If a goal is signalled by a strong activity in a sub-set of micro-columns in an associative cortex (A in Fig. 23.2), learning will consist of increasing the connective coefficients between this sub-set A and the sub-set B (in the motor or premotor cortex) which commands the appropriate muscular contraction.

These movements may produce several postural perturbations in other body segments. Displacement of a postural segment gives rise to an error message transmitted from the periphery to a specific cerebellar microzone (Fig. 23.2–2) which co-operates with the cerebral micro-columns (C) of the motor cortex that are able to correct the error.

These cerebello-cerebral connections can then guide activities in the corresponding micro-columns (C) and produce the appropriate cerebral commands for postural corrections to be made (Fig. 23.2–3). At this step, the postural adjustment is made in a closed loop mode by means of an error signal.

Within the cerebellar micro-zone that can participate in the corrections, two input signals interact on Purkinje cells: (a) mossy fibre activities and parallel fibre inputs conveying the signals from the cerebral cortex, which are involved in the anticipatory aspects of the command (Fig. 23.2–4); (b) error signals coming through the inferior olive from perturbed postural segments. This interaction will progressively shape the Purkinje cell response to the specific pattern of anticipatory inputs, until it suppresses the error signal. The movement will then be controlled in a feed-forward mode by the cerebellar micro-zone.

At this step, the micro-zones have acquired an internal model of the effects of the voluntary movements and in this sense, the cerebellum has learned a direct dynamics model of the skeleto-muscular apparatus. At the end of this learning phase, the appropriate motor commands are adequately tuned but the cerebral cortex is still in charge of the task (Fig. 23.2–5).

The learning of the inverse dynamics model

Cerebral loading is not necessary here because it corresponds to a redundant control of the motor commands expressed by a whole set of cortico-cortical interactions which have favoured the movement learning (Fig. 23.3–1). The cerebellar learning can suffice to produce the general command and progressively replace the cortico-cortical influences on the micro-columns (B) of the motor cortex (Fig. 23.3–2). The output activities of these columns will therefore be due only to the cerebellar influences provided by the thalamic inputs.

The second phase of learning process can take place if the differences

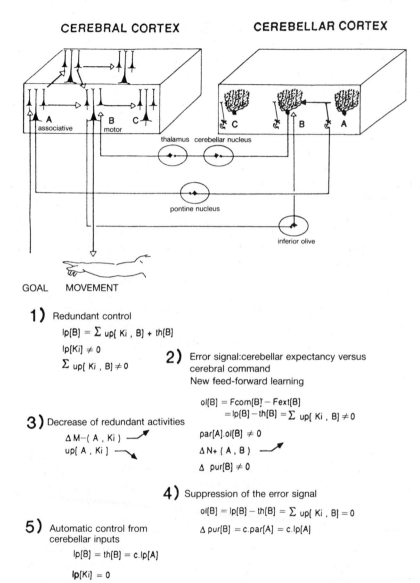

CEREBRAL CORTEX   **CEREBELLAR CORTEX**

A associative   B motor   C

thalamus   cerebellar nucleus

pontine nucleus

inferior olive

GOAL   MOVEMENT

1) Redundant control

$$lp[B] = \sum up[K_i , B] + th[B]$$

$$lp[K_i] \neq 0$$

$$\sum up[K_i , B] \neq 0$$

2) Error signal:cerebellar expectancy versus cerebral command

New feed-forward learning

$$ol[B] = Fcom[B] - Fext[B]$$
$$= lp[B] - th[B] = \sum up[K_i , B] \neq 0$$

3) Decrease of redundant activities

$$\Delta M-(A , K_i) \longrightarrow$$
$$up[A , K_i] \longrightarrow$$

$$par[A].ol[B] \neq 0$$

$$\Delta N+ (A , B) \longrightarrow$$

$$\Delta pur[B] \neq 0$$

4) Suppression of the error signal

$$ol[B] = lp[B] - th[B] = \sum up[K_i , B] = 0$$

$$\Delta pur[B] = c.par[A] = c.lp[A]$$

5) Automatic control from cerebellar inputs

$$lp[B] = th[B] = c.lp[A]$$

$$lp[K_i] = 0$$

Fig. 23.3. Cerebro-cerebellar co-operation for learning the inverse dynamics model of the skeleto-muscular apparatus. An error signal originating from the motor cortex corresponds to a redundant control exerted by both cerebral and cerebellar cortices. The cerebellar microzone progressively take over from the cortical control. As a result, learning becomes automatized, the process being stored in the cerebellar circuits (see text for abbreviations and details).

between the thalamic input and the motor cortex output give rise to an error signal which is sent to the inferior olive and then to the cerebellum (B) through the climbing fibre system. These signals will progressively change the input–output transfer function in the micro-zone and consequently, that thalamic input to the motor cortex. The micro-zones involved are probably different from those involved in the first phase of learning.

The cortico-cortical processes are slower than the cerebellar ones as the response of a column is a decision process elaborated through a progressive recruitment of neuronal activities within the column; whereas the input/output relations in the cerebellum are a more direct process with no recruitment delays. If the thalamic input to the motor cortex suffices for an appropriate command to occur, this command will inhibit the later, useless, cortical activities. The micro-columns influencing the motor cortex will thus progressively decrease their influence, because they are no longer able to produce the appropriate motor commands (Fig. 23.3–3).

The error signal disappears with the progressive decrease in the redundant cortical influences on the motor cortex (Fig. 23.3–4). As a result, learning is completely automatized and stored in the cerebellar circuits (Fig. 23.3–5). In this way, the cerebellum has learned a function that was previously performed by the cerebral cortex. This function corresponds to the inverse dynamics model of the skeleto-muscular apparatus formerly held in the cerebral cortex.

Conclusion

In this model, learning of the movement command is performed by a network that links two subsystems together: a cerebral sub-system which can learn a goal, and a second subsystem for quantitative adjustments. This model may explain (a) how adaptive control is progressively transferred from cerebral to cerebellar level during the acquisition of the co-ordination between posture and movement, and (b) how the whole movement could be automatized with a minimal load for the cerebral cortex. Each subsystem is essential for fast learning to occur and participates in the final result.

If we attempt to establish a parallel with artificial systems, the cerebral cortex can be said to be a multi-process but single-task 'central processing unit'. This unit needs a 'mass memory' that is provided by the extraordinary storage capacity available, thanks to the perpendicular arrangement of the cerebellar cortex. This cerebellar memory is a content-address, associative memory consisting of multiple cerebellar modules working in parallel in order to detect, memorize, and automize the repetitive tasks processed by the central unit.

Acknowledgements

We would like to thank Mrs J. Blanc for correcting the English version of the manuscript. This work was supported by French Ministry of Research and Technology grant 'Sciences de la Cognition'.

References

Albus, J. (1971). A theory of cerebellar function. *Mathematical Biosciences*, **10**, 25–61.

Alexandre, F., Burnod, Y., Guyot, F., and Haton, J. P. (1989). La colonne corticale, nouvelle unité de base pour les réseaux multicouches. *Compte-Rendus de l'Académie des Sciences*. Paris, **309**, III, 259–64.

Burnod, Y. (1989). *An adaptive neural network: the cerebral cortex*. Masson, Paris.

Chauvet, G. (1986). Habituation rules for a theory of the cerebellar cortex. *Biological Cybernetics*, **55**, 201–9.

Fujita, M. (1982). Adaptive filter model of the cerebellum. *Biological Cybernetics*, **45**, 195–206.

Holmes, G. (1939). The cerebellum of man. *Brain*, **1**, 1–30.

Houk, J. C. and Rymer, W. Z. (1981). Neural control of muscle length and tension. In *Handbook of physiology*, Section I, Vol. 2 (ed. V. B. Brooks), pp. 257–323.

Hubel, D. H., Wiesel, T. N., and Stryker, M. P. (1978). Anatomical demonstration of orientation columns in macaque monkey. *Journal of Comparative Neurology*, **177**, 361–80.

Ito, M. (1984). *The cerebellum and neural control*. Raven Press, New York.

Ito, M. (1989). Long term depression. *Annual Review of Neuroscience*, **12**, 85–102.

Ito, M. (1990). A new physiological concept on on cerebellum. *Revue Neurologique* (in press).

Ito, M., Sakurai, M., and Tongroach, P. (1982). Climbing fiber induced depression of both mossy fiber responsiveness and glutamate sensitivity of cerebellar Purkinje cells. *Journal of Physiology*, **324**, 113–34.

Kawato, M., Furukawa, K., and Suzuki, R. (1987). A hierarchical model for control and learning of voluntary movement. *Biological Cybernetics*, **57**, 169–85.

Leiner, H. C., Leiner, A. L., and Dow, R. S. (1989). Reappraising the cerebellum: What does the hindbrain contribute to the forebrain. *Behavioral Neuroscience*, **103**, 998–1008.

Massion, J. and Dufossé, M. (1988). Co-ordination between posture and movement: Why and How? *News in Physiological Sciences*, **3**, 88–93.

Marr, D. (1969). A theory of cerebellar cortex. *Journal of Physiology*, **202**, 437–70.

Minsky, M. and Papert, S. (1969). *Perceptrons*. MIT Press, Cambridge, MA.

Mountcastle, V. B. (1978). An organizing principle for cerebral function: the unit module and the distributed system. In *The mindful brain* (ed. F. O. Schmidt) pp. 257–323. MIT Press, Cambridge, MA.

Oscarsson, O. (1969). The sagittal organization of the cerebellar anterior lobe as revealed by the projection patterns of the climbing fiber system. In *Neurobiology of cerebellar evolution and development* (ed. R. Llinas) pp. 525–37. American Medical Association, Chicago.

Paillard, J. (1982). Apraxia and the neurophysiology of motor control. *Philosophical Transactions of the Royal Society*, London, B298, 111–34.

Rosenblatt, F. (1958). The perception: a probabilistic model for information storage and organization in the brain. *Psychological Review*, **65**, 386–408.

Shepherd, G. M. (1969). *The synaptic organization of the brain*. Oxford University Press.

Widrow, B. and Hopf, M. E. (1960). Adaptive switching circuits. *IRE Wescon Convention Record*, **4**, 96–104.

Epilogue

24

Knowing where and knowing how to get there

JACQUES PAILLARD

As a final comment, I would like to view the topic 'Brain and Space' from my own vantage point. I was first introduced to this field of research many years ago through the works of a neurologist, Henri Wallon, and those of a zoologist, Jean Piaget, who both became interested in the ontogenetic aspects of brain function. The former emphasized the importance of proprioceptive information as a foundation of both self and social identity through the development of emotional behaviour (Wallon 1949); the latter considered that the highest cognitive functions were rooted in basic sensorimotor machinery (Piaget 1971). As a psychobiologist by training, I became fascinated by these problems; by the question of how the spatial constraints that are specific to our terrestial environment have moulded our body architecture and its sensory and motor instruments; and in what way they have shaped our nervous system to cope with the quasi-euclidean space in which we live.

The neuroscientist who confronts the problem of 'brain and space' immediately faces a forest of question marks. How are spatial relationships encoded in the neural processing of sensory information and motor commands so as to provide a framework for our perceptions, and to orient and guide our actions? How are mental images of the outside world generated by the brain? How are the variety of symbolic and abstract representations of space, which pervade all our mental activities, built and stored in the neural tissue? How do these capacities emerge in the developing brain? What is inherited and what is acquired? How much can we learn about the healthy functioning brain from the study of spatial disorders? Few of these basic problems have been solved. But important new theoretical and experimental advances *have* been discussed during this meeting which point in the direction of future solutions. To that end, a convergent multi-disciplinary effort is mandatory.

Accordingly a deliberate emphasis has been put in this meeting on recent data stemming from an integrative approach in neuroscience. Such an approach is in my view indispensable for interfacing basic knowledge of neuronal mechanisms with our understanding of the living brain as a functional entity, generating its own mental representations and behaviour. It is only at this level of integration, for instance, that we may hope to relate spatial disorders resulting from brain damage to experimental behavioural data about space perception, motor performance, and developmental issues.

Spatial features may constrain the brain in many different ways. There is a remarkable and profuse variety of anatomical and functional solutions that living systems have evolved to overcome the many spatial problems raised by aerial, terrestrial, or aquatic locomotion in an environment dominated by the ubiquitous presence of the forces of gravity (Paillard 1971). Innumerable examples could be cited in many different functional domains. One of the most striking is a consequence of the erect posture of man, with the ensuing promotion of the forelimbs to sophisticated instruments of prehension. Another example is the development of binocular vision. In both cases, a corresponding deep transformation follows in the neural architectures of a larger brain (Paillard 1960; 1990).

With such a broad spectrum of spatial functions to study, conceptual guidelines are essential. Recent research has given rise to some interesting functional dichotomies which may stimulate further experimental and theoretical progress in the field.

What and where?

One of the most influential dichotomies which has arisen is the distinction between 'two visual systems', one for object perceptions and one for spatial location. This distinction was explicitly described in a series of articles published in *Psychologische Forschung* between 1967 and 1968 by Ingle (1967), Trevarthen (1968), Schneider (1969) and Held (1970). Trevarthen named the two systems 'focal' and 'ambient'. The focal system involved mainly the geniculo-striate pathways, whereas the ambient system was dependent on the superior colliculus. The model was dervied from a study of the visuomotor behaviour of the hamster by Schneider (1969). The study separated the role of collicular structures in orientation and localization from that of cortical visual areas in the perceptual discrimination and recognition of visual forms. It was later realized (Ungerleider and Mishkin 1982) that both systems were corticalized in primates and man. This dissociation has since been confirmed by neuroanatomical, neurophysiological, and neuropsychological evidence. The basic assumption is that visual formation is distributed from the primary areas of the striate cortex to the associative cortex along two main streams: one travels through the posterior parietal association cortex (see Andersen 1987; Stein 1989; and Chapter 11 in this volume) and subserves the function of knowing 'where'; the other mainly projects into the temporal association areas where object features are analysed, and thus constitutes the neural substrate of the function of knowing 'what'.

We have emphasized (Paillard 1971 and chapter 10, this volume), however, that an object contains its own network of spatial relationships. Thus, each channel has to compute a topographic representation of spatial features but differs in its basic encoding modes. One concerns the space of shape (*'l'espace des formes'*) and the other the space of locality (*'l'espace des lieux'*), thus reflecting two different processing modes. Subsequently, many other questions have sprung from this basic dissociation, which have in turn challenged the different disciplines in their own fields. Suffice it to mention a few.

Central versus peripheral vision

The functional distinction between foveal and ambient vision suggested by Trevarthen (1968) has its obvious anatomical and physiological foundations. The high spatial resolution and processing power of the fovea with the major distribution of the central retina along the geniculo-striate pathways can be contrasted with poor spatial discrimination outside the fovea and the main distribution of the peripheral retina to the extrageniculate pathways (including the colliculus). This anatomical contrast certainly supports the notion of a basic functional segregation.

Further evidence for a functional segregation is provided by the rod and cone equipment of the retina and their heterogeneous distribution over the retinotopic frame which, has long been recognized as subserving the segregation between spatial analysers (which are concentrated in foveal and parafoveal regions) and luminance detectors (which are widely distributed over the whole retina). The identification, in the cat, of two types of ganglial cells, X and Y, with sustained and transient modes of discharges respectively, and with a higher density of X cells in central vision and the number of Y cells increasing at the periphery, also reinforces the notion of a dual channel (see review in Howard 1982). The further identification of two main streams in the geniculo-striate pathways—one originating from the parvocellular part of the geniculate bodies (corresponding to the X system), and the other from the magnocellular part (corresponding to the Y system), with their distinct projections within the cortical colums of area 17—has been a useful guide in tracking the further distribution of these two visual channels through the multiple areas of the visual cortex, for their further processing by the association cortex (Livingston and Hubel 1985; de Yoe and van Essen 1988).

Interestingly, the segregation of a dorsal and ventral distribution of visual information, corresponding to the *'what'* and *'where'* dissociation mentioned previously appears to map on to the distinction between central and peripheral vision. The ventral branch (the *what* channel of the inferotemporal cortex) is mainly concerned with central vision (up to 10° of eccentricity) whereas the dorsal branch (the *where* channel of the inferior parietal association areas) receives most of its information from peripheral vision (Mishkin and Ungerleider 1982).

The search for a distinctive role of central versus peripheral vision in visuomotor coordination has been particularly rewarding (Paillard 1982). Here the reaching paradigm has been extensively used to study the visual requirements of spatially oriented behaviour. It lends itself to a clear segregation of functional segments, and provides an opportunity to separate and categorize the visual channels that are involved in the triggering and guidance of visuomotor behaviour. All these experiments have provided convincing evidence of the separate role of central and peripheral vision in providing, through separate channels, different types of error signal to guide the trajectory of the hand toward the target. To some extent, peripheral vision can be regarded as assisting the 'navigator' (in charge of the transport of the hand from its initial position toward the target) with the computing of the appropriate trajectory. Central vision may provide the 'pilot' with the cues necessary to achieve the smooth landing of the hand on the target.

Both functions are clearly separate. Navigator and pilot use different types of visual cue: movement and direction cues versus position and distance cues respectively, each referring its evaluation of spatial relationships to a different system of space coordinates.

Position versus movement cues

Like other sensory modalities, the visual system utilizes *tonic* and *phasic* modes of transduction. Tonic transducers provide information about stable features of the spatial environment, whereas transient channels signal what is going to change and the rate of changing. The two main streams of visual information (the what and where channels) are fed respectively by sustained and transient signals coming from the retina and thence convey position and movement cues separately. We have argued (Paillard and Amblard 1985) that these two distinct visual subsystems operate in a complementary way. Static vision is primarily mediated by the central retina: it is specially tuned for coding relative position, object shape, pattern, contour, and colour. Kinetic vision is the predominant concern of the peripheral retina: it is tuned for contrast sensitivity, and for velocity coding and directional selectivity; it detects the continuous motion of a stimulus and of image drift on the retina. Psychophysical studies (reviewed in Bonnet 1977) have illustrated the duality of the visual mechnanisms that subserve motion perception: one infers motion from the successive positions of a moving object, and the other perceives the direction in which the target signal is moving directly. The parallel computation of position and movement cues in two separate channels allows a somewhat redundant description of space relationships. Both descriptions may, theoretically, be complete and self-sufficient. In one channel, immobility and stationary features can be inferred from null-velocity signals, and the final position of a movement can be derived from the integral of its velocity. Velocity signals conveyed by the kinetic channel are, in that case, the key descriptors of a *movement space*. In the second channel, motion information can be derived from the static channel signalling discrete successive changes of the stimulus position, thereby defining primarily a *relative position space*.

Thus information about position is available directly from the static channel and indirectly from the integral of velocity provided by the kinetic channel. Conversely, velocity which is directly coded in the movement channel can also be indirectly evaluated by the position channel, as a derivative of the amplitude of location changes in relation to time. Two main descriptions of space are therefore available for the brain: one based on the coding of relative distance between stable points of the visual array, and the other based on the velocity and direction coding of moving features. The latter is probably the more primitive one from an evolutionary point of view. Detection of changes, incorporated in the logic of predator-prey relationships, has an obvious survival value for most species. Immobility has here a protective value and is clearly detected as 'no-movement' by a visual system endowed with the high temporal resolution power that is characteristic of the kinetic channel. In contrast, the static channel has evolved with the improvement of foveal vision; its high power of spatial resolution allows the fine-grain analysis of object features. As a consequence, the stabilization of the retinal frame with respect to the world frame evolved with the development of the mechanisms for both foveal grasping and saccadic displacement of the fovea, from one point of interest to another.

Like posture and movement, however, which clearly derive from separate control networks but function in tightly related synergy, both spatial systems are intimately associated in the interfacing of object-centred space with its environmental surround. Presumably, the stability of the visual frame may be directly derived from the retinal drift of covariant features that preserve the relative position of objects in the environmental frame: an authentic Gibsonian view recently revived and implicit in the model developed by Berthoz at the meeting (Chapter 6, this volume). Likewise, the preservation of object-constancy during movement presupposes a similar mechanism of evaluation and conservation of the relative distance between points of an invariant configuration together with a 'tag assignment' (place labelling) for non-spatial features (Strong and Whitehead 1989).

Direction versus distance coding

Separate control of the two dimensions of a vectorial coding of motor commands seems to be the rule at the later stages of motor programming. Directional coding is assumed to rely principally on address codes ('labelled lines') whereas amplitude coding is more dependent on intensity control by frequency codes (Paillard 1983). Most psychological studies of motor control emphasize the fact that directional change is much more demanding than amplitude change (Poulton 1981), and that the latter takes a minimum of time and can intervene during an ongoing movement without requiring reprogramming (Megaw 1972).

The dissociation of amplitude and directional requirements has been addressed in a series of recent experiments by Bard *et al.* (1990 and in press). Pointing and aiming tasks were used in young human subjects who were given separate feedback cues for the correction of distance and direction errors, with the following results. Distance accuracy required positional cues mainly processed by the central retina (up to 10° eccentricity). In contrast, directional accuracy depended principally on peripheral vision. These findings confirm earlier results from Beaubaton and Chapuis (1974) showing that central vision subserves the error-detecting mechanism involved in the homing-in phase of a pointing movement. It is also consistent with psychophysical data showing that the proximity of a stable reference does markedly improve the dynamic sensitivity of the location system which operates in the low velocity range (up to 10°/s). The sharp deceleration observed in the final phase of a pointing movement at the vicinity of a stationary target optimizes the functioning of this channel and provides the feedback loop with the relatively long delay (200 ms) it requires to effect a correction.

In contrast, directional errors are provided by movement cues processed by the dynamic channel. The peripheral retina is crossed by the image of the hand moving towards the fovea, which is itself strongly anchored to the target before and during the whole course of the movement. The correct trajectory is, therefore, one which is directed toward the fovea (Beaubaton *et al.* 1979). Thus we assume that movements which deviate from the required trajectory generate the directional error-signals that are needed for a feed-back loop to rectify the trajectory. This correction requires a rather short delay to operate, given that the pointing movement reaches its peak angular velocity, in terms of retinal trajectory, during the early part of the trajectory (at about 40° eccentricity for a pointing movement starting from the body midline toward a target located in the horizontal plane of gaze). Characteristic kinematic changes have been observed in the trajectory of aiming movements that are improved in their accuracy when vision is restricted to the early part of the trajectory (Teasdale *et al.* 1990), thus supporting the hypothesis of a fast intervening feedback loop. Fast visuomotor corrections have also been observed in postural regulation (Vidal *et al.* 1978).

Directionally sensitive neurons (preferentially tuned for movement toward and away from the fovea) have been described in the posterior parietal cortex (Molter and Mountcastle 1981) operating within a very broad velocity range (from 10 to 1000°/s). Moreover, similar neurons have been found in area MST that are distributed predominantly on a diagonal of the retinotopic frame. In the monkey this distribution seems to correspond to the sector of the visual field covered by reaching movements directed to a foveally fixated target. It has not yet been established whether the fast directional feedback loop operates on the motor cortex through a directional cortico-cortical pathway or, like the slow positional loops, through a parieto-cerebello-cortical circuit. Interestingly, two separate cortico-pontine circuits have been anatomically identified (Glickstein *et al.* 1980).

Vector versus location cues

It is a matter of debate whether our movements are directed in space in terms of a *vectorial coding* of our displacement (direction and distance) or in terms of a *locus calibration* within an internal space map. These modes, however, are not mutually exclusive and may depend on the requirement of the motor task and of the action system involved.

Those working in the oculomotor field seem ready to accept the generality of vectorial coding which, theoretically, seems to offer the most parsimonious solution to the problem of a neural description of space relationships, without need of a reference frame or of an abstract space map (Goldberg and Buschnell 1981). According to this view, motor error signals, of the type described at the collicular level for occular saccades, suffice for the description of a motor space from which a perceptual space could theoretically be derived.

In contrast, there is a substantial body of experimental data from ethological and psychological research which suggests that spatial orientation in animals and man relies heavily on their internal mapping of the environment. Most investigators of the locomotor space of rodents, for instance, accept Tolman's notion of *'cognitive spatial maps'* and now offer convincing evidence of a neural counterpart (see Part 4 of this volume). However, in this field, the distinction between 'maps' and 'routes', and between 'local' and 'taxon' systems (O'Keefe and Nadel 1978) allows for the coexistence of both processing modes of space relationships by the nervous system.

The elegant paradigm used by Goldberg and Bruce (1981) to determine whether, at the level of single unit activity, eye movements are coded in terms of a '*vector*' or as a '*locus*' to be reached in a space map provides rather strong evidence for a non-locus coding at the collicular level and in the frontal eye field. It does not rule out, however, the possibility of a place coding for eye movement, an hypothesis which seems to be supported by recent date at both of the anatomical levels mentioned above (Mays and Sparks 1980, Schlag and Schlag-Rey 1985 and Chapters 1 and 5 in this volume). The strategy elicited probably depends on context and task requirements.

It is still an open question whether this duality can be extended to reaching movements. Well-documented neurobehavioural data indicate that there is separate parametric control of direction and amplitude in movement programming, and therefore support the concept of a vectorial coding of motor commands. Nevertheless, there are alternative interpretations. These include the '*equilibrium point*' theory (Feldman 1974) and the '*mass spring*' model (Bizzi and Polit 1979, Polit and Bizzi 1979) which offer an elegant theoretical solution for the locus-coding basis of motor programming. These models have continued to attract considerable enthusiasm in the past fifteen years (Keele 1981), despite the persisting problem of providing it with a convincing neural explanation. Recent recording of spontaneous saccades in the supplementary eye field (Schlag and Schlag-Rey 1985), and with grasping and reaching arm movements in the inferior premotor area (Rizzolati *et al.* 1987) offer new opportunities for understanding the way in which the representation of a goal may structure the programming of an action.

Memorized versus perceived or registered location

Visually received information may be stored and used to guide behaviour in many different ways. Memory for *object* and *place* has long been dissociated by neuropsychology from the identification of the separate neural networks subserving each of them (Ungerleider and Mishkin 1982). Several subdivisions are recognized within the *where* and *what* functions (Maunsell and Van Essen 1987; Pandya and Yeterian 1984). Limiting our comments to the *where* problem, which has received relatively less attention in recent human studies than the problem of visual recognition disorders (but see de Renzi 1982), let us consider the following evidence as indicative of the richness of a still barely explored field.

The distinction between *perceived* and *registered* location has been successfully demonstrated by the blindsight phenomenon (Weiskrantz 1989): targets not perceived in the blind field of a hemianopic patient can nevertheless trigger a reaching program in the right direction. Thus, visual location cues are registered in maps that can be used directly by the motor system, without perceptual awareness of those targets. We later had the opportunity to describe an equivalent of the blindsight phenomenon in the tactile modality in a patient with a centrally deafferented arm (Paillard *et al.* 1983).

We were led to make a similar dissociation between *perceived* and *registered* location in a study on 'position sense' in healthy human subjects (Paillard and Brouchon 1968). The upper arm, with extended index finger, was displaced actively or passively. Blindfolded subjects were then asked to point with the index finger of the other hand to the presumed location of the displaced limb. They made three different constant errors, according to the displacement condition (active or passive) and to the time interval between displacement and pointing response (zero or 12 s). The consistency of these pointing errors led to the conclusion that the location of the target was *registered* in three different maps according to the nature of the proprioceptive information involved. These maps were, however, not *perceived* as different by the subjects who were unaware, within that particular range of movement, of any change of location.

A series of ingenious studies by Bridgeman *et al.* (1979, 1981) and by Wong and Mack (1981) have given convincing new evidence of the existence of separate maps of location in visual space. For example, a slightly moving target, whose perceived movement can be masked by saccadic suppression, is correctly reached at its (not perceived) new location by a pointing hand. Also, the illusory displacement of a target induced by a rapidly moving surrounding frame is ignored by the motor system, which points to the real physical position of the target at the same time as subjects verbally assess the perceived illusory position of the target on a metric scale. Interestingly, if pointing is slightly delayed for a few seconds in this last situation, subjects point to the illusory position as if the first location map used by the motor system had been a very limited 'short term memory' relative to the longer duration of the perceptual location map. Memory for object place defined within an egocentric frame of reference has only limited usefulness for mobile organisms, whereas specification of location with respect to fixed environmental cues in an allocentric reference system is stored for longer and thus is of more lasting value to the organism. Accordingly, a purely egocentric spatial label assigned to objects would then be restricted to orienting, triggering and guiding any ongoing activity which is directed to those objects that are in a stable spatial relationship with the body frame (whether gaze, head and/or body axis are predominantly involved).

Stark and Bridgeman (1983) have also shown that a discrepancy between an eye position signal and actual gaze direction, such as that which can be induced by pressing the eye while maintaining the gaze on the target leads to inaccurate pointing, even though subjects perceive the target in its correct physical location. This occurs provided that (and this reservation is particularly important) the visual background is structured. Here we are obviously facing a change of reference frames as gaze direction and eye position signal are independently represented: a perturbing signal can be inserted into either representation without affecting the other. Furthermore, the two frames use different spatial codes which are appropriate for retention over different time scales.

It has to be established which of the two systems is most appropriate for guiding an action, depending on the nature of the task and its context. This is particularly important for the retention time-scale of the allocentric perceived location which was observed in the pointing experiment described above, which was in the same range (8 to 12 s) as that observed by Thompson (1981) in his locomotor experiment with occluded vision. In both cases, a much longer term memory for location undoubtedly exists which relies on other types of central spatial representation, and probably on other coding modes.

Similarly, in our experiments on position sense (Paillard and Brouchon 1968, 1974), we observed that the calibration of final limb position (which resulted from active displacement and presumably from dynamic proprioceptive information) vanished within 12 s, to give way to a new stored location corresponding to static proprioceptive information which may persist unchanged for 20 minutes. Likewise, if required to remember the last position of their limb at the end of an experimental session, subjects can regain approximately the same position a day later. This merely emphasizes the variety of spatial memories that are to be disentangled by appropriate experimental procedures when studying the problem of encoding location cues, without even broaching the issue of a supramodal cognitive representation of space.

A second new field of investigation, recently introduced in the study of saccadic eye movements, concerns the dissociation between movements that are 'memory driven' versus 'stimulus driven', and their putative neural counterpart (Goldberg 1985). Our ability to trigger spatially oriented movement (such as an oculomotor saccade), either *reflexly* (in reaction to a visual stimulus displayed in the visual field, whether at an expected or an unpredicted locus), or *spontaneously* (as in the random exploration of a dark field when expecting the appearance of a target without knowing its location), or *voluntarily* (toward the memorized location of a target just extinguished) is differentially affected, depending on which neural structures are damaged (Leuck *et al.* 1990).

All these findings uncover new paradigms for exploring the way in which location cues are stored, and within which frameworks they are referred.

Reference frames versus co-ordinate systems

It is trivial to say that any description of a given state of matter is frame dependent. Spatial frameworks are incorporated in our perceptual and motor experiences. They are not, however, to be confused with the *system of co-ordinates* which abstractly represent them. When considering the latter, we immediately face the necessary distinction between *extrinsic* co-ordinates which are arbitrarily chosen by the observer for the convenience of his description, and *intrinsic* natural co-ordinates used by the nervous system to handle its spatial problems. These natural co-ordinates are not known. They can only be indirectly inferred according to our conceptual framework and our experimental strategy (Arbib 1981). The problem of *reference frames* was central for one session of the meeting (Part 2) and will not be further developed here. The general distinction between an *egocentric* and an *allocentric* frame of reference is generally accepted (Owen and Lee 1987). My personal view has always been that both are basically derived from the *geocentric* framework (within which all terrestrial living systems have been moulded (Paillard 1971)) and that they can not be studied independently. In fact, we have to consider that the framing of our visually guided behaviour in the 'locus space' depends on four fundamental referants organized around the invariant vertical orientation of gravity forces (see Fig. 24.1).

The *body frame* provides reference for posture and movements in all spatially oriented actions. The standing posture, which is actively maintained and species-specific, remains the main framework within which our environmental space is tailored for actions, and also the vertically oriented container for our perceptions (Paillard 1971).

The *object frame* refers here to the object-centred view of the observer. We know that the recognition of an object depends on its orientation with respect to the direction of gravity forces or on its relationship to the orientation of the body axis. The perceived orientation of both body and object may also be dependent on environmental landmarks.

The *world frame* includes both the object frame and the body frame as local spaces. Gravity forces also constrain the arrangement of physical matter around us. From our own limited living space, the surface of water is perceived as a horizontal plane, and the trees as growing vertically. Accordingly, the basic natural spatial constraints of our terrestrial environment, which have moulded our body architecture during the course of evolution, compel our organism to accommodate a quasi-Euclidean space.

Finally, the object and environmental frames are both derived from visual information that is first processed within the *retinal frame*. In most species with mobile eyes, this frame is automatically stabilized with respect

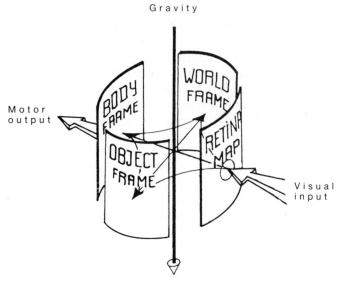

Fig. 24.1. The four fundamental reference frames organized around the invariant vertical orientation of gravity forces, which together subserve visually guided behaviour. See comments in the text.

to the horizon. The environmental framework is independently stabilized on the retina during the period of foveation of targets of interest and of gaze anchoring.

Thus, the ubiquitous geotropic constraint dominates the four references frames that are used in the visuomotor control of actions and perceptions, and thereby becomes a crucial factor in linking them together. Despite interesting research in cognitive psychology, little is known about the mode of interaction—synergistic or competitive—of these frames or the way in which they may supplement each other after experimental or pathological loss. (See, however, Chapter 13, this volume). Nevertheless, the impressive advance of our neuroanatomical knowledge of the hodology of intracortical connections may generate some new hypotheses for our understanding of spatial processing by the brain (see Fig. 24.2).

Neural versus computational mapping of space

The place taken by the modelling of space representation in this book (see Part 5) reflects what Francis Crick (1989) has described as 'the recent excitement about neural networks'. Undoubtedly, the remarkable properties of some newly discovered algorithms for 'neurone-like' networks

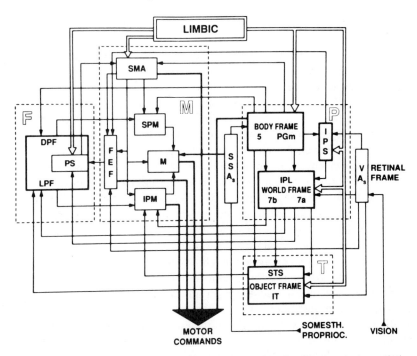

Fig. 24.2. Schematic diagram of major pathways connecting the three cortical association areas, frontal (F), parietal (P), and temporal (T), to the premotor and motor areas (M). It illustrates the following anatomical and functional connections: areas 5 and PGm provide information (mainly proprioceptive) for the elaboration of the body frame; area 7a supplies information (mainly visual) for the world frame; the retinal frame (receiving geniculo-striate afference) provides the visual information to both, parietal cortex (via the intraparietal sulcus IPS) and inferotemporal cortex (IT). Proprioceptive information about the body frame is mainly distributed to the dorsal region of the frontal areas, whereas multimodal information about object frame and world frame is chiefly supplied to ventral prefrontal areas.

Motor areas (M) are afferented by two different premotor zones: the inferior premotor area (IPM), which mainly contributes to guide actions in both object space and environmental frame within a stimulus-bound reactive mode; and the superior premotor area (SMA), which is mainly afferented with information about the body frame and internal states. The supplementary motor area (SMA) has an overall control over premotor and motor areas, as an instrument of internally and/or intentionally driven motor command, while inhibiting irrelevant stimulus-driven activity. Related areas in the schema include: VAs (visual areas), IPL (Inferior parietal lobule), SSAs (somatosensory areas), FEF (frontal eye field), DPF (dorsal prefrontal), LPF (lateral prefrontal), PS (sulcus principalis) (Paillard 1990).

trigger new ideas for our understanding of the computational properties of the brain. Despite the fact that the behaviour of computational networks, as yet, bears little resemblance to that of the brain (Paillard 1987), they may still be the most plausible candidates to support the claim that some complex operations (such as extracting categories that share common features from a complex array of incoming stimuli, or mapping a multidimensional representation of space) can be related directly to known properties of neural networks.

In a way, this new interest in computational networks is reminiscent of the cybernetic revolution of the fifties, when the astonishing power and versatility of servo-mechanisms seemed to promise a new era for biological engineering. Despite the considerable success of cybernetic concepts in the engineering field of automation and regulation, however, it has only made a rather meagre contribution to the modelling of brain circuitry. This is because there is neither a one way flow of control signals from receptor to muscles, nor a single region of the brain which, to the exclusion of others, controls the output system (as modern techniques of neuro-imaging clearly illustrate). The conceptual impact of cybernetics on biology has nevertheless been very important in giving verisimilitude to mechanical 'life-like' devices which are endowed with finality and goal-seeking properties. In a sense, modern neoconnectionism and neuromimetics are just within reach of allowing biology to exorcise the 'ghost' from the thinking machine in the same way that cybernetics once contributed to exorcise the 'finality ghost' from our sensorimotor machinery. From this vantage point, it is interesting to consider the vestibulo-ocular reflex (rightly considered crucial for the stabilization of gaze with respect to the environmental frame), which used to be a favourite topic for demonstrating the power of a cybernetic approach (Robinson 1981) and has now become the chosen focus for network modelling. In network modelling, a 'back propagation' algorithm (whose neural equivalent has not yet been identified) apparently approximates satisfactorily to what has been found by electrophysiological recording (Anastasio and Robinson 1990).

In a similar manner, electrophysiological studies of parietal cortex in the macque monkey, modelling of the activities of a subset of posterior parietal neurons (whose contribution to a mapping of the 'scene' frame is postulated) seems to mimic the behaviour of the hidden 'unit' of a computational network (Zisper and Andersen 1988).

Other examples can be found in the recent modelling of visual perception by 'neuron-like' computational networks (Feldman 1985; Strong and Whitehead 1987) which try to define the engineering requirements for object recognition, whereas brain-theorists (such as Lieblich and Arbib 1982) start from brain structure to propose solutions that are biologically plausible.

Bearing in mind the unbridled enthusiasm first generated by cybernetics, it is premature to specify the future contribution of computational models to our understanding of brain mechanisms. Here, the warning of Francois Jacob (1981) is apposite: evolutionary mechanisms are not a product of the logical brain of an engineer but are more likely to be the result of a 'bricolage genial'—the work of a tinkering genius. Thus, we must first understand the baffling ways in which biological systems have sometimes coped with the problems of adaptation before we too readily accept an engineering solution.

One final point is worth stressing when considering the difference between the ways in which computational networks and real brain circuitry operate. It is the absence, until recently, of an external loop that links output to input in most computer models (but see Grossberg and Kupferstein 1985 and Chapter 22 by Gilhodes *et al.* in this volume). In contrast, brain circuitry depends on a variety of motor–sensory loops that are the main instruments with which biological machines probe their environment and extract from the changing array of self-generated stimuli the regularities and covariances that assert the stability of the external world. Such regularities are printed in the neural circuitry of cortical modules through the stabilization of coactivated synapses (see discussion in Phillips *et al.* 1984). An internal representation of a stable predictable environmental framework thereby emerges, which gives coherence and unity to the spatial relationships that link the organism to its external world.

Where and how to get there?

This is a final comment directly related to the preceding remark on the role of sensorimotor loops as the basic source of knowledge acquired by mobile organisms about their environment. The notion of space is embodied in what is conventionally called *knowledge*. The distinction made by Piaget (1937) between '*savoir*' as the basis of operational intelligence and '*savoir faire*' as the basis of practical intelligence obviously overlaps with the often quoted distinction by Ryle (1949) between '*knowing what*' and '*knowing how*'. The '*what?*' and '*where?*' problem, which served as a point of departure for this epilogue, can now be divided into a subclass of behavioural activities which are clearly dissociated by pathology, and which are presumably dependent on separate neural networks for their achievement. Associated with *what?*, for example, is '*knowing how to use it*'. Associated with *where?* is '*knowing how to get there*'.

The disruption of 'knowing how to use it' is described in neurology as the syndrome of '*apractognosia of use*', recently related by Freud *et al.* (1989) to lesions of area 7b and of the second somaesthesic area. These two areas, with the inferior premotor areas, have also been implicated (see Fig. 24.2) in the preshaping of the digital grip in reaching movement (Jeannerod 1986; Rizolatti *et al.* 1987). Clearly, the repertoire of skills associated with the prehension of objects and tools concerns primarily movement oriented and directed in the '*object space*'. Interestingly, patients with frontal lesions may compulsively grasp and utilize any object presented to them as if they had become dependent upon sensory stimulation related to the perceptual identification of that object (Lhermitte 1983).

In contrast, as regards the dissociation between 'knowing where' and 'knowing how to get there', the primary distinction is that between a *perception of space* as interrelated positions in a central map of *'locus space'* and a *repertoire of motor programs*. The latter includes, for example, ocular saccades in the collicular vector map; they correspond to *sensori-motor path-structures* (see Paillard 1987 and Chapter 10 of this volume) which define the action to be performed in order to reach the target locus. The problem, then, is to know how far the *perception of space* can be dissociated from a *motor appropriation* of space; whether perception of objects, which is a 'reading' of their properties, is not, from its inception, an *action* performed on them. Finally, following the fascinating track which MacKay indicated (1966), we arrive at his concept of a 'state of conditional readiness', which characterizes the internal setting of 'potential actions', already envisaged as 'latent action programs' by Fessard (1970). These programs are specifically tuned to those components of incoming information that have acquired biological significance for the organism and that can be processed, recognized, and experienced as such.

The question then arises whether the considerable expansion of the representational capacities of the human brain, subsequent to the development of linguistic skills (perhaps even species-specific according to Thomas 1984), could take precedence over basic sensorimotor capacities and thereby mask the action-orientated evolutionary roots of the way in which spatial information is processed. Undoubtedly, more abstract representations of space do exist in humans that are not shared by other species, at least with the same degree of independence from action in space. This fact is reflected in the richness of man's spatial cognition, and is indirectly illustrated by the variety of spatial disorders studied by neuropsychologists (De Renzi 1982; Newcombe and Radcliff 1987, and see Radcliffe, Chapter 13 and Bisiach, Chapter 14, this volume). Be that as it may, the Piagetian assumption (Piaget 1971) that higher cognitive functions have their roots in simpler biological mechanisms cannot be dismissed. Complex higher mental activities evolve from solutions to basic problems in sensorimotor control.

Brain and space problems provide a productive ground for our understanding of how the cognitive machine can cohabit and cooperate with sensorimotor machinery (Paillard 1987). Further study of the way in which the sensorimotor and the representational framing of space progressively emerge from evolutionary constraints and develop ontogenetically within a body-centred space, in order to create a stable perceptual world, will provide a fertile arena for interdisciplinary exchange. Therein, biological, behavioural, and computational methods will each have a substantial contribution to make.

References

Anastasio, T. J. and Robinson, D. A. (1990). Distributed parallel processing in the vertical vestibulo-ocular reflex: learning networks compared to sensor theory. *Biological Cybernetics*, **63**, 161–7.

Andersen, R. A. (1987). Inferior parietal lobule function in spatial perception and visuomotor integration. In *Handbook of physiology, Section 1. The nervous system* (ed. V. B. Mountcastle), Vol. 5, pp. 485–518. American Physiological Society, Bethesda, MD.

Arbib, M. A. (1981). Perceptual structures and distributed motor control. In *Handbook of physiology*, Vol. 3, *Motor control* (ed. V. Brooks), pp. 1449–80. American Physiological Society, Bethesda, MD.

Bard, C., Hay, L., and Fleury, M. (1990). Timing and accuracy of visually directed movements in children: Control of direction and amplitude components. *Journal of Experimental Child Psychology*. (In press.)

Bard, C., Paillard, J., Fleury, M., Hay, L., and Larue, J. (1990). Positional versus directional control loops in visuomotor pointing. *C.P.C. European Bulletin of Cognitive Psychology*, **10**, 145–56.

Beaubaton, D. and Chapuis, N. (1974). Rôle des informations tactiles dans la précision du pointage chez le singe 'split-brain'. *Neuropsychologia*, **12**, 151–5.

Beaubaton, D., Grangetto, A., and Paillard, J. (1979). Contribution of positional and movement cues to visuomotor reaching in 'split brain' monkey. In *Structure and function of cerebral commissures* (ed. I. Steele-Russell, M. V. van Hof, and G. Berlucchi), pp. 371–84. Macmillan, London.

Bonnet, C. (1977). Visual motion detection models: Feature and frequency. *Perception*, **6**, 491–500.

Bizzi, E. A. and Polit, A. (1979). Processes controlling visually evoked movements. *Neuropsychologia*, **17**, 203–13.

Bridgeman, B., Lewis, S., Heit, G., and Nagle, M. (1979). Relation between cognitive and motor-oriented systems of visual position perception. *Journal of Experimental Psychology, Human Perception and Performance*, **5**, 692–700.

Bridgeman, B., Kirch, M., and Sperling, A. (1981). Segregation of cognitive and motor aspects of visual function using induced motion. *Perception of Psychophysics*, **29**, 336–42.

Conti, P. and Beaubaton, D. (1980). Role of the structural field and visual reafference in accuracy of pointing movements. *Perceptual and Motor Skills*, **50**, 239–44.

Crick, F. (1989). The recent excitement about neural networks. *Nature*, **337**, 129–32.

De Renzi, E. (1982). *Disorders of space exploration and cognition*. John Wiley & Sons, New York.

De Yoe, E. A. and Van Essen, D. C. (1988). Concurrent processing stream in monkey visual cortex. *Trends in Neuroscience*, **11**, 219–26.

Feldman, A. G. (1974). Change in the length of the muscle as a consequence of a shift in equilibrium in the muscle-load system. *Biofizika*, **19**, 534–8.

Feldman, J. A. (1985). Four frames suffice: a provisional model of vision and space. *The Behavioral and Brain Sciences*, **8**, 265–89.

Fessard, A. (1970). Approche neurophysiologique du problème de la mémoire. In *La Memoire* (ed. A.P.S.L.F.), pp. 459–98. P.U.F., Paris.

Freund, H. J. (1987). Abnormalities of motor behavior after cortical lesion in man. In *Handbook of physiology. Section I. The nervous system*. Vol. 5, Part 2 (ed. V. B. Mountcastle), Chapter 19, pp. 763–810. American Physiological Society. Bethesda, MD.

Glickstein, M., Cohen, J. L., Dixon, B., Gibson, A., Hollins, M., La Bossiere, E., and Robinson, F., (1980). Corticopontine visual projections in macaque monkeys. *Journal of Comparative Neurology*, **90**, 209–29.

Goldberg, G. (1985). Response and projection. A reinterpretation of the premotor concept. In *Neuropsychological studies of apraxia and related disorders* (ed. E. A. Roy), pp. 251–66. Elsevier, Amsterdam.

Goldberg, M. E. and Bruce, C. J. (1981). Frontal eye fields in the monkey: eye movements remap the effective coordinates of visual stimuli. *Society for Neuroscience Abstracts*, **7**, 131.

Goldberg, M. E. and Bushnell, M. C. (1981). Role of the frontal eye fields in visually guided saccades. In *Progress in oculomotor research* (ed. A. F. Fuchs and W. Becker). Elsevier, North Holland.

Grossberg, S. and Kupferstein, M. (1985). *Adaptive neural dynamics of ballistic eye movements*. North Holland Publishing Company, Amsterdam.

Held, R. (1970). Two modes of processing spatially distributed visual stimulation. In *The neurosciences second study program* (ed. F. O. Schmitt), pp. 317–24. MIT Press. Cambridge, MA.

Howard, I. P. (1982). *Human Visual Orientation*. John Wiley & Sons, New York.

Ingle, D. J. (1967). Two visual mechanisms underlying the behaviour of fish. *Psychologische Forschung*, **31**, 44–51.

Jacob, F. (1981). *Le jeu des possibles. Essai sur la diversité du vivant*. A. Fayard. Paris.

Jeannerod, M. (1972). Spatial behaviour and its alteration: old and new concepts. *International Journal of Mental Health*, **1**, 83–90.

Jeannerod, M. (1985). The posterior parietal area as a spatial generator. In *Brain mechanisms and spatial vision* (ed. D. J. Ingle, M. Jeannerod, and D. N. Lee), pp. 279–98. Martinus Nijhoff, Dordrecht.

Jeannerod, M. (1986). The formation of finger grip during prehension, a cortically mediated visuomotor pattern. *Behavioural Brain Research*, **19**, 99–116.

Keele, S. W. (1981). Behavioral analysis of movement. In *Handbook of Physiology. The nervous system*, Vol. 2, Motor control (ed. V. B. Brooks), Part 2, pp. 1391–414. Williams and Wilkins Company, Baltimore.

Lhermitte, F. (1983). 'Utilization behavior' and its relation to lesions of the frontal lobe. *Brain*, **106**, 237–45.

Lieblich, I. and Arbib, M. A. (1982). Multiple representations of space underlying behaviour. *The Behavioral and Brain Sciences*, **5**, 627–59.

Livingston, M. S. and Hubel, D. H. (1985). Specificity of cortico-cortical connections in monkey visual system. *Nature*, **304**, 531–4.

Lueck, C. J., Taniery, S., Crawford, T. J., Henderson, L., and Kennard, C. (1990). Antisaccades and remembered saccades in Parkinson's disease. *Journal of Neurology, Neurosurgery and Psychiatry*, **53**, 284–8.

MacKay, D. M. (1966). Cerebral organisation and the conscious control of action. In *Brain and conscious experience* (ed. J. C. Eccles), pp. 422–45. Springer Verlag, New York.

Maunsell, J. H. R. and Van Essen, D. C. (1987). The functional properties of the middle temporal visual area in the macaque monkey: representational biases and the relationship to callosal connections and myeloarchictectonic boundaries. *The Journal of Comparative Neurology*, **266**, 535–55.

Mays, L. E. and Sparks, D. L. (1980). Saccades are spatially not retinocentrically coded. *Science*, **208**, 1163–5.

Megaw, E. D. (1972). Directional errors and their correction in a discrete tracking task. *Ergonomics*, **15**, 633–43.

Mishkin, M. and Ungerleider, L. G. (1982). Contribution of striate inputs to the visuo-spatial functions of parieto-preoccipital cortex in monkeys. *Behavioural Brain Research*, **6**, 57–77.

Molter, B. C. and Mountcastle, V. B. (1981). The functional properties of light sensitive neurons of the posterior parietal cortex studied in waking monkeys: foveal sparing and opponent vector organization. *Journal of Neuroscience*, **1**, 3–26.

Newcombe, F. and Ratcliff, G. (1987). Visuospatial disorders. In *Disorders of visuospatial analysis. Handbook of neuropsychology* (ed. F. Boller and J. Grafman), Vol. 2. pp. 333–56. Elsevier, Amsterdam.

O'Keefe, J. and Nadel, L. (1978). *The hippocampus as a cognitive map*. Clarendon Press, Oxford.

Owen, B. M. and Lee, D. N. (1986). Establishing a frame of reference for action. In *Motor developments: Aspects of coordination and control* (ed. M. G. Wade and H. T. A. Whiting). Martinus Nijhoff, Dordrecht.

Paillard, J. (1960). The patterning of skilled movements. In *Handbook of physiology, Section 1, Neurophysiology* (ed. J. Field, H. V. Magoun, and V. E. Hall), Vol. 3 pp. 1679–708. American Physiological Society, Bethesda, MD.

Paillard, J. (1971). Les déterminants moteurs de l'organisation spatiale. *Cahiers de Psychologie*, **14**, 261–316.

Paillard, J. (1982). The contribution of central and peripheral vision to visually guided reaching. In *Analysis of visual behaviour* (ed. D. J. Ingle, M. A. Goodale, and R. J. Mansfield), pp. 367–85. MIT Press, Cambridge, MA.

Paillard, J. (1983). The functional labelling of neural codes. *Experimental Brain Research*, Suppl. 7, 1–19.

Paillard, J. (1987). Cognitive versus sensorimotor encoding of spatial information. In *Cognitive processing and spatial orientation in animal and man* (ed. P. Ellen and C. Thinus-Blanc), pp. 43–77. Martinus Nijhoff, Dordrecht.

Paillard, J. (1990). Basic neurophysiological structures of eye–hand coordination. In *Development of eye–hand coordination across the life span* (ed. C. Bard, M. Fleury, and L. Hay), pp. 26–74. South Carolina University Press, Columbia, SC.

Paillard, J. and Amblard, B. (1985). Static versus kinetic visual cues for the processing of spatial relationships. In *Brain mechanisms and spatial vision* (ed. D. J. Ingle, M. Jeannerod, and D. N. Lee), pp. 299–330. Martinus Nijhoff, The Hague.

Paillard, J. and Brouchon, M. (1968). Active and passive movements in the calibration of position sense. In *The neuropsychology of spatially oriented behaviour* (ed. S. J. Freedman), pp. 37–55. Dorsey Press, Illinois.

Paillard, J. and Brouchon, M. (1974). A proprioceptive contribution to the spatial encoding of position cues for ballistic movements. *Brain Research*, **71**, 273–84.

Paillard, J. Michel, F., and Stelmach, G. (1983). Localization without content: a tactile analogue of 'blind sight'. *Archives of Neurology (Chicago)*, **40**, 548–51.

Pandya, D. N. and Yeterian, E. H. (1984). Proposed neural circuitry for spatial memory. *Neuropsychologia*, **22**, 109–122.

Phillips, C. G., Zeki, S., and Barlow, H. B. (1984). Localization of function in the cerebral cortex. Past, present, future. *Brain*, **107**, 328–61.

Piaget, J. (1937). *La construction du réel chez l'enfant*. Delachaux et Niestle, Neuchâtel.

Piaget, J. (1971). *Biology and knowledge*. University of Chicago Press.

Piaget, J. and Inhelder, B. (1967). *The child's conception of space*. Norton, New York.

Polit, A. and Bizzi, E. (1979). Characteristics of the motor programs underlying arm movement in monkeys. *Journal of Neurophysiology*, **62**, 183–94.

Poulton, E. C. (1981). Human manual control. In *Handbook of Physiology. The nervous system*, Vol. 2, *Motor control* (ed. V. B. Brooks), Part 2, pp. 1337–89. American Physiological Society, Williams and Wilkins Company, Baltimore.

Rizzolatti, G., Gentilucci, M., Fogassi, L., Luppino, G., Matelli, N., and Panzoni-Maggi, S. (1987). Neurons related to goal directed motor acts in inferior area 6 of the macaque monkey. *Experimental Brain Research*, **67**, 220–4.

Robinson, D. A. (1981). The use of control systems analysis in the neurophysiology of eye movements. *Annual Review of Neuroscience*, **4**, 463–503.

Ryle, G. (1949). *The concept of mind*. Barnes and Noble, New York.

Schlag, J. and Schlag-Rey, M. (1985). Unit activity related to spontaneous saccades in frontal dorsomedial cortex of monkey. *Experimental Brain Research*, **5**, 208–11.

Schneider, G. E. (1969). Two visual systems: brain mechanisms for localization and discrimination area dissociated by tectal and cortical lesions. *Science*, **163**, 895–902.

Stark, L. and Bridgeman, B. (1983). Role of corollary discharge in space constancy. *Journal of Optical Society of America*, **55**, 371–80.

Stein, J. F. (1989). Representation of egocentric space in the posterior parietal cortex. *Quarterly Journal of Experimental Psychology*, **74**, 583–606.

Strong, G. W., and Whitehead, B. A. (1989). A solution to the tag-assignment problem for neural networks. *Behavioral and Brain Sciences*, **12**, 381–433.

Teasdale, N., Bard, C., Blouin, J., and Fleury, M. (1990). Visual feedback information in a rapid pointing task with varied deceleration requirements. North America Society for the Psychology of Sport and Physical Activity. Annual meeting. Abstracts. p. 14. Houston.

Thomas, G. J. (1984). Memory: time binding in organisms. In *Neuropsychology of Memory* (ed. L. R. Squire and N. Butters), pp. 374–84. Guilford Press, London.

Thompson, J. A. (1981). Is continuous visual monitoring necessary in visually guided locomotion? *Journal of Experimental Psychology: Human Perception and Performance*, **9**, 427–43.

Trevarthen, C. B. (1968). Two mechanisms of vision in primates. *Psychologische Forschung*, **31**, 299–337.

Ungerleider, L. G. and Mishkin, M. (1982). Two cortical visual systems. In *The analysis of visual behaviour* (ed. D. J. Ingle, M. A. Goodale, and R. J. W. Mansfield), pp. 549–86. MIT Press, Cambridge. MA.

Vidal, P. P., Gouny, M., and Berthoz, A. (1978). Rôle de la vision dans le déclenchement de réactions posturales rapides. *Archives Italiennes de Biologie*, **116**, 281–91.

Wallon, H. (1949). *Les origines du caractère chez l'enfant*, 2nd edn. Presses Universitaires de France, Paris.

Weiskrantz, L. (1989). Blindsight. In *Handbook of neuropsychology* (ed. F. Boller and J. Grafman), Vol. 2, pp. 375–85. Elsevier, Amsterdam.

Wong, E. and Mack, A. (1981). Saccadic programming and perceived location. *Acta Psychologica*, **48**, 123–31.

Zipser, D. and Andersen, R. A. (1988). A back propagation programmed network that stimulates the response properties of a subset of posterior parietal neurones. *Nature*, **331**, 679–684.

Author Index

Note: page numbers in italics refer to References.

Subject Index

attention 185–7
  direction of 239
  disturbance of 208–9, 239
  neglect 251–6
  parietal cortex and 29, 185–221
  searchlight theory 213

body schema 147–62
  automatic control 152–9
  kinaesthetic illusion 114–17
  limb position sense (static vs. dynamic) 53–4
  as partition of local visuomotor spaces 171
  perception of 148–52
  as a postural path structure 167–73

cerebellum
  modular organization 448–9, 456
  and motor learning 446–56
co-ordinate systems 4, 7, 186–215, 379–81, 471–2
  body-centred 49, 168, 185, 465
  Cartesian 278, 436
  egocentric 112
  Euclidean 85, 89, 380–83
  exocentric/allocentric 83
  hierarchy of 84
  internal/external 379
  object-centred 168, 465
  plurality of 84
  retinocentric 164
  retinotopic 214
  Riemannian 382
  transform of 382, 400

depth 166, 389–91
  astereognosis 207
  binocular impairment 264–5
  depth sensitive cells (VIP) 228–9
  stereopsis 395–7
direction
  of attention 239
  coding 466–7

directional firing of place cells 305–7
directional sensitivity (VIP) 239
direction/distance coding 466
fast correction 60–4
head direction cells (hippoc.) 316
of reaching 49–67
disorders, see spatial disorders

efference copy 38, 112, 167, 262, 267
  corollary discharge 5–82, 112, 420
  reafference 174–5
eye–head co-ordination 5, 14, 22, 30–1, 38–48, 50
  vestibulo-ocular reflex 14, 15, 86–8
eye movements
  anti-saccadic 20
  cognitively driven 20
  co-ordinates 381–3
  double step 60–3, 71, 77
  express saccades 20
  eye position 5, 7, 11–13, 38–47, 50, 74, 165, 469–70
  fixation neurons 23–6
  frontal eye field 7, 20, 56, 73, 77, 196
  gaze control 7–38, 85–8, 469–70
  gaze direction 127
  gaze signals 25, 29, 34, 50, 89–90
  goal directed 76
  and head position 38–48, 95
  intralaminar nuclei, thalamus 51, 73
  and location 177–8
  ocular motor disorders 258–70
  oculomotor range 22
  retinal error 5, 7, 9, 12, 70
  saccades 4–9, 20, 70, 164, 214–15, 381–3
  scan paths 168
  spatial programming of 70–7
  stabilization, VOR 14–15, 88
  supplementary eye field 468

finger grip
  grasping 62–3, 166, 475
  power/precision grip 166
  preshaping 381, 385
frame of reference 81–104
  allocentric 83

location
/direction specificity 321
/distance coding 466
and eye position 177–8
-local sign 152
memory for 211, 469–70
registered/perceived 176–7, 468
/shape space 168, 463
/vector cues 467–8
visual 3, 11, 13, 53, 126

maps
auditory 11, 22, 89
cognitive 273–93, 467
computational/projectional 173–4
and goal representation 291–2
and hippocampal neurons 296–301
implicit/explicit 391–2
Kohonen 405
motor 12, 168–71, 469
neuronal/computational 472–5
and place cells 299
proprioceptive 49, 52–4
retinal 434
space 1–78, 438–9, 472–5
spatio-temporal pattern of activity on
motor map 32–5
tecto-reticular motor 32–5
use of 285–92
visual 12, 14, 21, 51, 238
visuomotor 49–52
memory
auto-associative 360–3, 371
and Hebb synapses 360–2, 435
and the hippocampus 334–52
for location 469–70
long/short term 399
spatial 321–3, 334–48, 355–8, 364
static/dynamic 101
topographical 175, 246–7
visual 99
models (*see also* theories)
alpha/lambda 418–19
of coherence constraint 82
columnar model of the cortex 447–8
of compliance 418
of covariance 166, 174
dynamic and inverse dynamic 452–4
equilibrium point 407, 468
kinematic expectation 420
length–tension curves 426–8
local/taxon systems 174, 273, 296, 467
mass spring 468
of Moore–Penrose generalized inverse
382

of motor learning 446–56
neuromimetic 433–44
passive motion paradigm 407–8
robotic model 441–3
spatial 5–6
motor
appropriation of space 476
control 404–32
error 5–9, 22, 164, 214
-framing of space 163–82
-image 64–5
L, M, and S-units 412–21
layer 436–7
learning 446–56
map 4, 20–2, 32, 49–52
memory 114
passive paradigm 407–12
plan specification 420–2
relaxation networks 407–12
representation 440–1
space encoding 164–71
vector map 186, 434, 440
motor and premotor cortex
arcuate sulcus 14
area 4 (directional coding) 54, 136
area 6 14
frontal eye field 7, 20, 56, 73, 77, 196
inferior premotor area 468
supplementary eye field 468
motor learning
and cerebellum 446–58
cybernetic approach 449–50
dynamic model 452–4
inverse dynamic model 454
neural network approach 450–2
movement (*see* eye, head)
active/passive 178
active sight 214
active touch 214
centrifugal/centripetal 44–7
control 79, 182
cues 464–5
directional coding of 54, 136, 467
direction/distance 165, 466
kinematic/dynamic 133–8
latent action programs 476
learning and cerebellum 446–58
orientation 100–3
planning 138–43
position 464–5
reaching 49–67
-related discharges 30–2
self-motion perception 2, 15
spatiotopic 100–3
and strategies 83
and synergies 83, 167, 405
transform generation 290